Human Performance and Health in Sport and Exercise

Human Performance and Health in Sport and Exercise

Guest Editors

Barbara Gilic
Andrea Fusco

MDPI

Basel • Beijing • Wuhan • Barcelona • Belgrade • Novi Sad • Cluj • Manchester

Guest Editors
Barbara Gilic
Faculty of Kinesiology
University of Split
Split
Croatia

Andrea Fusco
Department of Medicine and
Aging Sciences
University "G. D'Annunzio"
of Chieti-Pescara
Chieti
Italy

Editorial Office
MDPI AG
Grosspeteranlage 5
4052 Basel, Switzerland

This is a reprint of the Special Issue, published open access by the journal *Applied Sciences* (ISSN 2076-3417), freely accessible at: https://www.mdpi.com/journal/applsci/special_issues/324H8MCJRF.

For citation purposes, cite each article independently as indicated on the article page online and as indicated below:

Lastname, A.A.; Lastname, B.B. Article Title. *Journal Name* **Year**, *Volume Number*, Page Range.

ISBN 978-3-7258-6526-0 (Hbk)
ISBN 978-3-7258-6527-7 (PDF)
https://doi.org/10.3390/books978-3-7258-6527-7

Contents

About the Editors

Barbara Gilic

Barbara Gilic is a postdoctoral fellow, teaching assistant, and researcher at the University of Split, Faculty of Kinesiology. Her scientific work is centered on health-related topics, with research interests spanning physical activity, physical literacy, and health literacy in various age groups and populations (e.g., persons with type 2 diabetes), as well as performance analysis in sport, particularly in sport climbing. She is the principal investigator of the Croatian Science Foundation project dealing with physical literacy, physical activity and fitness in primary school. She is the recipient of the Ministry of Science and Education Award for Scientific Production and the University of Split Award for Scientific Production, highlighting the significance and impact of her research contributions.

Andrea Fusco

Andrea Fusco is a researcher in Sport and Exercise Science at the Department of Medicine and Aging Sciences, University "G. d'Annunzio" of Chieti–Pescara, Italy. His research interests encompass training monitoring, sport and exercise performance testing, fatigue assessment, motor control, proprioception, and balance evaluation through digital and wearable technologies. He is also actively engaged in research on dual-career pathways for student-athletes, with a focus on the availability, quality and impact of support services within educational and sport systems. He has contributed to several national and European projects addressing athlete welfare, health promotion and performance optimization. His work aims to integrate methodological rigor with applied practice, supporting evidence-based approaches to athlete monitoring, health-oriented training, and dual-career development.

Preface

This Reprint brings together a selection of studies that examine the relationship between human performance and health across sport and exercise contexts. Its aim is to provide an integrated scientific overview of how physiological, biomechanical, psychological and behavioral factors contribute to both athletic development and long-term well-being. The scope of the Reprint extends from performance determinants and training load monitoring to adapted sport, recovery strategies and exercise applications in preventive and clinical settings. The motivation for making this collection comes from the growing need to align performance-oriented methodologies with evidence-based health considerations. Contemporary sport requires practitioners to balance optimization of competitive outcomes with the management of fatigue, injury risk and mental health. By consolidating diverse research approaches and populations, this Reprint offers a coherent reference for understanding these interdependent dimensions. The material is intended for researchers, sport scientists, clinicians, coaches and professionals involved in the assessment, training and support of athletes and physically active individuals. It is our hope that the studies presented here will contribute to advancing methodological rigor, informing applied practice and supporting healthier, more sustainable models of sport participation.

Barbara Gilic and Andrea Fusco
Guest Editors

applied sciences

MDPI

Editorial

Human Performance and Health in Sport and Exercise

Andrea Fusco [1], Barbara Gilic [2,*], Emanuel Festino [3] and Olga Papale [3]

[1] Department of Medicine and Aging Sciences, University "G. d'Annunzio" of Chieti-Pescara, 66100 Chieti, Italy; andrea.fusco@unich.it
[2] Faculty of Kinesiology, University of Split, 21000 Split, Croatia
[3] Department of Human Sciences, Society and Health, University of Cassino and Lazio Meridionale, 03043 Cassino, Italy; emanuel.festino@unicas.it (E.F.); olga.papale@unicas.it (O.P.)
* Correspondence: barbara.gilic@kifst.eu

1. Introduction

For people of all ages and genders, participating in physically demanding sports, whether competitive or recreational, has significant health benefits. According to research, playing sports on a regular basis strengthens bones and muscles, lowers the risk of developing chronic illnesses including diabetes, obesity, and high blood pressure, and improves cardiovascular health [1,2]. Furthermore, sports are important for mental health since they improve social integration and cognitive performance while lowering stress, anxiety, and depression [2]. However, because athletes must strain their bodies to the maximum, competitive sports frequently have a price tag, increasing the likelihood of injuries, exhaustion, and psychological discomfort [3]. A balanced approach to training and rehabilitation is also necessary because retired athletes often face long-term physical and mental health issues, such as joint issues, cardiovascular risks, and post-career identity conflicts [4].

Starting from the basics, assessing physical performance parameters is a fundamental aspect of sports and health science that provides directions to athletes, coaches, and researchers to understand and optimize training methodologies for strength, endurance, power, asymmetry in performance, preventing injuries, and enhancing competitive results [5]. Accordingly, a growing number of scientific investigations highlight the multiple methods available to quantify health, sport, and tactical performance, each focusing on different aspects of an individual's capabilities and skills. For example, critical information on a subject's endurance, recovery potential, and exercise prescription are provided by training load and physiological metrics, such as maximal oxygen consumption (VO_2max), lactate threshold, and heart rate variability (Contributions 1, 2, 3, 4). The importance of these parameters is evident across different sporting contexts and health settings.

This Special Issue includes 15 papers, comprising 12 original articles and 3 reviews, covering several parameters and variables used to quantify physical performance, from physiological and biomechanical determinants of athletic performance to strategies for optimizing recovery, injury prevention, and adapted sports participation. The findings in this Special Issue underscore the necessity of a multidimensional approach to evaluating sport performance, integrating physical, physiological, body composition, biomechanical, and recovery-based assessments, allowing for a more comprehensive understanding of athletic performance and overall health. In particular, these findings provide a scientific base for developing training methodologies tailored to specific sports and individual needs in different settings. The overview and general conclusions of papers published in this Special Issue will be presented in the following text.

2. An Overview of Published Articles

When it comes to performance analysis, Radaković et al. (Contribution 1) reported a strong correlation between cardiorespiratory fitness and performance in football players, where total match distance and high-intensity running are linked to aerobic capacity. Similarly, in handball, elite players display better reaction times and hand–eye coordination compared to sub-elite athletes, underlining the importance of psychomotor abilities in high-performance play (Contribution 5). Accordingly, analyzing movement dynamics, reaction speed, and gameplay effectiveness is crucial in high-level sports. Prieto-Lage et al. (Contributions 6, 7) explored padel and pickleball by showing that short rally durations and net proximity significantly influence point-winning strategies, providing indications on tactical training. Furthermore, as reported by Macedo et al. (Contribution 4), monitoring training load is important for quantifying the demand on psychological and physiological responses of athletes. Various external and internal load metrics, including GPS-based tracking, accelerometers, heart rate variability, and session rating of perceived exertion, are widely implemented in both team sports (e.g., soccer, rugby) and individual disciplines (e.g., endurance sports, resistance training); therefore, these tools enhance physical performance, injury risk assessment, training monitoring, and exercise management (Contribution 4).

Beyond traditional competitive sports, physiological assessments and training monitoring also play an important role in rehabilitation [6] and adapted exercise programs [7]. In para-sports, Álvarez-Hernández et al. (Contribution 2) demonstrated that para-footballers with cerebral palsy who have lower impairment levels achieve higher speeds and cover greater distances, indicating potentially greater match performance. Generally, these considerations emphasize the role of physiological monitoring in optimizing training programs, ensuring that athletes, both in competitive sports or rehabilitation settings, achieve high adaptation and performance.

Together with physical performance, anthropometric characteristics can also influence health performance, sport success, and injury occurrence [8]. For example, a retrospective study conducted by Ginszt et al. (Contribution 8) analyzed the relationship between climbing experience, anthropometric data, and the best result in sport climbing achieved by male sport climbers in bouldering and lead climbing, suggesting that lower body mass and lower body height are correlated with the better performance in sport climbing. On the same topic, Śliż et al. (Contribution 5) examined handball players and found that body fat percentage, fat-free mass, and total body water influence reaction time, movement time, and response accuracy.

Several studies in the present Special Issue investigated the impact of different specific training regimens on health and physical performance (Contributions 2, 4, 9, 10). In fact, the research conducted by Gavala-González et al. (Contribution 9) on adolescent rowers reveals that specific ergometer-based training enhances power output more effectively than general strength exercises, demonstrating the importance of a sport-specific training program. Furthermore, the improvement in velocity, command, and deception metrics may also be attributed to external facilitator, as shown by Crotin et al. (Contribution 10) in baseball players through the use of intra-abdominal pressure belts, suggesting innovative tools for enhancing performance. Finally, regarding sport-specific skills, Busuttil et al. (Contribution 11) investigated tennis coaching practices, examining how tennis coaches perceive and approach the development of grip positions, a foundational skill in tennis. The findings suggest that teaching grip positions early in training, using physically constraining tools, could improve stroke development while reducing the risk of overtraining injuries.

However, although exercise training and sports participation have been recognized for their positive impact on health, by contributing to physical and mental well-being across different age groups and performance levels, achieving peak performance often requires significant sacrifices, exposing subjects to risks such as injuries, chronic fatigue, and mental health challenges like anxiety, depression, exercise addiction, and body dissatisfaction [9]. Additionally, it is worth noting that beyond physical training, athletes and physically active subjects' quality of life is influenced by sleep hygiene, dietary habits, and mental health, all playing integral roles in athletic success and health performance achievements (Contributions 11, 12, 13). In line with these influencing factors, Migliaccio et al. (Contribution 14) showed the importance of sleep hygiene for the health and performance of physically active individuals, demonstrating how good sleep hygiene, sleep quality and quantity, and a regular sleep routine are associated with a range of benefits for health and performance including recovery, less risk of injuries, enhanced concentration and attention, improved coordination and muscle strength, mental well-being, and reduced risk of chronic diseases. Similarly, dietary strategies play an important role in recovery. As demonstrated by Bozbay et al. (Contribution 12), pomegranate–black carrot juice supplementation significantly improved mineral metabolism and fatty acid profiles, indicating that an antioxidant-rich dietary intervention can help reduce exercise-induced oxidative stress and promote more efficient recovery.

Beyond high-performance sports and elite athletes, sport and structured physical activity plays a fundamental role in prevention [10] and management [11] of non-communicable diseases, particularly in childhood and adolescent populations, having a big impact on public health [12]. In fact, Uvacsek et al. (Contribution 15) investigated sport and physical activity participation among school-aged Hungarian children, examining the differences in engagement based on weight groups. Their findings revealed that overweight and obese children had almost the same participation rates in sport activities as children in other weight classifications, reinforcing the importance of daily physical education in schools and governmental support of sport in fostering engagement in exercise and reducing obesity risk.

Accordingly, whether in competitive, recreational, home, or green settings, engaging in structured physical activity and sports promotes cardiovascular fitness, muscular strength, and psychophysiological well-being independently from age and clinical condition [13]. In fact, Papamichail et al. (Contribution 13) examined the impact of exercise on balance, functional ability, and depression in a patient with progressive supranuclear palsy, showing significant improvements in mental well-being. This is further confirmed from a study conducted by Gavala-González (Contribution 3) on breast cancer survivors engaging in rowing, indicating improvements in cardiovascular function and overall fitness, underscoring the role of structured exercise as not only essential for athletic performance, but also for clinical populations to recover and long-term health benefits.

3. Conclusions

In conclusion, the studies in this Special Issue collectively highlight the importance of a multidimensional approach to assessing and enhancing health and sport performance. By integrating physical, physiological, body composition, biomechanical, and recovery-based assessments, researchers and practitioners can gain deeper understandings into the factors influencing both athletic achievement and overall health. Moreover, these papers underscore the significance of tailored training methodologies, holistic athlete monitoring, and the valuable role that structured exercise plays in prevention, rehabilitation, and performance optimization. As such, the body of work presented in this Special Issue provides a foundation for advancing best practice in sport, exercise, and health, benefiting athletes, coaches, clinical populations, and overall society.

We extend our gratitude to all contributors whose efforts have enriched this collection and look forward to further advancements in the topic of human performance and health in sport and exercise.

Author Contributions: Conceptualization, A.F., B.G., E.F. and O.P., methodology, A.F., B.G., E.F. and O.P., formal analysis, A.F., B.G., E.F. and O.P., writing—original draft preparation, A.F., B.G., E.F. and O.P., writing—review and editing, A.F., B.G., E.F. and O.P. All authors have read and agreed to the published version of the manuscript.

Funding: This research received no external funding.

Conflicts of Interest: The authors declare no conflicts of interest.

List of Contributions:

1. Radaković, R.; Katanić, B.; Stanković, M.; Masanovic, B.; Fišer, S.Ž. The Impact of Cardiorespiratory and Metabolic Parameters on Match Running Performance (MRP) in National-Level Football Players: A Multiple Regression Analysis. *Appl. Sci.* **2024**, *14*, 3807. https://doi.org/10.3390/app14093807.
2. Álvarez-Hernández, S.; Castillo, D.; Villa-Vicente, J.G.; Yanci, J.; Marqués-Jiménez, D.; Rodríguez-Fernández, A. Analyses of Physical and Physiological Responses during Competition in Para-Footballers with Cerebral Palsy: A Systematic Review. *Appl. Sci.* **2024**, *14*, 3812. https://doi.org/10.3390/app14093812.
3. Gavala-González, J.; Real-Pérez, M.; Gamboa-González, J.; Fernández-García, J.C. Effects of Rowing on Cardiac Function in Breast Cancer Survivors: Sliding Seat Rowing vs. Fixed Seat Rowing. *Appl. Sci.* **2024**, *14*, 6239. https://doi.org/10.3390/app14146239.
4. Macedo, A.G.; Almeida, T.A.F.; Massini, D.A.; de Oliveira, D.M.; Espada, M.C.; Robalo, R.A.M.; Hernández-Beltrán, V.; Gamonales, J.M.; Vilela Terra, A.M.S.; Pessôa Filho, D.M. Load Monitoring Methods for Controlling Training Effectiveness on Physical Conditioning and Planning Involvement: A Narrative Review. *Appl. Sci.* **2024**, *14*, 10465. https://doi.org/10.3390/app142210465.
5. Śliż, M.; França, C.; Martins, F.; Marszałek, P.; Gouveia, É.R.; Przednowek, K. Psychomotor Abilities, Body Composition and Training Experience of Elite and Sub-Elite Handball Players. *Appl. Sci.* **2025**, *15*, 176. https://doi.org/10.3390/app15010176.
6. Prieto-Lage, I.; Reguera-López-de-la-Osa, X.; Durán-Rodríguez, N.; Silva-Pinto, A.J.; Argibay-González, J.C.; Gutiérrez-Santiago, A. Assessing the Probability of Winning a Point in Men's Padel: A Comprehensive Analysis. *Appl. Sci.* **2024**, *14*, 6642. https://doi.org/10.3390/app14156642.
7. Prieto-Lage, I.; Reguera-López-de-la-Osa, X.; Juncal-López, A.; Silva-Pinto, A.J.; Argibay-González, J.C.; Gutiérrez-Santiago, A. Notational Analysis of Men's Singles Pickleball: Game Patterns and Competitive Strategies. *Appl. Sci.* **2024**, *14*, 8724. https://doi.org/10.3390/app14198724.
8. Ginszt, A.; Zieliński, G.; Dolina, A.; Stachyra, E.; Zaborek-Łyczba, M.; Łyczba, J.; Gawda, P.; Ginszt, M. Anthropometric Parameters and Body Composition in Elite Lead Climbers and Boulderers—A Retrospective Study. *Appl. Sci.* **2024**, *14*, 5603. https://doi.org/10.3390/app14135603.
9. Gavala-González, J.; Porras-García, M.E.; Fernández-García, J.C.; Real-Pérez, M. Effects of Specific Training Using a Rowing Ergometer on Sport Performance in Adolescents. *Appl. Sci.* **2024**, *14*, 3180. https://doi.org/10.3390/app14083180.
10. Crotin, R.L.; Conforti, C. A Case Study Exploring the Effects of a Novel Intra-Abdominal Pressure Belt on Fastball and Change-Up Velocity, Command, and Deception Among Collegiate Baseball Pitchers. *Appl. Sci.* **2024**, *14*, 10471. https://doi.org/10.3390/app142210471.
11. Busuttil, N.A.; Roberts, A.H.; Dunn, M.; Hyunh, M.; Middleton, K.J. Perceptions and Practices of Accredited Tennis Coaches When Teaching Foundational Grip Development. *Appl. Sci.* **2024**, *14*, 7127. https://doi.org/10.3390/app14167127.

12. Bozbay, K.; Çinar, V.; Akbulut, T.; Aydemir, I.; Yasul, Y.; Aytac, K.Y.; Ozkaya, A.; Russo, L.; Fusco, A.; Migliaccio, G.M. Effects of Exercise and Pomegranate–Black Carrot Juice Interventions on Mineral Metabolism and Fatty Acids. *Appl. Sci.* **2024**, *14*, 7284. https://doi.org/10.3390/app14167284.
13. Papamichail, P.; Michalas, M.; Krokos, D.; Balamoutsou, M.; Karkoula, P.; Lyros, E.; Sakellari, V.; Christakou, A. The Effectiveness of Exercise Programs on Balance, Functional Ability, Quality of Life, and Depression in Progressive Supranuclear Palsy: A Case Study. *Appl. Sci.* **2024**, *14*, 8368. https://doi.org/10.3390/app14188368.
14. Migliaccio, G.M.; Di Filippo, G.; Sancassiani, F.; Padulo, J.; Russo, L. Boost Your Brainpower: 24 Daily Sleep Hacks for Active Lifestyles. *Appl. Sci.* **2024**, *14*, 6701. https://doi.org/10.3390/app14156701.
15. Uvacsek, M.; Wágner, B.; Simkó, G. Sport and Physical Activity Participation by Weight Groups in School-Aged Hungarian Children. *Appl. Sci.* **2024**, *14*, 6575. https://doi.org/10.3390/app14156575.

References

1. Warburton, D.E.R.; Bredin, S.S.D. Health Benefits of Physical Activity. *Curr. Opin. Cardiol.* **2017**, *32*, 541–556. [CrossRef] [PubMed]
2. Reiner, M.; Niermann, C.; Jekauc, D.; Woll, A. Long-Term Health Benefits of Physical Activity—A Systematic Review of Longitudinal Studies. *BMC Public Health* **2013**, *13*, 813. [CrossRef] [PubMed]
3. Gouttebarge, V.; Aoki, H.; Lambert, M.; Stewart, W.; Kerkhoffs, G. A History of Concussions Is Associated with Symptoms of Common Mental Disorders in Former Male Professional Athletes across a Range of Sports. *Phys. Sportsmed.* **2017**, *45*, 443–449. [CrossRef] [PubMed]
4. Mannes, Z.L.; Waxenberg, L.B.; Cottler, L.B.; Perlstein, W.M.; Burrell II, L.E.; Ferguson, E.G.; Edwards, M.E.; Ennis, N. Prevalence and Correlates of Psychological Distress among Retired Elite Athletes: A Systematic Review. *Int. Rev. Sport Exerc. Psychol.* **2019**, *12*, 265–294. [CrossRef] [PubMed]
5. Hughes, D.C.; Ellefsen, S.; Baar, K. Adaptations to Endurance and Strength Training. *Cold Spring Harb. Perspect. Med.* **2018**, *8*, a029769. [CrossRef] [PubMed]
6. Hutchinson, D.S.; Skrinar, G.S.; Caitlin, C. The Role of Improved Physical Fitness in Rehabilitation and Recovery. *Psychiatr. Rehabil. J.* **1999**, *22*, 355. [CrossRef]
7. Maud, P.; Foster, C. Physiological Assessment of Human Fitness. In *Human Kinetics*; Human Kinetics: Champaign, IL, USA, 2006.
8. Melloni, M.A.S.; De Almeida Ávila, J.; Páscoa, M.A.; De Oliveira Barbeta, C.J.; Cirolini, V.X.; Gonçalves, E.M.; Guerra-Júnior, G. Can Anthropometric, Body Composition, and Bone Variables Be Considered Risk Factors for Musculoskeletal Injuries in Brazilian Military Students? *BMC Musculoskelet. Disord.* **2018**, *19*, 377. [CrossRef]
9. Festino, E.; Papale, O.; Di Rocco, F.; De Maio, M.; Cortis, C.; Fusco, A. Effect of Physical Activity Behaviors, Team Sports, and Sitting Time on Body Image and Exercise Dependence. *Sports* **2024**, *12*, 260. [CrossRef]
10. Budreviciute, A.; Damiati, S.; Sabir, D.K.; Onder, K.; Schuller-Goetzburg, P.; Plakys, G.; Katileviciute, A.; Khoja, S.; Kodzius, R. Management and Prevention Strategies for Non-Communicable Diseases (NCDs) and Their Risk Factors. *Front. Public Health* **2020**, *8*, 574111. [CrossRef]
11. Saqib, Z.A.; Dai, J.; Menhas, R.; Mahmood, S.; Karim, M.; Sang, X.; Weng, Y. Physical Activity Is a Medicine for Non-Communicable Diseases: A Survey Study Regarding the Perception of Physical Activity Impact on Health Wellbeing. *Risk Manag. Healthc. Policy* **2020**, *13*, 2949–2962. [CrossRef] [PubMed]
12. Haskell, W.L.; Blair, S.N.; Hill, J.O. Physical Activity: Health Outcomes and Importance for Public Health Policy. *Prev. Med.* **2009**, *49*, 280–282. [CrossRef] [PubMed]
13. Papale, O.; Festino, E.; Condello, G.; Di Rocco, F.; De Maio, M.; Cortis, C.; Fusco, A. Psychophysiological Data Harmonization for the Sustainability of Outdoor Activities. *Sustainability* **2023**, *15*, 15838. [CrossRef]

applied sciences

MDPI

Article

Anthropometric Profile, Body Composition and Somatotype of Elite ILCA 7 Class Sailors—Differences Across General Competitive Success Levels

Luka Pezelj [1,*], Jan G. Bourgois [2,3], Mirjana Milić [4], Josip Maleš [4] and Israel Caraballo [5]

1 Faculty of Maritime Studies, University of Split, 21000 Split, Croatia
2 Sport Science Laboratory Jacques Rogge, Department of Movement and Sports Sciences, Faculty of Medicine and Health Sciences, Ghent University, Watersportlaan 2, 9000 Ghent, Belgium; jan.bourgois@ugent.be
3 Centre of Sports Medicine, Ghent University Hospital, Corneel Heymanslaan 10, 9000 Ghent, Belgium
4 Faculty of Kinesiology, University of Split, 21000 Split, Croatia; mirjana.milic@kifst.hr (M.M.); jmales@unist.hr (J.M.)
5 Department of Physical Education, Faculty of Education Sciences, University of Cadiz, 11519 Puerto Real, Spain; israel.caraballo@uca.es
* Correspondence: luka.pezelj@pfst.hr

Abstract: Setting up anthropometric profiles for elite athletes in each sport, sport discipline, or specific sport positions could be a key element of sport selection processes. The main purpose of this study was to determine the anthropometric characteristics, body composition, and somatotype profiles of elite international ILCA 7 class sailors and to determine the differences contributing to different levels of competitive success. The subject sample included 97 elite ILCA 7 class sailors. A set of 25 anthropometric variables was applied. The sailors were divided into three groups according to their level of general competitive success according to the World Sailing Rankings. Differences between elite ILCA 7 sailors, separated into Higher, Medium, and Lower groups based on their success, were found in terms of age, body mass, muscle mass, trunk muscle mass, leg muscle mass, biepicondilar humerus width, sum of skinfolds, triceps skinfold, supraspinale skinfold, medial calf skinfold, and endomorphy rating. The most successful group of sailors was, on average, 4.9 years older than the least successful group. More highly successful sailors were also found to have an average of 2.73 kg more muscle mass but an 8.81 mm lower sum of skinfolds than those in the lower success group. Considering the average values of somatotype categories, ILCA 7 sailors fit the endomorphic–mesomorph somatotype category (3.23 ± 0.99–4.81 ± 0.90–2.25 ± 0.86). This research clearly identifies the anthropometric profile of elite ILCA 7 sailors, which can significantly contribute to a more informed choice of sailing class. Given the results of this research, current ILCA 7 sailors can easily compare their own anthropometric parameters with elite ILCA 7 sailors and eventually adjust their training process to obtain a more desirable anthropometric profile.

Keywords: dinghy sailing; elite athletes; fitness testing; morphological characteristics; Olympic sailing; yachting; sport performance; body composition; Tanita; skinfolds; world sailing rankings

1. Introduction

Athletes, coaches, and sports scientists are interested in the structure and function of the human body, especially in relation to athletic performance. The physical and physiological characteristics of elite athletes are very different between different sports, sports disciplines, and specific sports positions. Certain physiques are found more often in some high-performance sports (or disciplines) and specific sports positions than others. In this context, anthropometry is important and is often included as a tool to aid understanding of the relationship between body structure and performance [1].

Olympic sailing is a multifaceted sport where numerous factors, such as boat handling, technical and tactical skills, and physical and physiological characteristics, determine performance. Sailing has a long Olympic history (since 1900, except for 1904), and the importance of physical and physiological characteristics for this sport has increased due to a higher international competition level, but also as a consequence of the changes in sailing classes and racing format made by World Sailing after each Olympic cycle [2,3]. Sailing at the Paris 2024 Olympics consisted of 10 events, covering six yacht classes (single- or double-handed crew; gender) and comprising a total of 10 sailor positions/functions, each requiring specific physical and physiological characteristics. A sailor's anthropometric profile is one of the criteria employed in selecting a sailing class, since optimal anthropometric requirements differ between yacht classes [4]. Some studies have shown that a high level of performance in Olympic sailing is generally associated with greater body mass, stature, and femur length [5–7]. When sailing, the sailor uses their body as a lever to control the boat and to increase an up-righting moment, as sideways wind forces acting on the sails cause a leeward tilting moment on the boat [2,7]. Sailors may perform this technical gesture for up to 94% of their total sailing time [8].

The ILCA 7 dinghy is one of the Olympic yacht classes, making its Olympic debut as a monohull in Atlanta 1996. It is considered one of the most physically and mentally demanding single-handed classes in the world. Dinghy sailors need to carefully control the balance of the boat in continuously varying wind and wave conditions. The technique involving ILCA 7 sailors sitting on the deck and leaning over the side to create an up-righting moment through a windward displacement of the ensemble center of gravity of the boat and sailor is a characteristic movement, known as hiking [9]. Based on the sailor-to-yacht weight ratio, a classification system for Olympic sailors was introduced to simplify monitoring of physical requirements [2]. ILCA 7 sailors are identified as dynamic side deck hikers because they hike in a very dynamic way due to a high sailor-to-yacht weight ratio [2]. The righting moment that is generated while hiking is a function of the sailor's body weight and their position relative to the centerline of the boat (i.e., body height). In this context, anthropometric characteristics, body composition, and the somatotype of an ILCA 7 sailor are very important determinants of ILCA 7 sailing success. Size is only an advantage if extra weight does not add more to the resistance of the yacht than it contributes to the propulsive forces of the dinghy.

The changes that occur in the context of sports give rise to a constant evolution of ideal anthropometric characteristics. It is therefore essential that the reference databases are kept up to date. The relationship between sports performance and anthropometric characteristics, including body composition and somatotype, has been the subject of study in a number of different sports disciplines [10–16]. Regarding the ILCA 7 sailing class, previous studies provide only limited information about the anthropometric characteristics of elite sailors [11,17–21]. A detailed analysis of the anthropometric characteristics, body composition, and somatotype of a large elite cohort of ILCA 7 sailors has not yet been conducted.

Therefore, this study aims to (1) quantify the anthropometric characteristics, body composition, and somatotype of international elite ILCA 7 class sailors, and (2) determine the differences in anthropometric profiles across general competitive levels.

2. Methods

2.1. Sample and Study Design

The anthropometric characteristics, body composition, and somatotype of 97 elite ILCA 7 class sailors (mean chronological age: 22.95 ± 3.40 years, varying from 17.15 to 32.55 years) were measured before the start of the ILCA 7 World Championship (IWC), 2017, in Split, Croatia. The competition included 147 sailors. The 97 sailors who participated in the study represented 66% of the total number of participants in the competition. The IWC was the most important competition for ILCA 7 sailors in 2017, including the best-ranked sailors in the world, among whom were the Olympic, world, and continental medal winners. Therefore, based on training and performance, participants in this study can be categorized as World Class and International Elite level (Trier 5 & 4), according to the Participation Classification Framework of McKay et al. (2022) [22].

All sailors participated in the study voluntarily. Participants were provided with detailed information about all experimental procedures, and written informed consent was obtained prior to their participation. The study was approved by the Scientific Committee of the Faculty of Kinesiology in Split and conducted with the support of the Executive Committee of the ILCA Association. The study met the requirements of the Declaration of Helsinki (1964) and the ethical standards of sports and exercise research.

All measurements were performed by a well-trained expert anthropometrist, assisted by a recorder who was also familiar with the anthropometric techniques, in the morning hours before the first training session in the week before the competition. For all measurements, the subjects wore dry underwear and were barefoot. All measurements were conducted within 30 min for each sailor.

The sailors were divided into three groups according to their level of general competitive success: more successful (1), medium successful (2), and less successful (3) groups. We determined this competitive success criterion from the ranking in the World Sailing Rankings (WSR). The WSR is formed by collecting the points from the six most successful competitions for each sailor in the 12 months from the publication of the table. For this study, we used the WSR table for the ILCA 7 class published on 04 September 2017, the last one before the IWC started. The group of sailors with a higher level of general success (1) included the subjects ranked among the first 30 sailors according to the WSR (N = 15), the group of sailors with a medium level of general success (2) included the subjects ranked from the 31st to the 60th place of the WSR (N = 20), and the group of sailors with a lower level of general success (3) included the subjects ranked lower than the 61st place of the WSR (N = 62). The threshold values for the groups were determined in collaboration with coaching experts and elite sailors.

2.2. Anthropometric Measures, Body Composition, and Somatotype

The measuring techniques were mainly based on the procedures and batteries of measurements used and described in previous studies by Pezelj et al. (2016; 2024) [17,18].

All anthropometric measurements were conducted following the International Society for the Advancement of Kinanthropometry (ISAK) protocol [23] on the dominant side of the body, as suggested in the original instructions for using the Heath–Carter method for somatotype calculation [24]. The following anthropometric dimensions were measured: (1) Length development: stature and sitting height; (2) Breadth development: biepicondylar humerus width and biepicondylar femur width; (3) Muscle development: upper arm girth flexed and tensed and calf girth; (4) Fat development: triceps skinfold, subscapular skinfold, supraspinale skinfold and medial calf skinfold.

Bioelectric impedance analysis (BIA) is a rapid and non-invasive method for evaluating body composition. Bioimpedance measurements were performed using a Tanita BC-418

(Tanita Corp., Tokyo, Japan) device, which uses a constant current source with a high-frequency current (50 kHz, 90 μA), following the recommendations given by Kyle et al. [25]. BIA was used to determine the following body composition measures: *body mass, fat range, muscle mass, trunk muscle mass, arms muscle mass, legs muscle mass, fat mass, trunk fat mass, arms fat mass*, and *legs fat mass*. The BIA measurement was taken when subjects were barefoot and only wearing dry underwear. All jewelry, watches, or any other pieces of clothing were removed. The GMON software was used to conduct measurements where the "body type" value was set for all subjects to "sports mode," and the "clothing weight" value was set to 0.0 kg.

Based on the anthropometric measurements and BIA measures, body mass index and sum of skinfolds were calculated, and somatotype (endomorphy, mesomorphy, and ectomorphy) was determined in accordance with the Heat–Carter method [24]. Cut-off values for the endomorphy rating were set from 0.5 to 16, for the mesomorphy rating from 0.5 to 12, and for the ectomorphy rating from 0.5 to 9 [26].

2.3. Statistical Analysis

Data analysis included the calculation of basic statistical indicators: mean, standard deviation, median, minimum value, maximum value, and determination of measures of sensitivity of result distribution: skewness, kurtosis, and maximum distance between relative cumulative theoretical frequency (normal) and relative cumulative empirical frequency (obtained by measuring). The results of the Kolmogorov–Smirnov test of the observed variables indicated that neither of the variables exceeds the cut-off value of this test, which is 0.14 for the observed sample. These findings indicated that the variables did not deviate significantly from a normal distribution and that all variables were suitable for further parametric statistical analysis. The differences between groups of sailors were determined using a one-way analysis of variance (ANOVA). Further, post hoc analyses of differences between the three groups of ILCA 7 sailors were made using Fisher's LSD test. To determine the effect sizes of the differences found, squared eta ($\eta 2$) coefficients were calculated and interpreted according to the criterion of Gamst et al. (2008) [27]. Data were analyzed using the STATISTICA software package (ver. 14.00).

3. Results

Table 1 presents descriptive indicators of all the measured variables: arithmetic mean, standard deviation, median, and minimum and maximum results. The sensitivity analysis was based on coefficients of asymmetry and peakedness of distributions, whereas the Kolmogorov–Smirnov test was used to test the normality of distributions.

Table 1. Descriptive statistics of anthropometric and somatotype variables of ILCA 7 sailors (N = 97).

Variables	Mean ± SD	M	Min	Max	Skew	Kurt	MaxD
Age (yrs)	22.95 ± 3.40	22.29	17.15	32.55	0.70	−0.12	0.136
Stature (cm)	181.76 ± 5.28	182.40	167.90	194.40	−0.22	−0.25	0.08
Sitting height (cm)	96.65 ± 3.27	96.70	88.00	105.00	0.07	0.05	0.04
Body mass (kg)	80.68 ± 3.87	81.40	67.10	91.40	−0.65	1.99	0.12
Body mass index (kg/m^2)	24.40 ± 1.60	24.50	20.30	28.20	−0.10	0.19	0.07
Fat range (%)	10.99 ± 3.57	11.20	2.00	18.80	−0.06	−0.20	0.04
Muscle mass (kg)	68.43 ± 3.78	68.40	57.00	77.10	−0.30	0.35	0.04
Trunk muscle mass (kg)	36.81 ± 2.33	36.80	30.70	42.20	0.14	−0.07	0.07
Arms muscle mass (kg)	8.62 ± 0.65	8.60	6.70	10.20	−0.05	0.12	0.06
Legs muscle mass (kg)	23.01 ± 1.17	23.10	19.40	25.80	−0.43	1.02	0.09
Fat mass (kg)	8.89 ± 3.02	8.90	1.60	16.30	0.07	−0.17	0.05

Table 1. *Cont.*

Variables	Mean ± SD	M	Min	Max	Skew	Kurt	MaxD
Trunk fat mass (kg)	4.79 ± 2.05	4.80	1.30	10.30	0.22	−0.44	0.06
Arms fat mass (kg)	0.99 ± 0.28	1.00	0.40	1.80	0.17	−0.14	0.12
Legs fat mass (kg)	3.21 ± 0.84	3.30	1.10	7.10	0.82	3.85	0.10
Biepicondilar humerus width (cm)	6.97 ± 0.39	6.95	6.00	7.70	0.05	−0.60	0.08
Biepicondilar femur width (cm)	9.33 ± 0.50	9.35	7.95	10.65	−0.31	0.45	0.08
Upper arm girth flexed and tensed (cm)	35.69 ± 1.80	35.65	30.65	41.30	0.13	0.80	0.08
Calf girth (cm)	38.37 ± 1.59	38.20	34.00	42.65	−0.09	0.14	0.06
Sum of skinfolds (mm)	45.13 ± 12.64	44.10	21.30	85.13	0.94	0.96	0.10
Triceps skinfold (mm)	9.31 ± 2.65	8.90	4.90	18.70	0.96	1.11	0.09
Subscapular skinfold (mm)	11.32 ± 3.70	10.40	6.10	28.20	1.95	5.68	0.13
Supraspinale skinfold (mm)	13.48 ± 5.65	12.10	5.00	34.70	1.15	1.57	0.11
Medial calf skinfold (mm)	11.02 ± 3.83	10.67	4.20	21.90	0.68	0.11	0.07
Endomorphy rating	3.23 ± 0.99	3.03	1.35	6.31	0.78	0.50	0.08
Mesomorphy rating	4.81 ± 0.90	4.70	2.74	7.56	0.43	0.35	0.08
Ectomorphy rating	2.25 ± 0.86	2.25	0.56	4.46	0.17	−0.46	0.05

Notes: SD—standard deviation, M—median, Min—minimum value, Max—maximum value, Skew—Skewness, Kurt—kurtosis, MaxD—maximum distance between relative cumulative theoretical frequency (normal) and relative cumulative empirical frequency obtained by measuring, and limit value of KS test for N = 97 is 0.14.

Coefficients of asymmetry for variables *subscapular skinfold* and *supraspinale skinfold* indicate a slightly positive asymmetry. Coefficients of peakedness indicate a somewhat lower sensitivity of the *legs fat mass* and *subscapular skinfold* variables. Although the kurtosis and skewness values indicate a weak sensitivity of the aforementioned variables used, the KS test found that there is no significant deviation from the normal distribution.

Table 2 presents the descriptive parameters (arithmetic means and standard deviations), results of univariate analysis of differences (ANOVA; coefficient of analysis of variance and significance of differences), and results of the *post-hoc* analysis of differences carried out using *Fisher's LSD test* (significance of differences).

Significant differences in arithmetic means between the three groups of elite sailors according to the general competitive success criterion were found for *age, body mass, muscle mass, trunk muscle mass, leg muscle mass, biepicondilar humerus width, sum of skinfolds, triceps skinfold, supraspinale skinfold, medial calf skinfold* and *endomorphy rating* between the groups of elite sailors according to the general competitive success criterion.

Post-hoc analysis revealed significant differences between groups of sailors at different levels of general competitive success in the variables *age* (higher vs. medium and higher vs. lower), *body mass* (higher vs. lower and medium vs. lower), *muscle mass* (higher vs. lower and medium vs. lower), *trunk muscle mass* (higher vs. lower and medium vs. lower), *arm muscle mass* (medium vs. lower), *legs muscle mass* (higher vs. lower and medium vs. lower), *biepicondilar humerus width* (higher vs. lower), *sum of skinfolds* (higher vs. lower and medium vs. lower), *triceps skinfold* (higher vs. lower and medium vs. lower), *supraspinale skinfold* (medium vs. lower), *medial calf skinfold* (higher vs. lower), and *endomorphy rating* (higher vs. lower and medium vs. lower).

The effect size of these differences was high for the variable age, moderate for the variables muscle mass, trunk muscle mass, legs muscle mass, sum of skinfolds and triceps skinfold, and low for body mass, biepicondilar femur width, supraspinale skinfold, medial calf skinfold, and endomorphy rating.

Table 2. Analysis of variance (ANOVA) and *post-hoc* analysis between groups of ILCA 7 sailors' different levels of general success.

Variables	LEVEL OF SUCCESS			ANOVA		Post-Hoc LSD Test (Between Groups)		
	Higher (N = 15)	Medium (N = 20)	Lower (N = 62)	F	*p*=	*p*= *		
	Mean ± SD	Mean ± SD	Mean ± SD			1–2	1–3	2–3
Age (yrs)	26.79 ± 2.89	23.35 ± 2.86	21.89 ± 2.98	16.96	**0.000**	**0.001**	**0.001**	0.06
Stature (cm)	182.97 ± 2.89	183.09 ± 4.78	181.04 ± 5.78	1.63	0.20	0.95	0.21	0.13
Sitting height (cm)	97.65 ± 3.56	96.80 ± 2.89	96.36 ± 3.29	0.97	0.38	0.45	0.17	0.60
Body mass (kg)	82.17 ± 1.62	82.14 ± 2.80	79.85 ± 4.31	4.25	**0.02**	0.98	**0.03**	**0.02**
Body mass index (kg/m^2)	24.53 ± 0.55	24.44 ± 1.11	24.35 ± 1.89	0.08	0.92	0.88	0.70	0.83
Fat range (%)	10.39 ± 3.34	10.53 ± 2.80	11.29 ± 3.85	0.59	0.56	0.91	0.39	0.41
Muscle mass (kg)	70.21 ± 3.37	70.07 ± 3.19	67.48 ± 3.76	6.08	**0.003**	0.91	**0.010**	**0.006**
Trunk muscle mass (kg)	38.03 ± 2.42	37.72 ± 2.07	36.22 ± 2.20	6.19	**0.003**	0.69	**0.005**	**0.010**
Arms muscle mass (kg)	8.71 ± 0.50	8.86 ± 0.42	8.52 ± 0.72	2.28	0.11	0.52	0.29	**0.047**
Legs muscle mass (kg)	23.47 ± 0.75	23.49 ± 1.10	22.74 ± 1.20	4.81	**0.010**	0.95	**0.03**	**0.011**
Fat mass (kg)	8.50 ± 2.64	8.67 ± 2.34	9.06 ± 3.30	0.28	0.76	0.87	0.52	0.62
Trunk fat mass (kg)	4.44 ± 2.12	4.58 ± 1.67	4.94 ± 2.16	0.48	0.62	0.84	0.40	0.50
Arms fat mass (kg)	1.05 ± 0.20	1.02 ± 0.24	0.98 ± 0.31	0.45	0.64	0.74	0.38	0.59
Legs fat mass (kg)	3.11 ± 0.49	3.18 ± 0.62	3.25 ± 0.97	0.20	0.82	0.81	0.55	0.73
Biepicondilar humerus width (cm)	7.16 ± 0.33	7.05 ± 0.43	6.89 ± 0.37	3.65	**0.03**	0.36	**0.014**	0.12
Biepicondilar femur width (cm)	9.30 ± 0.51	9.47 ± 0.43	9.29 ± 0.51	1.05	0.35	0.33	0.91	0.15
Upper arm girth flexed and tensed (cm)	35.47 ± 1.40	36.00 ± 1.16	35.65 ± 2.04	0.43	0.65	0.39	0.73	0.45
Calf girth (cm)	38.42 ± 1.65	38.79 ± 1.73	38.23 ± 1.53	0.96	0.39	0.49	0.67	0.17
Sum of skinfolds (mm)	39.18 ± 10.90	40.75 ± 8.89	47.99 ± 13.28	4.79	**0.010**	0.71	**0.014**	**0.02**
Triceps skinfold (mm)	8.10 ± 1.98	8.39 ± 1.92	9.90 ± 2.83	4.63	**0.012**	0.75	**0.02**	**0.02**
Subscapular skinfold (mm)	10.31 ± 2.54	10.73 ± 3.68	11.76 ± 3.91	1.25	0.29	0.74	0.18	0.28
Supraspinale skinfold (mm)	11.67 ± 4.55	11.39 ± 3.87	14.59 ± 6.11	3.52	**0.03**	0.89	0.07	**0.03**
Medial calf skinfold (mm)	9.11 ± 3.98	10.24 ± 2.66	11.74 ± 3.95	3.56	**0.03**	0.38	**0.02**	0.12
Endomorphy rating	2.81 ± 0.85	2.86 ± 0.75	3.45 ± 1.04	4.47	**0.014**	0.87	**0.02**	**0.02**
Mesomorphy rating	4.82 ± 0.68	4.98 ± 0.82	4.76 ± 0.93	0.44	0.65	0.62	0.81	0.35
Ectomorphy rating	2.23 ± 0.37	2.26 ± 0.70	2.25 ± 0.99	0.01	0.99	0.92	0.94	0.95

Notes: SD—standard deviation, F—Analysis of variance coefficient, *p*=—level of statistical significance, *p*= *—level of statistical significance of Fisher LSD post-hoc test between groups of ILCA 7 sailors with different levels of general success (1-higher, 2-medium, 3-lower), bolded values $p < 0.05$.

Table 3 presents the classification of the ILCA 7 sailors according to the somatotype category. The frequency and percentage of each somatotype category were calculated for the total sample.

Out of the 13 possible somatotype categories, elite ILCA 7 sailors fit eight. Just over 75% of the total sample of elite sailors fit the somatotype categories with the dominant mesomorphic component, 41.24% of which fit the endomorphic mesomorph category.

Figure 1 depicts a graphic representation of the somatotype ratings of ILCA 7 class sailors divided into three groups according to their level of general competitive success: *higher level* (square), *medium level* (rhomb), and *lower level* (triangle).

Table 3. Frequency and ratio of somatotype categories of ILCA 7 sailors (N = 97).

Somatotype Categories	Frequency	Ratio (%)
Central	7	7.22
Mesomorphic endomorph	3	3.09
Mesomorph-endomorph	10	10.31
Endomorphic mesomorph	40	41.24
Balanced mesomorph	23	23.71
Ectomorphic mesomorph	10	10.31
Mesomorph-ectomorph	3	3.09
Ectomorphic endomorph	1	1.03

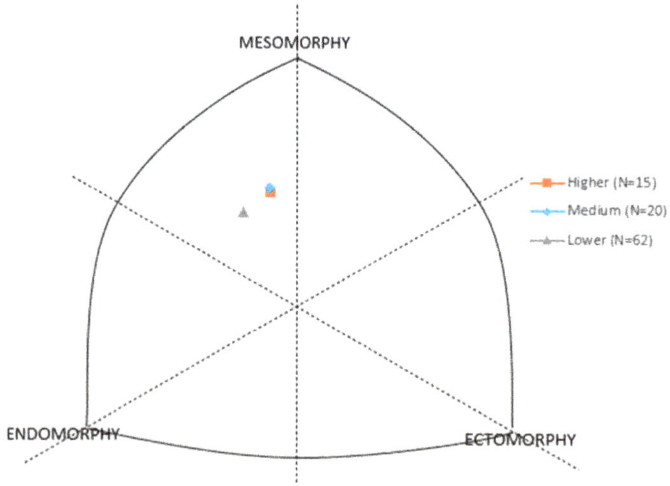

Figure 1. Somatochart.

4. Discussion

Olympic sailing is a multifaceted sport for which body size and mass are criteria for selecting an Olympic sailing class and are undoubtedly performance-related factors. However, scientific literature on anthropometrical data, body composition, and the somatotype of elite sailors is scarce. In this context, this study of World Class and International Elite level (Trier 5 & 4) ILCA 7 sailors produced two major findings: (a) for the first time, the anthropometric profile, body composition, and somatotype of 97 elite ILCA 7 class sailors have been determined, and (b) significant differences between more, medium, and less-successful elite ILCA 7 sailors have been found in terms of their anthropometric parameters, body composition, and somatotype.

4.1. ILCA 7 Sailors Anthropometric Parameters and Body Composition Comparison to Previous ILCA 7 Findings

Many studies have reported at least some of the anthropometric parameters of ILCA 7 sailors [19,20,28–33]. The mean values for the stature of ILCA 7 sailors are within ±1 cm of the measurements for our international elite sample. This is particularly interesting because the previous studies are not homogeneous in terms of the age and level of sailing performance of ILCA 7 sailors. Almost all identical mean values for *body mass* (81.18–81.88 kg) were found in scientific literature that analyzed sailors who participated in the Olympic Games [28,29,31,32]. On the other hand, a range of 76.26–78.60 kg in *body mass* values was found in studies that analyzed national elite-level sailors [19,20,28,30]. Similar values for *body mass index*, like those in this research, are reported in the literature [29,31], but also somewhat lower values in the range of *body mass index* 23.01–23.70 kg/m^2 have been reported [20,21,28].

As far as the authors are aware, only two scientific papers have analyzed the anthropometric profile of ILCA 7 sailors more extensively, but on a relatively small sample of national-level sailors (N = 7 and 9) [19,20]. Croatian ILCA 7 sailors had similar values for *stature*; smaller values for *body mass, sitting height, body mass index, upper arm girth flexed, and tensed,* and *calf girth;* but higher values for *biepicondilar humerus width* and *biepicondilar femur width* [20]. Spanish ILCA 7 sailors showed similar values for *body mass* and *upper arm girth flexed and tensed*, smaller values for *calf girth,* and higher values for *stature, biepicondilar humerus width,* and *biepicondilar femur width.*

Although body composition results obtained using different methods are difficult to compare, they will be presented in this paper informatively. Our study determined a fat range of 10.99 $\pm$ 3.57% and a muscle mass of 68.43 $\pm$ 3.57 kg (BIA). Manzanares et al. (2023) reported for six elite sailors an average muscle mass of 68.07 kg and a fat range of 14% [29]. In Croatian ILCA 7 sailors, fat ranges of 10.19% (Heath–Carter method) and 15.16% (Durnin–Wormesley method) were reported, depending on the method used [20], and Spanish ILCA 7 sailors showed a fat range of 13.9% (Heath–Carter method) [19].

4.2. ILCA 7 Sailors Anthropometric Parameters and Body Composition Comparison to Other Sailing Class Sailors' Parameters

As is the case for the ILCA 7 class, detailed anthropometric studies on sailors in any Olympic or other sailing classes are lacking.

The ILCA 6 dinghy is an Olympic class only for women, but also a developmental class for younger male sailors. The ILCA 6 dinghy uses the same hull but a more flexible and slightly shorter lower mast, with a sail area 18% smaller than that of the ILCA 7. Fifteen ILCA 6 male sailors (18.01 yrs) showed smaller values for *stature, sitting height, body mass, body mass index, upper arm girth flexed and tensed,* and *calf girth* [20] compared to our ILCA 7 male sailors. The same differences were found in ILCA 6 female sailors, with smaller values for *stature, body mass,* and *body mass index* in elite- [19,29,31] or national-level [21,28] ILCA 6 female sailors.

The 470 is a double-handed Olympic class where the helmsman is classified as a side-deck hiker—just like an ILCA 7 sailor—and the crew are characterized as trapeze sailors [2]. 470 sailors (helmsman and crew) have smaller *body mass* and *body mass index* values. Smaller values for *stature* were found in helmsmen, while similar *stature* values were determined in the crew [21,28,31,34]. The 49er is also a double-handed Olympic class, but none of the crew is categorized as a side-deck hiker. Anthropometric values for a 49er helmsman are lower for *stature, body mass,* and *body mass index* in all analyzed research, but results are not homogeneous for crew members. The anthropometric values of a 49er crew vary from 178 to 190.6 cm in *stature* and 76.3 to 85.3 kg in *body mass,* while *body mass index* is similar to that of ILCA 7 sailors [19,28,31]. Nacra 17 is a double-handed Olympic class that has to be sailed as a man and woman pair, where both helmsman and crew are trapeze sailors. Smaller values of *stature, body mass,* and *body mass index* have been determined in Nacra 17 helmsmen, and smaller values of *body mass* and *body mass index* and higher values of *stature* have been determined in Nacra 17 crew [31].

More detailed anthropometric research was conducted on Finn class sailors [17,18,35]. The Finn class is the former Olympic heavyweight single-handed dinghy (i.e., an Olympic Class until 2021) and—similar to the ILCA 7 class—is a "classic" dinghy where the helmsman can be classified as a side deck hiker [2]. The main difference between the ILCA 7 and the Finn class is the weight of the hull and the almost 30% bigger sail area of the Finn class dinghy. Compared to ILCA 7 sailors, who are dynamic side deck hikers due to the high sailor-to-yacht weight ratio, Finn sailors are classified as static side deck hikers due to a low sailor-to-yacht weight ratio [2]. Given the above context, it is not surprising that Finn sailor have greater values for all anthropometric and body composition values (*stature, body mass, body mass index, fat range, muscle mass, trunk muscle mass, arms muscle mass, legs muscle mass, fat mass, trunk fat mass, arms fat mass, legs fat mass, biepicondilar humerus width, biepicondilar femur width, upper arm girth flexed and tensed, calf girth, sum of skinfolds, triceps skinfold, subscapular skinfold, supraspinale skinfold* and *medial calf skinfold*) compared to ILCA 7 sailors [17,18,35].

4.3. ILCA 7 Sailors Somatotype

The lack of scientific research on the body structure of ILCA 7 sailors is also evident with respect to somatotype. Both studies that determined somatotype and this study found that the mesomorphic component is a dominant feature in ILCA 7 sailors [19,20]. The somatotype category "endomorphic mesomorph" was found across Spanish ILCA 7 sailors [19], while Croatian ILCA 7 sailors were classified as "balanced mesomorph" [20].

In our study, more than 75% of elite ILCA 7 sailors have a dominant mesomorphic somatotype component and can be categorized as "*endomorphic mesomorph*" somatotypes. Similar distributions were also observed in elite Finn class sailors [18]. Generally, the mesomorphic component is dominant for sailors in all sailing classes where somatotype was calculated: Finn [18,19], ILCA 6 [20], Formula [11], Optimist [36], RSX [19], and Olympic classes 470 & 49er [19]. The *endomorphic mesomorph* somatotype is common to ILCA 7 and Finn class sailors [18], while the *balanced mesomorph* somatotype is more common in ILCA 6, Formula, and 49er classes [11,19,20], and the *ectomorphic mesomorph* somatotype in RSX and 470 classes [19]. The dominant mesomorphic somatotype component of ILCA 7 sailors could be explained by the theory that size only confers an advantage if extra weight does not add more to the resistance of the yacht than it contributes to the propulsive forces of the dinghy; therefore, optimal leverage (stature) and ballast mass (body mass) are needed to be an efficient ILCA 7 sailor.

A mesomorphic somatotype component is dominant in various high-performance athletes in sports such as soccer [37], rowing [38], table tennis [39], track cyclist [40], canoe and kayak paddlers [15], 100 m sprinters [10,41] track and field [41], swimming [41], and basketball [12]. However, ILCA 7 sailors share the same *endomorphic mesomorph* somatotype category with sprint-track cyclists [40], rowers [42], kayakers [12], and water polo players [43].

4.4. Differences of ILCA 7 Sailors According to Level of Success

In our study, significant differences were found between the ILCA 7 sailors' higher, medium, and lower successful groups in terms of *age, body mass, muscle mass, trunk muscle mass, legs muscle mass, biepicondilar humerus width, sum of skinfolds, triceps skinfold, supraspinale skinfold, medial calf skinfold* and *endomorphy rating*. However, age was the only variable that differentiated the higher and medium successful groups, while for all other measured variables, the two groups (higher and medium successful) were quite homogeneous. Experience can be a key element of sport excellence, especially in an individual sport such as sailing, where tactics and race anticipation play a decisive role. The fact that in this research, WSR was used as a criterion to classify ILCA 7 sailors can be favorable for the more experienced sailors. WSR takes into account the six best regatta ratings within the last twelve months. It can be assumed that more experienced athletes are able to keep a higher level of performance over a longer period under potentially different environmental race conditions. So, the difference in age between the higher and lower successful groups can be justified by the years of sailing experience. Physical maturity may have also influenced the results, as some sailors included in the study were younger than the typical age at which full physical development is attained. Although the difference in age between the medium and lower successful groups is not significant, it is also very indicative.

The lower successful group of ILCA 7 sailors has smaller values for *body mass*, *muscle mass*, *trunk muscle mass*, and *leg muscle mass*, and higher values of *sum of skinfolds*, *triceps skinfold*, and *endomorphy rating* compared to the higher and medium successful groups. Similar results have been determined in Finn class sailors [18], and therefore, the same conclusion of the findings could be repeated in the ILCA 7 class. The homogeneity of ILCA 7 sailors in the parameters of longitudinal and transverse skeletal dimensions might reflect the selection process for the sailing class, whereas the determined impact and analyses of differences in the dimensions of soft tissue might reflect an adaptive process [18]. As previously noted, optimal stature appears to be a well-established factor in maximizing leverage efficiency in the ILCA 7 sailing class. Sailors of shorter stature may experience a mechanical disadvantage due to reduced leverage, while taller sailors may benefit from improved leverage but potentially at the cost of increased energy expenditure and a lower muscle mass to body mass ratio. While bone length and width dimensions are not changeable, muscle and fat mass and their distribution are likely to be affected by a long-term build-up training program. It appears to take some time to adapt the body to the more successful ILCA 7 sailor model, which has more muscle mass and a lower endomorphy rating. Additionally, the "adaptation process" may be significantly influenced by nutritional factors and shaped by individual genetic predispositions. Higher values of *muscle mass* and lower *endomorphy ratings* have been reported at professional levels compared to the amateur level Formula class sailors [11].

4.5. Limitations of the Study

In this study, only the BIA method was used to analyze body composition. It is well known that hydration levels can significantly influence impedance readings. Dehydration or overhydration can lead to incorrect estimates of fat mass or lean mass. Although the measurement protocol was the same for all sailors, the hydration status was not controlled for by any method. Among the other body composition methods, e.g., Heath–Charter or Durnin–Womersley, BIA was chosen as it is the fastest method for estimating body composition. Given the advancing understanding of body composition, future research should consider integrating a broader set of anthropometric parameters to enhance the accuracy and applicability of various body composition assessment methods.

The group sizes of the sailors, categorized based on overall success in this study, were unequal, which may have influenced the statistical power of the analysis. Although squared eta (η^2) coefficients were calculated, alternative methods such as Welch's ANOVA, which accounts for unequal variances, could also be employed. Where feasible, future research should aim to balance group sizes to improve the robustness of statistical comparisons.

Only anthropometric parameters were assessed, limiting the ability to directly analyze the influence of functional and motor abilities on competitive performance. While morphological variables may offer indirect insights into these influences, a more comprehensive evaluation of performance in sailing requires the inclusion of assessments targeting functional and motor capacities. Although the implementation of such tests prior to major competitions may present challenges, as coaches and athletes may be reluctant to engage in potentially strenuous assessments during critical preparation periods, collaboration among researchers, coaches, athletes, and class officials is essential to explore viable approaches. Incorporating both morphological and functional data could yield valuable insights, with substantial implications for the development of specific sailing classes and the enhancement of performance within the sport more broadly.

Age and training history may confound the analysis; therefore, it is advisable to include additional demographic data, such as sailing history (e.g., previously sailed classes, years spent in the specific sailing class, etc.), as well as non-sailing fitness information, including types of cross-training activities and other relevant pursuits that could influence anthropometric parameters.

The World Sailing Ranking (WSR) serves as a general indicator of sailing performance, representing a composite measure of performance over a two-year period in the ILCA 7 class. Unlike the outcome of a single regatta, the WSR is less susceptible to situational variables such as wind speed, water conditions, and other environmental factors that may dominate during a specific competition week. Nevertheless, it remains important to examine potential differences in morphological characteristics across varying levels of situational competitive success. Any study focused on a single regatta would inherently be influenced by the aforementioned environmental variables, and its findings should be interpreted in the context of prevailing wind conditions and other relevant race parameters.

5. Conclusions

The anthropometric profile, body composition, and somatotype of world-class and elite international ILCA 7 sailors have been defined, and differences between sailors of different levels of success were determined. To the best of the authors' knowledge, this study included the largest cohort of international elite ILCA 7 sailors or sailors of any other Olympic sailing class.

Although anthropometric measures, body composition, and somatotype provide valuable information about the optimal profile of elite ILCA 7 sailors, body structure profiling is not complete without the determination of functional and motor abilities. Thus, future studies on elite ILCA 7 sailors should focus on the relationship between body structure and function.

The WSR can be seen as a measure of general sailing success. Its strength is that it is less dependent on situational "on water" conditions, such as wind speed, sea state, and other environmental conditions that were dominant during a specific competition. However, it is advisable that similar research could be replicated, considering results from a single competition, and hopefully analyzing and considering sailing performance under different wind conditions.

The present study can help coaches and young sailors in the process of choosing the ideal sailing class. In the sport of sailing, there are many sailing classes, and six of them are in the Olympic program. Choosing the ideal sailing class that best fits the athlete's anthropometric profile could be a crucial first step in a sailor's career. This research clearly determines the anthropometric profile, body composition, and somatotype of elite ILCA 7 sailors, which can significantly contribute to a more informed choice of sailing class. Given the results of this research, current ILCA 7 sailors can easily compare their own anthropometric parameters with elite ILCA 7 sailors and eventually adjust the training process to obtain a more desirable anthropometric profile.

Author Contributions: Conceptualization, L.P., J.G.B. and M.M.; methodology, L.P., J.G.B. and M.M.; field research, L.P., M.M. and J.M.; writing—original draft preparation, L.P., J.G.B., M.M., J.M. and I.C.; visualization, L.P. and J.G.B.; writing—review and editing, L.P., J.G.B., M.M., J.M. and I.C. All authors have read and agreed to the published version of the manuscript.

Funding: This research received no external funding.

Institutional Review Board Statement: This study was conducted in accordance with the general ethical principles of conducting research with human participants and approved by the Scientific Committee and by the Dean of the Faculty of Kinesiology, University of Split (4 September 2017). 2181-205-01-1-17-054.

Informed Consent Statement: Informed consent was obtained from all subjects involved in the study.

Data Availability Statement: The data presented in this study are available on request from the corresponding authors.

Acknowledgments: The authors gratefully acknowledge the support and help of the International Laser Class Association and the Sailing Club Mornar, Split.

Conflicts of Interest: The authors declare no conflicts of interest.

References

1. Bourgois, J.; Claessens, A.L.; Vrijens, J.; Philippaerts, R.; Van Renterghem, B.; Thomis, M.; Janssens, M.; Loos, R.; Lefevre, J. Anthropometric characteristics of elite male junior rowers. *Br. J. Sports Med.* **2000**, *34*, 213–216. [CrossRef] [PubMed]
2. Bojsen-Møller, J.; Larsson, B.; Magnusson, S.P.; Aagaard, P. Yacht type and crew-specific differences in anthropometric, aerobic capacity, and muscle strength parameters among international Olympic class sailors. *J. Sports Sci.* **2007**, *25*, 1117–1128. [CrossRef] [PubMed]
3. Tan, B.; Aziz, A.R.; Spurway, N.C.; Toh, C.; Mackie, H.; Xie, W.; Wong, J.; Fuss, F.K.; Teh, K.C. Indicators of maximal hiking performance in Laser sailors. *Eur. J. Appl. Physiol.* **2006**, *98*, 169–176. [CrossRef] [PubMed]
4. Plyely, M.J.; Davis, G.M.; Shepard, R.J. Body Profile of Olympic Class Sailors. *Phy. Sport.* **1985**, *13*, 152–167. [CrossRef]
5. De Vito, G.; Di Filippo, L.; Felici, F.; Marchetti, M. Hiking Mechanics in Laser Athletes. *Med. Sci. Res.* **1993**, *21*, 859–860.
6. Allen, J.B.; De Jong, M.R. Sailing and sports medicine: A literature review. *Br. J. Sports Med.* **2006**, *40*, 587–593. [CrossRef]
7. Caraballo, I.; González-Montesinos, J.L.; Alías, A. Performance factors in dinghy sailing: Laser class. *Int. J. Environ. Res. Public Heal.* **2019**, *16*, 4920. [CrossRef]
8. Legg, S.J.; Miller, A.B.; Slyfield, D.; Smith, P.; Gilberd, C.; Wilcox, H.; Tate, C. Physical Performance of Elite New Zeland Olympic Class Sailors. *J. Sports Med. Phys. Fit.* **1997**, *37*, 41–49.
9. Bourgois, J.G.; Dumortier, J.; Callewaert, M.; Celie, B.; Capelli, C.; Sjøgaard, G.; De Clercq, D.; Boone, J. Tribute to Dr Jacques Rogge: Muscle activity and fatigue during hiking in Olympic dinghy sailing. *Eur. J. Sport Sci.* **2017**, *17*, 611–620. [CrossRef]
10. Barbieri, D.; Zaccagni, L.; Babić, V.; Rakovac, M.; Mišigoj-Duraković, M.; Gualdi-Russo, E. Body composition and size in sprint athletes. *J. Sports Med. Phys. Fit.* **2017**, *57*, 1142–1146. [CrossRef]
11. Cortell-Tormo, J.; Pérez-Turpin, J.; Cejuela-Anta, R.; Chinchilla-Mira, J.; Marfell-Jones, M. Anthropometric profile of male amateur vs professional formula windsurfs competing at the 2007 European championship. *J. Hum. Kinet.* **2010**, *23*, 97–101. [CrossRef]
12. Gutnik, B.; Zuoza, A.; Zuozienė, I.; Alekrinskis, A.; Nash, D.; Scherbina, S. Body physique and dominant somatotype in elite and low-profile athletes with different specializations. *Medicina* **2015**, *51*, 247–252. [CrossRef] [PubMed]
13. Hébert-Losier, K.; Zinner, C.; Platt, S.; Stöggl, T.; Holmberg, H.-C. Factors that Influence the Performance of Elite Sprint Cross-Country Skiers. *Sports Med.* **2016**, *47*, 319–342. [CrossRef]
14. Sanchez-Munoz, C.; Muros, J.J.; Zabala, M. World and Olympic mountain bike champions anthropometry, body composition, and somatotype. *J. Sports Med. Phys. Fit.* **2018**, *58*, 843–851. [CrossRef] [PubMed]
15. Coufalová, K.; Busta, J.; Cochrane, D.J.; Bíly, M. Morphological Characteristics of European Slalom Canoe and Kayak Paddlers. *Int. J. Morphol.* **2021**, *39*, 896–901. [CrossRef]
16. Ginszt, A.; Zieliński, G.; Dolina, A.; Stachyra, E.; Zaborek-Łyczba, M.; Łyczba, J.; Gawda, P.; Ginszt, M. Anthropometric Parameters and Body Composition in Elite Lead Climbers and Boulderers—A Retrospective Study. *Appl. Sci.* **2024**, *14*, 5603. [CrossRef]
17. Pezelj, L.; Marinović, M.; Milavić, B. Morphological Characteristics of Elite U23 Sailors—Finn European Championship, Split 2015. *Sport Sci.* **2016**, *9*, 116–120.
18. Pezelj, L.; Milavić, B.; Milić, M. Anthropometric and Somatotype Profile of Elite Finn Class Sailors. *J. Funct. Morphol. Kinesiol.* **2024**, *9*, 121. [CrossRef]
19. Sanchez, L.R.; Banos, V.M. Anthropometric profile and somatotype of sailors of the spanish pre-olympic sailing team. *SPORT TK Rev. Euroam. De Cienc. Del Deporte* **2018**, *7*, 117–122.
20. Marinović, M. Morphological Characteristics of the Seaman in Class Laser and Laser Radial. *Hrvat. Športskomed. Vjesn.* **2001**, *16*, 16–20.
21. Pan, D.; Zhong, B.; Guo, W.; Xu, Y. Physical fitness characteristics and performance in single-handed dinghy and 470 classes sailors. *J. Exerc. Sci. Fit.* **2022**, *20*, 9–15. [CrossRef] [PubMed]

22. McKay, A.K.A.; Stellingwerff, T.; Smith, E.S.; Martin, D.T.; Mujika, I.; Goosey-Tolfrey, V.L.; Sheppard, J.; Burke, L.M. Defining Training and Performance Caliber: A Participant Classification Framework. *Int. J. Sports Physiol. Perform.* **2022**, *17*, 317–331 [CrossRef]
23. Stewart, D.; Marfell-Jones, M.J.; Olds, T.; De Ridder, J.H. *International Standards for Anthropometric Assessment*; Society for the Advancement of Kinanthropometry (ISAK): Lower Hutt, New Zealand, 2011.
24. Carter, J.E.L. *The Heath-Carter Anthropometric Somatotype—Instruction Manual*; San Diego State University, Department of Exercise and Nutritional Science: San Diego, CA, USA, 2002.
25. Kyle, U.G.; Bosaeus, I.; De Lorenzo, A.D.; Deurenberg, P.; Elia, M.; Gómez, J.M.; Heitmann, B.L.; Kent-Smith, L.; Melchior, J.-C.; Pirlich, M.; et al. Bioelectrical impedance analysis—Part II: Utilization in clinical practice. *Clin. Nutr.* **2004**, *23*, 1430–1453 [CrossRef] [PubMed]
26. Carter, J.E.L.; Heath, B. *Somatotyping—Development and Applications*; Cambridge University Press: Cambridge, UK, 1990.
27. Gamst, G.; Meyers, L.S.; Guarino, A.J. *Analysis of Variance Designs: A Conceptual and Computational Approach with SPSS and SAS* Cambridge University Press: New York, NY, USA, 2008.
28. Pan, D.; Sun, K.; Liu, X. Anthropometric and physiological profiles of highly trained sailors in various positions and level. *Sci. Rep.* **2024**, *14*, 1–9. [CrossRef]
29. Manzanares, A.; Encarnación-Martínez, A.; Chicoy-García, I.; Segado, F. Performance profile of elite ILCA class sailors. Differences between men and women. *Arch. de Med. del Deport.* **2023**, *40*, 194–199. [CrossRef]
30. Cunningham, P.; Hale, T. Physiological responses of elite Laser sailors to 30 minutes of simulated upwind sailing. *J. Sports Sci. J Sports Sci.* **2007**, *25*, 1109–1116. [CrossRef]
31. Skrypchenko, S.; Hamad, H.; Joksimović, M.; Singh, R.M.; Yarymbash, K.; Lastovkin, V. Significance of anthropometric characteristics of Olympic sailors and their functional position in boat for relation to racing success. *Rev. De Educ. Fisica* **2022**, *11*, 83–102.
32. Zubac, D.; Valić, Z.; Ivančev, V. Setting sail for Paris 2024: Retrospective analysis of world-class ILCA 7 Olympic sailors cardiorespiratory fitness (2015–2020). *Exp. Physiol.* **2024**, 1–8. [CrossRef]
33. Winchcombe, C.; Goods, P.; Binnie, M.; Doyle, M.; Fahey-Gilmour, J.; Peeling, P. Workload demands of laser class sailing regattas. *Int. J. Perform. Anal. Sport* **2021**, *21*, 663–678. [CrossRef]
34. Sánchez-Oliver, A.J.; Caraballo, I.; Pérez-Bey, A.; Sánchez-Gómez, Á.; Domínguez, R. Anthropometric characteristics of young elite sailors based on performance level. *J. Exerc. Sci. Fit.* **2022**, *21*, 125–130. [CrossRef]
35. Pezelj, L.; Milavic, B.; Erceg, M. Respiratory parameters in elite finn-class sailors. *Montenegrin J. Sports Sci. Med.* **2019**, *8*, 5–9 [CrossRef]
36. Palomino-Martín, A.; Quintana-Santana, D.; Quiroga-Escudero, M.E.; González-Muñoz, A. Incidence of anthropometric variables on the performance of top optimist sailors. *J. Hum. Sport Exerc.* **2017**, *12*, 41–57. [CrossRef]
37. Petri, C.; Campa, F.; Holway, F.; Pengue, L.; Arrones, L.S. ISAK-Based Anthropometric Standards for Elite Male and Female Soccer Players. *Sports* **2024**, *12*, 69. [CrossRef]
38. Busta, J.; Hellebrand, J.; Kinkorová, I.; Macas, T. Morphological and hand grip strength characteristics and differences between participants of the 2022 world rowing championship. *Front. Sports Act. Living* **2023**, *5*, 1115336. [CrossRef] [PubMed]
39. Pradas, F.; De La Torre, A.; Carrasco, L.; Muñoz, D.; Courel-Ibáñez, J.; González-Jurado, J.A. Anthropometric Profiles in Table Tennis Players: Analysis of Sex, Age, and Ranking. *Appl. Sci.* **2021**, *11*, 876. [CrossRef]
40. Muros-Molina, J.J.; Mateo-March, M.; Zabala, M.; Sánchez-Muñoz, C. Anthropometric differences between world-class professional track cyclists according to speciality (endurance vs. sprint). *J. Sports Med. Phys. Fit.* **2022**, *61*, 1481–1488. [CrossRef]
41. Stanković, D.; Pavlović, R.; Petković, E.; Raković, A.; Puletić, M. The Somatotypes and Body Composition of Elite Track and Field Athletes and Swimmers. *Artic. Int. J. Sports Sci.* **2018**, *8*, 67–77. [CrossRef]
42. Mikulić, P.; Vučetić, V.; Matković, B.; Oreb, G. Morphological Characterstics and Somatotype of Elite Croatian Rowers. *Hrvat Športskomed. Vjesn.* **2005**, *20*, 15–19.
43. Suárez, M.H.V.; Fiol, C.F.; Suárez, N.R.; Iturriaga, F.M.A.; Valeiras, J.A.A. Características antropométricas, composición corporal y somatotipo en jugadores de élite de waterpolo. *Rev. Bras. De Ciências Do Esporte* **2010**, *32*, 184–197. [CrossRef]

applied sciences

Article

Psychomotor Abilities, Body Composition and Training Experience of Elite and Sub-Elite Handball Players

Maciej Śliż [1,*], Cintia França [2,3,4], Francisco Martins [2,3,5], Patryk Marszałek [1], Élvio Rúbio Gouveia [2,3,6] and Krzysztof Przednowek [1]

1 Institute of Physical Culture Sciences, Medical College of Rzeszów University, University of Rzeszów, 35-959 Rzeszów, Poland; pmarszalek@ur.edu.pl (P.M.); krprzednowek@ur.edu.pl (K.P.)
2 Department of Physical Education and Sport, University of Madeira, 9020-105 Funchal, Portugal; cintia.franca@staff.uma.pt (C.F.); joao.martins@staff.uma.pt (F.M.); erubiog@staff.uma.pt (É.R.G.)
3 LARSYS, Interactive Technologies Institute, 9020-105 Funchal, Portugal
4 Research Center in Sports Science, Health Sciences, and Human Development (CIDESD), 5000-801 Vila Real, Portugal
5 Research Unit for Sport and Physical Activity (CIDAF), Faculty of Sports Sciences and Physical Education, University of Coimbra, 3004-504 Coimbra, Portugal
6 CIPER, Faculty of Human Kinetics, University of Lisbon, 1649-004 Lisbon, Portugal
* Correspondence: msliz@ur.edu.pl

Abstract: Background: Handball is characterized by fast and dynamic movements requiring appropriate psychomotor abilities and body mass composition. High levels of reaction and movement time can be crucial factors influencing quick reactions and in-time decision-making at the handball court. The aim of this study was to assess psychomotor abilities among elite and sub-elite Polish and Portuguese male and female handball players at the different levels of competition. **Methods**: Computer Test2Drive systems were used to assess reaction time, movement time and percentage of correct responses of 199 handball players (60 females). **Results**: Statistically significant correlation was noted between SIRT cr and the Elite group (r = 0.44) and between the CHORT cr and all groups (r = 0.33). A statistical correlation between CHORT MT and total body water (r = 0.44) was also noted in Elite handball players. **Conclusions**: High level of psychomotor abilities and body composition seems to have impact on the competitive level in male and female handball players.

Keywords: handball; psychomotor abilities; reaction time; decision making; movement time; body composition

1. Introduction

Modern elite handball is characterized by 60 min of repeated accelerations, sprints, jumps, shots, rapid changes of direction, and a high number of physical confrontations with opponent players [1,2]. Therefore, handball is a complex, multi factorial [3] dynamic sport discipline, where each team tries to score goals with different technical, tactical and physiological demands [4,5]. It is a kind of competitive sport that requires processing a significant amount of information at the same time [6], combined with possessing knowledge to correctly respond in a timely manner [7]. Therefore, modern handball results may depend on numerous factors [8,9] such as reaction time, movement time, decision-making or body composition [10,11]. The scientific research of Curiţianu et al. [12] can be an example showcasing that players' reaction speed has an impact on the number of effective quick attacks. Similarly, Ohnjec et al. [13] have shown, by quantifying 60 matches for the World Women's Handball Championship in 2003, that the possibility of a fast break is determined by reaction speeds. Also Krawczyk [14] showed that top-level goalkeepers wait until the last second before reacting to the opponent's shot, which makes their decisions more effective. Moreover, high demands on the retention time and range of perception, and the multitude of visual stimuli and moving objects in the central as well as the peripheral field of vision at the same time makes handball a sport with a high need for perceptual competence in its players [15]. Approximately sixty per cent of offensive actions have a standard duration between 21 and 35 s, while seventeen per cent of them are short actions with a duration of less than twenty seconds [16,17]. Anticipation abilities and quick reaction time can be crucial in handball at different competitive levels [14,18–20]. The optimal reaction time for athletes is between 140 and 160 milliseconds [21]. This can also be used to assess psychophysical state and technical and tactical skills [22]. Although the basic physical and motor elements are important, physical training alone seems to not be enough for sporting success. So, psychomotor abilities like coordination and perception can play an important role in enabling players to successfully perform and respond to complex tasks [23]. In addition, success in motor coordination depends on individual perception (i.e., the ways in which a person perceives a given situation). Bideau [24] showed that professional handball goalkeepers' success depends on their ability to anticipate and shorten their reaction time. Related conclusions presented by Krawczyk et al. [14] show that handball goalkeepers exhibit high abilities in reaction time and motor time in terms of simple reaction time and choice reaction time. Moreover, Śliż et al. [25] showed statistically significant reaction and movement time differences between female handball players on different levels of competition. Furthermore, the female players from the Polish Women's Superliga exhibited the fastest reaction time according to the simple reaction time, choice reaction time and spatial anticipation test. Nevertheless, psychomotor abilities differentiate players by position, especially short-term memory capacity and reaction time [26]. Przednowek et al. [27] revealed that, in the majority of psychomotor tests, the first-division handball players had a shorter reaction time than players competing in lower leagues. It is also necessary to take note of the fact that appropriate anthropometric characteristics and body composition of male and female handball players at different training levels is very important in current handball [9–11,28–33]. The importance of adequate anthropometric characteristics and body composition was shown in a study by Martinez-Rodriguez et al. [34], who presented that female handball players have a proportion of fat mass of around 20%, with a slightly lower proportion in elite players. For male players, the proportion of fat mass is significant at around 14%, with a higher proportion in non-elite players.

Therefore, there are many scientific works about the relationship between body components and reaction time in team sports at the different gender, age, level of league and training competition characteristics [35–40]. A similar investigation published by Śliż et al. 2023 [9] showed that the level of selected motor abilities might be affected by some parameters of body composition.

Summarizing, a crucial matter of concern in handball can be finding a solution between body composition, training experience, reaction time, movement time and correct responses [41].

2. Aim

This study's aim was two fold: (i) to assess psychomotor abilities such as reaction time, movement time, correct responses in male and female handball players from the Elite and Sub-Elite Polish and Portuguese handball leagues during 2023/2024 season, (ii) analyze the relationship between body composition, training experience and psychomotor abilities in different levels of competition in Polish and Portuguese female and male handball players. Furthermore, the aim of this research was also to identify whether there was a correlation between reaction time, movement time and correct response according to sex, age, body fat, body mass, fat-free mass, body height and total body water of male and female handball groups (Elite and Sub-Elite).

3. Material

Participants

The study group consisted of 199 handball players (60 female and 139 male) (Table 1) associated in the Polish and Portuguese Handball Federation (female average age: 29.3 ± 5.4 and male average age: 24.3 ± 3.9). The group of male and female handball players was divided into Elite and Sub-Elite athletes, according to the National division in which their team compete. The Elite group of female and male handball players were professionals and competed in the top national league, while the Sub-Elite group were semi-professionals playing in the second national league. Therefore, 68 Elite and 71 Sub-Elite male handball players were examined. Also, the female handball players consisted of 21 Elite and 39 Sub-Elite handball players. All female and male handball players participated in different competitive levels (Elite and Sub-Elite competition) in Poland and Portugal. Before the beginning of the tests, we received permission from the handball clubs to allow the players to participate in the scientific research. All the male and female handball players studied were Elite and Sub-Elite group who were tested during the Portuguese (March 2024) and Polish (April 2024) national competitions.

Table 1. Characteristic of Polish and Portuguese female and male handball players.

Group	Female Handball	Male Handball
N	60	139
Age	29.3 ± 5.4	24.3 ± 3.9
Body Height (cm)	180.6 ± 6.7	186.0 ± 7.0
Body Weight (kg)	78.9 ± 9.1	103.1 ± 15.2
BMI	29.3 ± 4.6	24.2 ± 2.1

N—number of participants, BMI—Body Mass Index.

4. Methods

4.1. Psychomotor Abilities Assessment

Test2Drive is a modern device that is clear and intuitive for the test participant. The tests are conducted using an online-connecting computer equipped with a touch monitor. The use of the touchscreen monitor makes it possible to replace the elaborate traditional apparatus, which significantly reduces the examination time. The entire examination with a complete battery of tests is carried out at one station. All tests of the Test2Drive system were preceded by a practice phase after which the test participant proceeded to the main test. Immediately after the examination, the participant had access to the reports and protocols of the results. The system is standardized with tables of norms. The report includes raw scores, as well as normalized results presented on a sten scale. Figure 1 shows 6 tests assessing psychomotor ability such as reaction time, movement time and correct response in SIRT, CHORT, HECOR, SPANT, PUT and PAMT tests. The compatibility and effectiveness of Test2Drive are confirmed by previous studies, making it an effective replacement for conventional psychological tests [21,42–44]. Simple reaction time (SIRT)—in a standing position, the participant's task is to move the forefinger from one box on the screen to another in response to a stimulus. All stimuli are identical, presented at random intervals. The test measures reaction time (from the stimulus to lifting the finger from the resting field) and movement time (movement time to the reaction field). The median reaction time and median motor time are therefore evaluated. Choice reaction time (CHORT)—in a standing position, varying responses are required of the participant—depending on the displayed pattern, the participant must touch the appropriate box or hold back from reacting. In addition to reaction and movement time, an important variable is the percentage of correct reactions, indicating the effectiveness of inhibition processes. HECOR (hand–eye coordination) measures eye–hand coordination. The participant has to press the box under the presented stimulus. The test is a development of the idea of the classic Piórkowski apparatus. The variables are reaction time and movement time. SPANT (spatial anticipation test) was also designed to measure eye–hand coordination. The SPANT test involves tapping a box at the intersection of the row and column indicated by the signal. In these tests, the variables are reaction time, movement time and the percentage of correct responses. SPANT is the most complex task testing psychomotor performance. PUT (pop-up test) is based on Anna Treismann's trait-integration concept. The task involves searching a set of elements for an object defined by a conjunction of features. It allows for the assessment of visual search speed and attentiveness. The participant was instructed to select the black triangle pointing either vertically upward or downward. If no such triangle appeared, the participant was to click the "NONE" button located in the bottom-right corner to proceed to the next stage. The perception–anticipation of movement test (PAMT) involves evaluating the movement of objects and making decisions at the right moment. The result of the test is the percentage of correctly performed tasks. The participant was required to touch an object using the index finger in such a way that it would avoid collision with other objects while moving horizontally across the board. The tests were selected to correspond to the specifics of the profession that female and male handball players face. During a handball match, handball players make a significant number of decisions in offensive and defensive actions where reaction time can be key to achieve the individual and team goal.

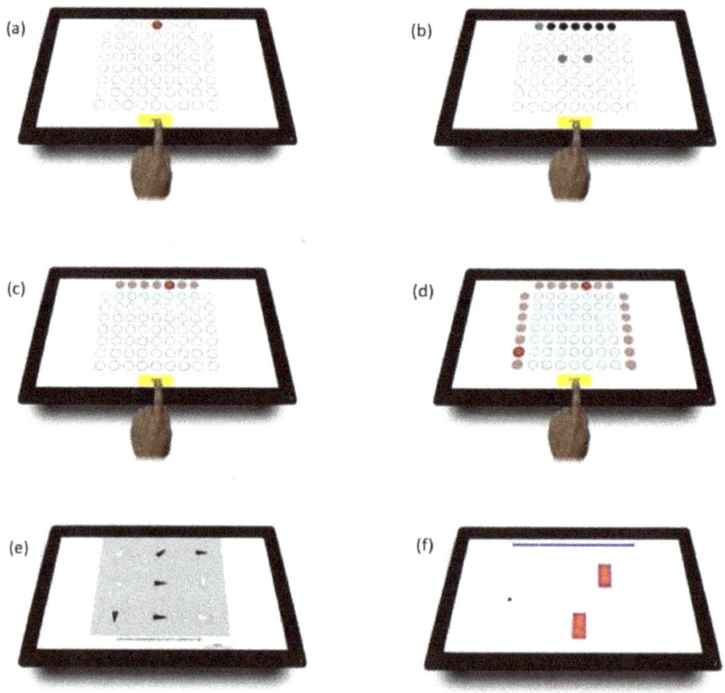

Figure 1. Reaction panel of the Test2Drive system: (**a**) SIRT, (**b**) CHORT, (**c**) HECOR, (**d**) SPANT, (**e**) PUT, (**f**) PAMT.

4.2. Statistical Analysis

Descriptive statistics were presented as mean ± standard deviation. A Shapiro–Wilk test was performed on all analyzed groups, which showed that the distribution of the data deviated from normal. Accordingly, the Mann–Whitney test was performed to identify statistically significant differences between Elite and Sub-Elite athletes. In addition, Spearman rank correlations were used to determine the relationship between the various components of body composition, experience and psychomotor performance. All statistical procedures were performed using IBM SPSS Statistics 29.0 software (SPSS Inc., Chicago, IL, USA), and the significance level was set at 5%. Scatter plots for selected variables were prepared in R Studio (version 4.3.3).

The G*Power 3.1 software was used to estimate the minimal sample size. For the Mann–Whitney test, a total number of N = 74 (37 in each group research and control) were required to detect the effect size of 0.80 at the 0.05 significance level and power 0.95.

5. Results

Table 2 presents specific selected psychomotor abilities in the group of Elite and Sub-Elite female handball players. In all tests performed, there were no statistically significant differences in reaction time and movement of players at different competitive levels. Analysis of the results obtained in the SIRT test showed that the reaction time is at a highly comparable level (Elite 333.48 ± 33.89, Sub-Elite 333.92 ± 36.23). Similar results were noted assessing correct responses in the SIRT test, in which the correct answers were Elite: 98.81 ± 2.69, Sub-Elite: 98.95 ± 2.88. Therefore, no statistically significant differences were seen in the SIRT test results obtained. However, faster reaction time in individual tests was characterized by female players. Such an example was observed in the CHORT test, in which a difference was noted between the test groups in reaction time in favor of the Elite group (658.95 ± 64.35 vs. 668.89 ± 57.38). Despite the difference in the results obtained, no statistical significance was observed. The HECOR test also showed that female handball players in the Elite group (393.14 ± 46.99) obtained shorter reaction times than the Sub-Elite group (405.58 ± 60.04). In two further tests (SPANT, PAMT) assessing reaction time, movement time and correct responses, the results obtained are at a very similar level and no statistical significance was noted between the study groups. The only statistically significant differences were observed in the PUT test, where the decisiveness of incorrect answers was assessed. The mean value for the Elite group was 95.43 ± 3.30, while the Sub-Elite group scored 94.11 ± 3.97 ($p = 0.0048$).

Table 3 presents specific selected psychomotor abilities in the group of Elite and Sub-Elite male handball players. In the group of handball players studied, in most cases no statistically significant differences were seen between the Elite and Sub-Elite male handball players. In addition, better results were observed for movement time in the SIRT, CHORT and HECOR tests. In the SIRT test, the average movement time for the Elite group was 227.24 ± 44.16 and for the Sub-Elite group it was 183.90 ± 37.87 ($p = 0.0004$). In the CHORT test, the Elite group also scored worse (239.86 ± 47.29) compared to the Sub-Elite group (197.49 ± 43.34), which was also statistically significant ($p = 0.0002$). A similar trend was also observed for the HECOR test, where the average movement time for the Elite group was 269.33 ± 51.58 versus the Sub-Elite group: 225.61 ± 35.59 ($p = 0.0001$).

Table 2. Numeral characteristics of psychomotor abilities of female handball players.

Variable		Total			Elite			Sub-Elite			e.s	*p*
		Mean	Min	Max	Mean	Min	Max	Mean	Min	Max		
SIRT	RT [ms]	333.76 ± 35.12	262.00	451.00	333.48 ± 33.89	262.00	383.00	333.92 ± 36.23	272.00	451.00	−0.05	0.3382
	MT [ms]	221.29 ± 35.16	162.00	331.00	227.24 ± 44.16	162.00	331.00	218.00 ± 29.19	166.00	283.00	−0.08	0.6123
	cr [%]	98.90 ± 2.80	85.00	100.00	98.81 ± 2.69	90.00	100.00	98.95 ± 2.88	85.00	100.00	0.03	0.8724
CHORT	RT [ms]	665.36 ± 59.60	509.00	793.00	658.95 ± 64.35	509.00	779.00	668.89 ± 57.38	577.00	793.00	0.10	0.5245
	MT [ms]	238.66 ± 42.01	161.00	382.00	239.86 ± 47.29	190.00	382.00	238.00 ± 39.44	161.00	305.00	0.05	0.7595
	cr [%]	94.59 ± 5.03	79.00	100.00	94.62 ± 4.20	83.00	100.00	94.58 ± 5.50	79.00	100.00	0.05	0.7357
HECOR	RT [ms]	401.15 ± 55.65	306.00	671.00	393.14 ± 46.99	306.00	486.00	405.58 ± 60.04	332.00	671.00	0.08	0.5988
	MT [ms]	261.31 ± 39.48	199.00	413.00	269.33 ± 51.58	214.00	413.00	256.87 ± 30.80	199.00	314.00	−0.08	0.2490
	cr [%]	99.32 ± 1.73	95.00	100.00	99.29 ± 1.79	95.00	100.00	99.34 ± 1.71	95.00	100.00	0.01	0.9437
SPANT	RT [ms]	614.20 ± 94.50	433.00	893.00	615.86 ± 113.46	433.00	893.00	613.29 ± 83.89	448.00	809.00	0.01	0.9312
	MT [ms]	293.80 ± 69.53	178.00	552.00	299.29 ± 90.76	193.00	552.00	290.76 ± 55.66	178.00	406.00	0.06	0.6561
	cr [%]	89.07 ± 10.40	40.00	100.00	88.81 ± 13.41	40.00	100.00	89.21 ± 8.50	65.00	100.00	−0.08	0.6319
PUT	cr [%]	94.58 ± 3.77	88.00	100.00	95.43 ± 3.30	88.00	100.00	94.11 ± 3.97	88.00	100.00	−0.19	0.2341
	cr [%] avr RT	1915.07 ± 384.46	1341.00	3120.00	2046.14 ± 473.76	1384.00	3120.00	1842.63 ± 308.60	1341.00	3021.00	−0.24	0.1273
	cr % inr RT	1335.76 ± 191.20	986.00	1868.00	1424.14 ± 199.43	986.00	1868.00	1286.92 ± 170.07	1024.00	1859.00	−0.44	0.0048 *
PAMT	cr [%]	87.73 ± 8.14	67.00	100.00	85.43 ± 9.01	67.00	100.00	89.00 ± 7.44	72.00	100.00	0.22	0.1574

SIRT—Simple Reaction Time, CHORT—Choice Reaction Time, HECOR—Hand-Eye Coordination Test, SPANT—Spatial Anticipation Test, PUT—Perception and Attention test, PAMT—Anticipation test, RT—reaction time, MT—movement time, cr—correct response, *p*—probability of testing, *—statistical significance.

Table 3. Numeral characteristics of psychomotor abilities of male handball players.

Variable		Total			Elite			Sub-Elite			e.s	*p*
		Mean	Min	Max	Mean	Min	Max	Mean	Min	Max		
SIRT	RT [ms]	337.73 ± 36.43	199.00	503.00	333.48 ± 33.89	262.00	383.00	334.24 ± 36.66	199.00	447.00	−0.05	0.2493
	MT [ms]	197.35 ± 43.61	111.00	345.00	227.24 ± 44.16	162.00	331.00	183.90 ± 37.87	111.00	319.00	−0.34	0.0004 *
	cr [%]	99.21 ± 2.11	90.00	100.00	98.81 ± 2.69	90.00	100.00	99.30 ± 1.94	90.00	100.00	0.02	0.8255
CHORT	RT [ms]	658.61 ± 82.06	238.00	886.00	658.95 ± 64.35	509.00	779.00	652.61 ± 81.27	238.00	811.00	−0.08	0.3888
	MT [ms]	212.49 ± 48.94	96.00	367.00	239.86 ± 47.29	190.00	382.00	197.49 ± 43.34	100.00	315.00	−0.36	0.0002 *
	cr [%]	94.87 ± 7.52	46.00	100.00	94.62 ± 4.20	83.00	100.00	94.79 ± 6.56	62.00	100.00	−0.08	0.4234
HECOR	RT [ms]	403.97 ± 38.48	262.00	529.00	393.14 ± 46.99	306.00	486.00	406.24 ± 34.78	316.00	483.00	0.10	0.3263
	MT [ms]	243.33 ± 48.30	147.00	432.00	269.33 ± 51.58	214.00	413.00	225.61 ± 35.59	147.00	302.00	−0.42	0.0001 *
	cr [%]	97.34 ± 13.78	0.00	100.00	99.29 ± 1.79	95.00	100.00	98.24 ± 9.82	20.00	100.00	0.07	0.4532
SPANT	RT [ms]	607.63 ± 91.23	421.00	818.00	615.86 ± 113.46	433.00	893.00	606.45 ± 90.38	438.00	812.00	−0.01	0.8773
	MT [ms]	249.76 ± 67.22	135.00	564.00	299.29 ± 90.76	193.00	552.00	238.63 ± 56.71	135.00	505.00	−0.19	0.0532
	cr [%]	92.30 ± 10.82	10.00	100.00	88.81 ± 13.41	40.00	100.00	91.62 ± 12.56	10.00	100.00	−0.03	0.7480
PUT	cr [%]	95.71 ± 4.10	69.00	100.00	95.43 ± 3.30	88.00	100.00	95.65 ± 3.90	81.00	100.00	−0.03	0.44123
	cr [%] avr RT	1909.64 ± 388.21	1106.00	3164.00	2046.14 ± 473.76	1384.00	3120.00	1884.72 ± 353.44	1118.00	3164.00	−0.05	0.1559
	cr [%] inr RT	1263.96 ± 176.98	925.00	1895.00	1424.14 ± 199.43	986.00	1868.00	1243.08 ± 148.20	925.00	1631.00	−0.07	0.4685
PAMT	cr [%]	84.09 ± 8.21	61.00	100.00	85.43 ± 9.01	67.00	100.00	84.01 ± 8.67	61.00	100.00	0.01	0.9180

SIRT—Simple Reaction Time, CHORT—Choice Reaction Time, HECOR—Hand–Eye Coordination Test, SPANT—Spatial Anticipation Test, PUT—Perception and attention test, PAMT—Anticipation test, RT—reaction time, MT—movement time, cr—correct response, *p*—probability of testing, *—statistical significance.

Table 4 presents correlation between specific selected psychomotor abilities, body composition components and training experience in the group of Elite and Sub-Elite male handball players. All statistically significant results are marked with an asterisk, and the numbers represent Spearman's rank correlation coefficients (r). It was observed that correct answers in the HECOR cr positively correlated (r = 0.27) with body mass and body height (r = 0.31) in the Sub-Elite group. In addition, a negative correlation coefficient was observed in HECOR cr with training experience in all the groups (r = −0.23), whereas SPANT cr showed a correlation with training experience in the Elite group (r = −0.30). A statistical significance was also noted in the male study group between PUT cr and fat-free mass (kg) (r = 0.18), and also between PAMT cr and body height (r = 0.19). No statistically significant correlations were observed for the SIRT and CHORT test.

Table 4. Correlation analysis between body composition, body height, training experience and correct answers among male handball players.

Variable	Group	SIRT cr [%]	CHORT cr [%]	HECOR cr [%]	SPANT cr [%]	PUT cr [%]	PAMT cr [%]
Body Fat [%]	Total	NS	NS	NS	NS	NS	NS
	Elite	NS	NS	NS	NS	NS	NS
	Sub-Elite	NS	NS	NS	NS	NS	NS
Body mass [kg]	Total	NS	NS	NS	NS	NS	NS
	Elite	NS	NS	NS	NS	NS	NS
	Sub-Elite	NS	NS	0.27 *	NS	NS	NS
Fat-Free Mass [kg]	Total	NS	NS	NS	NS	0.18*	NS
	Elite	NS	NS	NS	NS	NS	NS
	Sub-Elite	NS	NS	NS	NS	NS	NS
Body Height	Total	NS	NS	NS	NS	NS	0.19 *
	Elite	NS	NS	NS	NS	NS	NS
	Sub-Elite	NS	NS	0.31 *	NS	NS	NS
Total Body Water [L]	Total	NS	NS	NS	NS	NS	NS
	Elite	NS	NS	NS	NS	NS	NS
	Sub-Elite	NS	NS	NS	NS	NS	NS
Training Experience [years]	Total	NS	NS	−0.23 *	NS	NS	NS
	Elite	NS	NS	NS	−0.30*	NS	NS
	Sub-Elite	NS	NS	NS	NS	NS	NS

cr—correct response; *—statistical significance ($p < 0.05$); NS—not statistically significant; Values represent Spearman's rank correlation coefficient (r).

Table 5 shows the correlation analysis between body composition, body height, training experience and correct response. Correlations of moderate strength were noted between the SIRT cr and Elite group (r = 0.44) and between CHORT cr and all the groups (r = 0.33). In most cases, a negative correlation was also observed in SIRT cr with body height in all the groups (r = −0.26) and the Elite group (r = −0.38), as well as in SIRT cr with total body water in all the groups (r = −0.26). Correlation of high strength, however, was observed between SPANT cr and body fat percentage in the Elite group (r = −0.58) and in the whole group (r = −0.37). Comparable occurrence was observed between SPANT cr and body mass (kg) and fat-free mass (kg) with strong correlation. Moreover, a statistical significance in PAMT cr it was also observed with body mass (kg) and fat-free mass (kg) and training experience in all groups (r = −0.38). No statistically significant correlations were observed for the HECOR and PUT tests.

Table 5. Correlation analysis between body composition, body height, training experience and correct answers among female handball players.

Variable	Group	SIRT cr [%]	CHORT cr [%]	HECOR cr [%]	SPANT cr [%]	PUT cr [%]	PAMT cr [%]
Body Fat [%]	Total	NS	0.33 *	NS	−0.37 *	NS	NS
	Elite	NS	NS	NS	−0.58 *	NS	NS
	Sub-Elite	NS	NS	NS	NS	NS	NS
Body Mass [kg]	Total	NS	NS	NS	−0.54 *	NS	−0.48 *
	Elite	NS	NS	NS	−0.78 *	NS	−0.54 *
	Sub-Elite	NS	NS	NS	NS	NS	NS
Fat-Free Mass [kg]	Total	NS	NS	NS	−0.46 *	NS	−0.56 *
	Elite	NS	NS	NS	−0.66 *	NS	−0.58 *
	Sub-Elite	NS	NS	NS	NS	NS	−0.49 *
Body Height	Total	−0.26 *	NS	NS	NS	NS	NS
	Elite	−0.38 *	NS	NS	NS	NS	NS
	Sub-Elite	NS	NS	NS	NS	NS	NS
Total Body Water [L]	Total	−0.26 *	NS	NS	NS	NS	NS
	Elite	NS	NS	NS	NS	NS	NS
	Sub-Elite	NS	NS	NS	NS	NS	NS
Training Experience [years]	Total	NS	NS	NS	NS	NS	−0.38 *
	Elite	0.44 *	NS	NS	NS	NS	NS
	Sub-Elite	NS	NS	NS	NS	NS	NS

cr—correct answers; *—statistical significance ($p < 0.05$); NS—not statistically significant; Values represent Spearman's rank correlation coefficient (r).

Table 6 shows the correlations analysis between body composition, body height, age and movement time in male handball players. A weak to moderate correlation was observed in CHORT MT (r = −0.30) and SPANT MT (r = −0.26) with age in the Sub-Elite group. While the HECOR MT test showed a statistically significant correlation with body fat % (r = −0.20) in all the groups of players, fat-free mass (kg) also saw a significant correlation (r = −0.26) in the Sub-Elite group.Moreover, in the same test, there was also a moderate correlation with total body water (r = −0.37). No statistically significant correlations were observed for the SIRT test.

Table 6. Correlation analysis between body composition, body height, age and movement time among male handball players.

Variable	Group	SIRT MT [ms]	CHORT MT [ms]	HECOR MT [ms]	SPANT MT [ms]
Body Fat [%]	Total	NS	NS	−0.20 *	NS
	Elite	NS	NS	NS	NS
	Sub-Elite	NS	NS	NS	NS
Body Mass [kg]	Total	NS	NS	NS	NS
	Elite	NS	NS	NS	NS
	Sub-Elite	NS	NS	NS	NS
Fat-Free Mass [kg]	Total	NS	NS	NS	NS
	Elite	NS	NS	NS	NS
	Sub-Elite	NS	NS	−0.26 *	NS
Body Height	Total	NS	NS	NS	NS
	Elite	NS	NS	NS	NS
	Sub-Elite	NS	NS	NS	NS
Total Body Water [L]	Total	NS	NS	−0.19 *	−0.18 *
	Elite	NS	NS	NS	NS
	Sub-Elite	NS	NS	−0.37 *	NS
Age [years]	Total	NS	NS	NS	NS
	Elite	NS	NS	NS	NS
	Sub-Elite	NS	−0.30 *	NS	−0.26 *

MT—movement time; *—statistical significance ($p < 0.05$); NS—not statistically significant; Values represent Spearman's rank correlation coefficient (r).

Table 7 shows the correlation analysis between body composition, body height, age and movement time in female handball players. A moderate correlation was observed between CHORT MT and total body water (r = 0.44) in Elite handball players. Meanwhile, HECOR MT correlated with age in the Sub-Elite group (r = −0.39). Moreover, SPANT MT showed a correlation with fat-free mass (r = −0.30) and total body water (r = −0.30) in all the groups. No significant relationships were shown for the SIRT test.

Table 7. Correlation analysis between body composition, body height, age and movement time among female handball players.

Variable	Group	SIRT MT [ms]	CHORT MT [ms]	HECOR MT [ms]	SPANT MT [ms]
Body Fat [%]	Total	NS	NS	NS	NS
	Elite	NS	NS	NS	NS
	Sub-Elite	NS	NS	NS	NS
Body Mass [kg]	Total	NS	NS	NS	NS
	Elite	NS	NS	NS	NS
	Sub-Elite	NS	NS	NS	NS
Fat-Free Mass [kg]	Total	NS	NS	NS	−0.30 *
	Elite	NS	NS	NS	NS
	Sub-Elite	NS	NS	NS	NS
Body Height	Total	NS	NS	NS	NS
	Elite	NS	NS	NS	NS
	Sub-Elite	NS	NS	NS	NS
Total Body Water [L]	Total	NS	NS	NS	−0.30 *
	Elite	NS	0.44 *	NS	NS
	Sub-Elite	NS	NS	NS	NS
Age [years]	Total	NS	NS	NS	NS
	Elite	NS	NS	NS	NS
	Sub-Elite	NS	NS	−0.39 *	NS

MT—movement time; *—statistical significance ($p < 0.05$); NS—not statistically significant; Values represent Spearman's rank correlation coefficient (r).

The correlation analysis between body composition, body height, age and reaction time in male handball players was presented in Table 8. A weak-to-moderate correlation was observed between SIRT reaction time and body mass (r = 0.32), fat-free mass (r = 0.28) and total body water (r = 0.31) in the Sub-Elite group. Meanwhile, SIRT reaction time correlated in the Elite group with total body water (r = 0.24). It is noteworthy that, in the HECOR test in relation to the Sub-Elite group, the highest values for correlation were determined with fat-free mass and total body water in all the groups as well as in the Sub-Elite group. A correlation was also observed with body fat (r = 0.28) in the Elite group.Moreover, a weak correlation was observed in PUT reaction time with body height (r = −0.14) in all groups. No meaningful relationship were observed for the CHORT reaction time, SPANT reaction time and PUT reaction time tests.

Table 9 shows the correlation analysis between body composition, body height, age and reaction time in female handball players. A weak-to-moderate correlation was observed in CHORT reaction time with body mass (r = 0.27) and age (r = 0.27) in all handball groups and in PUT reaction time with body fat percentage (r = 0.59) in the Elite group, as also with age (r = 0.30) in all groups. Moreover, in PUT k reaction time, a correlation was observed with fat-free mass in the Elite group (r = 0.52) and in all the groups (r = 0.33). Furthermore, a correlation was also observed for total body water in the Elite group (r = 0.56) and all the groups (r = 0.36), as well as for age (r = 0.32) in all the groups. No relationships were observed for the SIRT reaction time, HECOR reaction time and SPANT reaction time tests.

Table 8. Correlation analysis between body composition, body height, training experience and reaction time among male handball players.

Variable	Group	SIRT RT [ms]	CHORT RT [ms]	HECOR RT [ms]	SPANT RT [ms]	PUT RT [ms]	PUT k RT [ms]
Body Fat [%]	Total	NS	NS	NS	NS	NS	NS
	Elite	NS	NS	0.28 *	NS	NS	NS
	Sub-Elite	NS	NS	NS	NS	NS	NS
Body Mass [kg]	Total	0.16 *	NS	NS	NS	NS	NS
	Elite	NS	NS	NS	NS	NS	NS
	Sub-Elite	0.32 *	NS	0.25 *	NS	NS	NS
Fat-Free Mass [kg]	Total	NS	NS	0.22 *	NS	NS	NS
	Elite	NS	NS	NS	NS	NS	NS
	Sub-Elite	0.28 *	NS	0.43 *	NS	NS	NS
Body Height	Total	NS	NS	NS	NS	NS	−0.14 *
	Elite	NS	NS	NS	NS	NS	NS
	Sub-Elite	NS	NS	NS	NS	NS	NS
Total Body Water [L]	Total	NS	NS	0.21 *	NS	NS	NS
	Elite	0.24 *	NS	NS	NS	NS	NS
	Sub-Elite	0.31 *	NS	0.43 *	NS	NS	NS
Age [years]	Total	NS	NS	NS	NS	NS	NS
	Elite	NS	NS	NS	NS	NS	NS
	Sub-Elite	NS	NS	NS	NS	NS	NS

RT—reaction time; *—statistical significance ($p < 0.05$); NS—no statistical significance; Values represent Spearman's rank correlation coefficient (r).

Table 9. Correlation analysis between body composition, body height, training experience and reaction time among female handball players.

Variable	Group	SIRT RT [ms]	CHORT RT [ms]	HECOR RT [ms]	SPANT RT [ms]	PUT RT [ms]	PUT k RT [ms]
Body Fat [%]	Total	NS	NS	NS	NS	0.33 *	NS
	Elite	NS	NS	NS	NS	0.59 *	NS
	Sub-Elite	NS	NS	NS	NS	NS	NS
Body Mass [kg]	Total	NS	0.27 *	NS	NS	NS	NS
	Elite	NS	NS	NS	NS	NS	NS
	Sub-Elite	NS	NS	NS	NS	NS	NS
Fat-Free Mass [kg]	Total	NS	NS	NS	NS	NS	0.33 *
	Elite	NS	NS	NS	NS	NS	0.52 *
	Sub-Elite	NS	NS	NS	NS	NS	NS
Body Height	Total	NS	NS	NS	NS	NS	NS
	Elite	NS	NS	NS	NS	NS	NS
	Sub-Elite	NS	NS	NS	NS	NS	NS
Total Body Water [L]	Total	NS	NS	NS	NS	NS	0.36 *
	Elite	NS	NS	NS	NS	NS	0.56 *
	Sub-Elite	NS	NS	NS	NS	NS	NS
Age [years]	Total	NS	0.27 *	NS	NS	0.30 *	0.32 *
	Elite	NS	NS	NS	NS	NS	NS
	Sub-Elite	NS	NS	NS	NS	NS	NS

RT—reaction time; *—statistical significance ($p < 0.05$); NS—not statistically significant; Values represent Spearman's rank correlation coefficient (r).

Figure 2 presents the correlations between body mass [kg], body fat [%] and percentage of correct answers in the SPANT Cr [%] test. The blue dots on the chart illustrate the individual results of the athletes, while the red line represents the overall trend line, showing the general tendency. Among elite female athletes, a statistically significant negative correlation ($p < 0.05$) was observed for both of the above cases. High strength correlations, for body mass (r = −0.78) and body fat (r = −0.58), indicate that an increase in body mass and body fat content decreases the number of correct answers on the SPANT cr test.

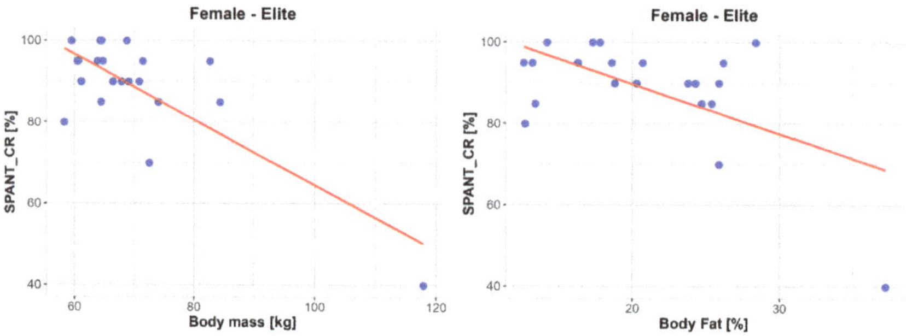

Figure 2. Scatter plot of SPANT test results in a group of professional female players: relationship between body fat, body mass, and the number of correct answers (CR). Blue dots represent individual results of the athletes, while the red line indicates the overall trend line showing the general tendency.

6. Discussion

The purpose of this study was to assess psychomotor abilities in male and female handball players from the Elite and Sub-Elite Polish and Portuguese handball leagues during the 2023/2024 season. Moreover, the aim of this evaluation was to analyze the relationship between body composition, training experience and psychomotor abilities at different levels of competition in Polish and Portuguese male and female handball players. Additionally, this study sought to identify potential correlations between reaction time, movement time and correct responses across male and female handball players in both Elite and Sub-Elite groups, with respect to variables such as sex, age, body fat percentage, body mass, fat-free mass, body height and total body water. Handball is considered to be a sport that requires the player to be constantly ready and maintain attention during offensive and defensive actions [5], even though there are shorter or longer breaks, as the sport is dominated by sudden and rapid changes in the direction and position of the players [1,2,15,45]. Therefore, appropriate development of psychomotor abilities in combination with appropriate physique and body composition of male and female handball players seems to be important in this competitive team sport.

In recent years, the problem of psychomotor abilities in team games of professional and amateur sport in the wide sense has been repeatedly undertaken by scientists all over the world. There are scientific investigations in the literature related to the assessment of reaction time, movement time, eye–hand coordination and anticipation in team sports [9,20,26,27]. Furthermore, there are also scientific publications in the literature connected to the relationship between body components and reaction time in the different level of competition [25,27,46]. Therefore, the aim of this study was to investigate the relationship between body composition, training experience and psychomotor abilities among female and male handball players of different competitive levels.

Through the analysis of the psychomotor performance assessment tests, it can be seen that the group of Elite male handball players with more training experience achieved a better result in the SPANT cr ($r = -0.30$) psychomotor test. This shows that, the more experience athletes have, the better percentage of correct answers handball players achieve. Similar results were presented by Jackson and Mogan [47], in which their analysis showed that players at a higher level of competition are characterized by a greater level of anticipation as compared to amateurs. The same conclusions were also presented in a study by Przednowek et al. [27], where the fastest reaction time occurred among those practicing sport with the longest seniority (more than 14 years), while better performance in movement time (MT) was seen among the study group with a seniority of 10–14 years. These results raise the hypothesis that more experienced handball players should have greater anticipatory abilities and correct response than the group with lower seniority. However, in a study of Shelton et al. [48] on female handball players, the authors investigated differences in reaction speed to situations depending on the sporting level represented. Furthermore, Ando et al. [49] showed that reaction time decreased with repeated exercise, which suggests that, the more experienced the player, the shorter the reaction time is.

As already mentioned, many scientific publications aimed to evaluate the relationship between reaction time and movement time with body composition parameters [1,9,37,39,46,50,51]. The results of the handball players showed a statistically significant relationship between the SPANT cr test and selected body mass components ($p < 0.05$). A negative correlation was observed with the body fat percentage in the Elite group (r = −0.58), in the whole group of female athletes (r = −0.37), as well as with body weight (kg) and lean body mass (kg). Studies have shown that, the lower the level of body fat, the higher the number of observed and correct answers. This suggests that body fat level may affect correct decision-making during a handball match. A parallel situation took place in the test in PAMT cr with body mass (kg) and fat-free mass (kg) in all the groups. This shows that, the higher the body mass, the fatter, the lower the number of correct responses.

Moreover, in HECOR MT test was observed a statistical correlation with body fat percentage in all male groups, as well as a correlation with fat-free mass and total body water (kg) in the Sub-Elite group. Meanwhile, in the group of female handball players, SPANT MT correlated with fat-free mass and total body water. Such conclusions are confirmed by the studies of other researchers. Skurvydas et al. [46] observed that the group of participants with a higher level of BMI had a significantly longer reaction time. Moreover, they noticed significant differences between the reaction time of the mid- and high-BMI groups [46]. Meanwhile, in the research of Arabaci et al. [50], the authors noticed that lower leg fat percentages and fat mass in taekwondo athletes affected the reaction time in a positive way. Moreover, Poliszczuk et al. [51], in their research on reaction time and body tissue composition of upper limbs in young female basketball players, found a correlation between movement time and the FFM [kg] (r = −0.62), as with PMM [kg] (r = −0.63) parameters.

Referring to the results obtained in a group of female and male handball players at the different levels of competition, it should be concluded that even small differences in body mass composition can have a substantial influence on the speed of in-time decision-making on the pitch, anticipation of the opponent's movement and reaction time and movement time during each offensive and defensive action in handball.

This scientific study has some limitations that need to be taken into account during its interpretation. The number of male handball players is very similar, but only 60 were tested in the female group, divided into Elite and Sub-Elite groups. We also did not have a balanced number between male and female handball players. A larger sample would have ensured greater consistency and range of results presented.

Regarding the female sample size in this study, it is important to note that the relatively small number of female participants could impact the broader applicability of the results. Therefore, future research with a larger and more diverse sample of female participants is necessary to enhance the generalizability of the results and provide more comprehensive insights into the psychomotor abilities, body composition and training experience of female handball players across various levels of competition.

The findings of this study on psychomotor abilities, body composition and training experience of Elite and Sub-Elite handball players have several practical implications for handball coaches, particularly in the context of optimizing player performance. For example, this study suggests that body fat percentage, fat-free mass and total body water may influence reaction time, movement time and correct responses. Coaches can use this information to identify players who may benefit from adjustments in their body composition, such as implementing specific conditioning training to reduce body fat or increase lean muscle mass. Elite players, who have accumulated more years of experience, may demonstrate superior reaction time and movement efficiency compared to Sub-Elite players. Therefore, training programs for Sub-Elite players could focus on accelerating the development of these psychomotor abilities, with an emphasis on speed and decision-making under pressure. Lastly, by systematically tracking changes in body composition and their potential impact on psychomotor performance, coaches can refine training system, providing athletes with individualized feedback to optimize their physical and mental capabilities.

7. Conclusions

Based on the analysis of the data, the following hypotheses were formulated:

1. The results seems to indicate that, the higher the level of body mass, body fat and total body water, the lower the level of correct responses in psychomotor performance assessment tests.
2. There is a relationship between SPANT cr and training seniority among the male handball Elite group. This demonstrates that, the greater the level of experience of the players, the lower the percentage of correct responses of the male handball players.
3. A statistical correlation was observed between movement time in the HECOR test and body fat in the Elite and Sub-Elite male handball players; moreover, fat-free mass and total body water (kg) correlated in the Sub-Elite group.

Author Contributions: Conceptualization, K.P., É.R.G. and M.Ś.; Investigation, K.P., É.R.G., M.Ś. and F.M.; Methodology, K.P., É.R.G. and M.Ś.; Project administration, K.P. and M.Ś.; Software, K.P. and M.Ś.; Supervision, K.P., É.R.G. and M.Ś.; Visualization, C.F., F.M. and M.Ś.; Writing original draft, K.P., M.Ś., F.M., C.F. and P.M.; Writing, review and editing, K.P., F.M., C.F., M.Ś. and P.M. All authors have read and agreed to the published version of the manuscript.

Funding: The scientific paper was financed from the statutory resources of the University of Rzeszow.

Institutional Review Board Statement: Not applicable.

Informed Consent Statement: This study was conducted in accordance with the Declaration of Helsinki and the protocol was approved by the Ethics Committee of the University of Rzeszow/Poland (resolution 10 February 2020). Before the study, written informed consent to participate in the study was obtained from all the participants.

Data Availability Statement: The original contributions presented in this study are included in the article. Further inquiries can be directed to the corresponding author.

Conflicts of Interest: The authors declare no conflicts of interest.

References

1. Michalsik, L.B.; Aagaard, P.; Madsen, K. Technical activity profile and influence of body anthropometry on playing performance in female elite team handball. *J. Strength Cond. Res.* **2015**, *29*, 1126–1138. [CrossRef] [PubMed]
2. Karcher, C.; Buchheit, M. On-court demands of elite handball, with special reference to playing positions. *Sports Med.* **2014** *44*, 797–814. [CrossRef] [PubMed]
3. Milanović, D.; Vuleta, D.; Ohnjec, K. Performance indicators of winning and defeated female handball teams in matches of the 2012 Olympic Games Tournament. *J. Hum. Kinet.* **2018**, *64*, 247–253. [CrossRef] [PubMed]
4. Čavala, M.; Trninić, V.; Jašić, D.; Tomljanović, M. The influence of somatotype components and personality traits on the playing position and the quality of top Croatian female cadet handball players. *Coll. Antropol.* **2013**, *37*, 97–100.
5. Smolarczyk, M. Decreasing number of distance shooting in handball–trend of nowadays male handball competition. *Biomed Hum. Kinet.* **2023**, *15*, 83–88. [CrossRef]
6. Mayer, J.; Thiel, A. Presenteeism in the elite sports workplace: The willingness to compete hurt among German elite handball and track and field athletes. *Int. Rev. Sociol. Sport* **2018**, *53*, 49–68. [CrossRef]

. Janelle, C.M.; Hillman, C.H. Expert performance in sport. *Expert Perform. Sports Adv. Res. Sport Expert.* **2003**, *2*, 19–47.
. Florkiewicz, B.; Fogtman, S.; Kszak-Krzyżanowska, A.; Zwierko, T. The ability to maintain attention during visuomotor task performance in handball players and non-athletes. *Cent. Eur. J. Sport Sci. Med.* **2014**, *7*, 99–106.
. Sliz, M.; Pasko, W.; Dziadek, B.; Ziajka, A.; Poludniak, N.; Marszalek, P.; Krawczyk, G.; Przednowek, K. Relationship between body composition and cognitive abilities among young female handball players. *J. Phys. Educ. Sport* **2023**, *23*, 1650–1659.
0. Čižmek, A.; Ohnjec, K.; Vučetić, V.; Gruić, I. Morphological differences of elite Croatian female handball players according to their game position. *Hrvat. Športskomedicinski Vjesn.* **2010**, *25*, 122–127.
1. Bon, M.; Pori, P.; Šibila, M. Position-related differences in selected morphological body characteristics of top-level female handball players. *Coll. Antropol.* **2015**, *39*, 631–639. [PubMed]
2. Curiţianu, I.; Neamţu, M. A comparative study on the evolution of left wings, right wings and pivots at male handball teams HCM Constanta and FC Barcelona in "Champions League" 2011–2012. *Procedia-Soc. Behav. Sci.* **2014**, *116*, 3859–3863. [CrossRef]
3. Ohnjec, K.; Vuleta, D.; Milanović, D.; Gruić, I. Performance indicators of teams at the 2003 World Handball Championship for Women in Croatia. *Kinesiology* **2008**, *40*, 69–79.
4. Krawczyk, P.; Bodasinski, S.; Bodasinska, A.; Słupczynski, B. Level of psychomotor abilities in handball goalkeepers. *Balt. J. Health Phys. Act.* **2018**, *10*, 7. [CrossRef]
5. Bilge, M. Game analysis of Olympic, World and European Championships in men's handball. *J. Hum. Kinet.* **2012**, *35*, 109–118. [CrossRef]
6. Spieszny, M.; Walczyk, L. *Piłka Ręczna: Program Szkolenia Dzieci i Młodzieży*; Centralny Ośrodek Sportu, Pion Programowo-Sportowy: Warszawa, Poland, 2001.
7. Spieszny, M.; Św, W.O. Trening młodych piłkarzy. Kształtowanie sprawności fizycznej oraz przygotowanie psychiczne. *Acta Sci. Acad. Ostroviensis Nauk. WSBiP W Ostrowcu Świętokrzyskim* **2003**, *12*, 21–36.
8. Belcic, I.; Ocic, M.; Dukaric, V.; Knjaz, D.; Zoretic, D. Effects of One-Step and Three-Step Run-Up on Kinematic Parameters and the Efficiency of Jump Shot in Handball. *Appl. Sci.* **2023**, *13*, 3811. [CrossRef]
9. Dhillon, J.S. Comparison of psychomotor abilities among handball players: A comparative study. *Int. J. Physiol. Nutr. Phys. Educ.* **2019**, *4*, 2291–2296.
0. Krawczyk, P.; Bodasiński, S. Psychomotor abilities as predictors of actions of handball goalkeepers during saves. *Pol. J. Sport Tour.* **2022**, *29*, 15–22. [CrossRef]
1. Tarnowski, A. The Test2Drive system in driver assessments: Relationships between theory, law and practice. *Przegląd Psychol.* **2021**, *64*, 157–167. [CrossRef]
2. Miller, R.A.; Rogers, R.R.; Williams, T.D.; Marshall, M.R.; Moody, J.R.; Hensarling, R.W.; Ballmann, C.G. Effects of protective American football headgear on peripheral vision reaction time and visual target detection in Division I NCAA football players. *Sports* **2019**, *7*, 213. [CrossRef] [PubMed]
3. Nuri, L.; Shadmehr, A.; Ghotbi, N.; Attarbashi Moghadam, B. Reaction time and anticipatory skill of athletes in open and closed skill-dominated sport. *Eur. J. Sport Sci.* **2013**, *13*, 431–436. [CrossRef] [PubMed]
4. Bideau, B.; Multon, F.; Kulpa, R.; Fradet, L.; Arnaldi, B.; Delamarche, P. Using virtual reality to analyze links between handball thrower kinematics and goalkeeper's reactions. *Neurosci. Lett.* **2004**, *372*, 119–122. [CrossRef] [PubMed]
5. Śliż, M.; Przednowek, K.H.; Kapuściński, P.; Dziadek, B.; Godek, Ł.; Warchoł, K.; Zieliński, J.; Przednowek, K. Characteristics of the level of psychomotor abilities of female handball players. *BMC Sports Sci. Med. Rehabil.* **2022**, *14*, 83. [CrossRef]
6. Blecharz, J.; Wrześniewski, K.; Siekańska, M.; Ambroży, T.; Spieszny, M. Cognitive factors in elite handball: Do players' positions determine their cognitive processes? *J. Hum. Kinet.* **2022**, *82*, 213–221. [CrossRef]
7. Przednowek, K.; Śliż, M.; Lenik, J.; Dziadek, B.; Cieszkowski, S.; Lenik, P.; Kopeć, D.; Wardak, K.; Przednowek, K.H. Psychomotor abilities of professional handball players. *Int. J. Environ. Res. Public Health* **2019**, *16*, 1909. [CrossRef] [PubMed]
8. Cavedon, V.; Zancanaro, C.; Milanese, C. Anthropometric prediction of DXA-measured body composition in female team handball players. *PeerJ* **2018**, *6*, e5913. [CrossRef]
9. Granados, C.; Izquierdo, M.; Ibáñez, J.; Ruesta, M.; Gorostiaga, E.M. Are there any differences in physical fitness and throwing velocity between national and international elite female handball players? *J. Strength Cond. Res.* **2013**, *27*, 723–732. [CrossRef]
0. Ziv, G.; Lidor, R. Physical characteristics, physiological attributes, and on-court performances of handball players: A review. *Eur. J. Sport Sci.* **2009**, *9*, 375–386. [CrossRef]
1. Lidor, R.; Falk, B.; Arnon, M.; Cohen, Y.; Segal, G.; Lander, Y. Measurement of talent in team handball: The questionable use of motor and physical tests. *J. Strength Cond. Res.* **2005**, *19*, 318–325. [CrossRef] [PubMed]
2. Šibila, M.; Pori, P. Position-related differences in selected morphological body characteristics of top-level handball players. *Coll. Antropol.* **2009**, *33*, 1079–1086.
3. Milanese, C.; Piscitelli, F.; Lampis, C.; Zancanaro, C. Effect of a competitive season on anthropometry and three-compartment body composition in female handball players. *Biol. Sport* **2012**, *29*, 199–204. [CrossRef]

34. Martínez-Rodríguez, A.; Martínez-Olcina, M.; Hernández-García, M.; Rubio-Arias, J.Á.; Sánchez-Sánchez, J.; Sánchez-Sáez, J.A. Body composition characteristics of handball players: Systematic review. *Arch. Med. Deporte* **2020**, *37*, 52–61.
35. Nikolaidis, P.T.; Ingebrigtsen, J. Physical and physiological characteristics of elite male handball players from teams with a different ranking. *J. Hum. Kinet.* **2013**, *38*, 115–124. [CrossRef]
36. Masanovic, B. Comparative study of anthropometric measurement and body composition between junior basketball and volleyball players from Serbian national league. *Sport Mont* **2018**, *16*, 19–24. [CrossRef]
37. Masanovic, B.; Popovic, S.; Bjelica, D. Comparative study of anthropometric measurement and body composition between basketball players from different competitive levels: Elite and sub-elite. *Pedagog. Psychol. Med-Biol. Probl. Phys. Train. Sports* **2019**, *4*, 176–181. [CrossRef]
38. Farley, J.B.; Stein, J.; Keogh, J.W.; Woods, C.T.; Milne, N. The relationship between physical fitness qualities and sport-specific technical skills in female, team-based ball players: A systematic review. *Sport. Med.-Open* **2020**, *6*, 18. [CrossRef] [PubMed]
39. Ari, E.; Sözen, H. The relationship between anaerobic power, reaction time and body composition parameters of young soccer players. *Kinesiol. Slov.* **2021**, *27*, 108–120.
40. Turkeri, C.; Ozturk, B.; Buyuktas, B.; Ozturk, D. Comparison of Balance, Reaction Time, Attention and BMI Values in Individual and Team Sports. *J. Educ. Learn.* **2019**, *8*, 119–128. [CrossRef]
41. Trejo-Silva, A.; Gomez-Ruano, M.A.; Feu, S.; Brazo-Sayavera, J. Analysis of offensive performance during exclusions in female senior handball. *Int. J. Perform. Anal. Sport* **2022**, *22*, 684–700. [CrossRef]
42. Czapska, K. Intellectual processes and psychomotor performance of professional drivers in conventional psychological tests and Test2Drive. *Pol. J. Aviat. Med. Psychol.* **2015**, *21*, 30–39.
43. Schmiedek, F.; Lövdén, M.; Lindenberger, U. On the relation of mean reaction time and intraindividual reaction time variability. *Psychol. Aging* **2009**, *24*, 841. [CrossRef] [PubMed]
44. Verbruggen, F.; Logan, G.D. Response inhibition in the stop-signal paradigm. *Trends Cogn. Sci.* **2008**, *12*, 418–424. [CrossRef] [PubMed]
45. Martins, F.; França, C.; Sarmento, H.; Przednowek, K.; Śliż, M.; Campos, P.; Lopes, H.; Marques, A.; Gouveia, É.R. Analyzing the effects of competitive fatigue on body composition and functional capacities of youth elite handball players. *Montenegrin J. Sports Sci. Med.* **2024**, *13*, 71–77. [CrossRef]
46. Skurvydas, A.; Gutnik, B.; Zuoza, A.; Nash, D.; Zuoziene, I.; Mickeviciene, D. Relationship between simple reaction time and body mass index. *HOMO* **2009**, *60*, 77–85. [CrossRef] [PubMed]
47. Jackson, R.C.; Mogan, P. Advance visual information, awareness, and anticipation skill. *J. Mot. Behav.* **2007**, *39*, 341–351. [CrossRef] [PubMed]
48. Shelton, J.; Kumar, G.P. Comparison between auditory and visual simple reaction times. *Neurosci. Med.* **2010**, *1*, 30–32. [CrossRef]
49. Ando, S.; Kida, N.; Oda, S. Practice effects on reaction time for peripheral and central visual fields. *Percept. Mot. Skills* **2002**, *95*, 747–751. [CrossRef]
50. Arabacı, R.; Çankaya, C.; Çatıkkaş, F.; Şahin, S. Assessment body composition and leg reaction time of elite taekwondo athletes. *Sport Sci.* **2011**, *6*, 139–147.
51. Poliszczuk, T.; Mańkowska, M.; Poliszczuk, D.; Wiśniewski, A. Symmetry and asymmetry of reaction time and body tissue composition of upper limbs in young female basketball players. *Pediatr. Endocrinol. Diabetes Metab* **2013**, *19*, 132–136.

applied sciences

MDPI

Article

A Case Study Exploring the Effects of a Novel Intra-Abdominal Pressure Belt on Fastball and Change-Up Velocity, Command, and Deception Among Collegiate Baseball Pitchers

Ryan L. Crotin [1,2,3,*] and Christian Conforti [4]

1 RC13 Sports, Phoenix, AZ 85050, USA
2 Human Performance Laboratories, Department of Kinesiology, Louisana Tech University, Ruston, LA 71272, USA
3 Sports Performance Research Institute New Zealand, Auckland University of Technology, Auckland 1010, New Zealand
4 Toronto Blue Jays (MLB), Toronto, ON M5V 1J1, Canada; cconfor@alumni.uwo.ca
* Correspondence: rlcrotin@gmail.com

Abstract: Baseball pitchers must reduce batters' decision-making ability, locating pitches in zones where batters make weak contact. The purpose of this case study was to investigate potential pitching performance improvements when wearing a specialized intra-abdominal pressure (IAP) belt. Thirteen collegiate pitchers were randomly assigned to three bullpens of 40 pitches with visual encouragement from an integrated LED screen and a portable radar. Pitchers wore their typical belt, an IAP belt at regular length, and the IAP belt with a two-inch cinch for separate bullpen conditions. Fastball and change-up velocities, their average differences in velocity, and strike-throwing percentages were indexed and analyzed. A repeated measures ANOVA with an a priori of 0.05 and Tukey's post hoc analyses evaluated significant differences amongst the case study population across pitch velocity, command, and deception, which was measured as the average velocity difference between fastballs and change-ups. Given the small sample size, subject-specific data were presented and showed the majority of pitchers threw faster, had greater accuracy, and displayed greater velocity ranges between fastballs and change-ups. The subject-specific results in this case study indicated that most pitchers improved performance across velocity, command, and deception metrics with the use of an intra-abdominal pressure belt designed to be worn in competition.

Keywords: ulnar collateral ligament; Tommy John Surgery; shoulder; elbow

1. Introduction

Pitching performance is uniquely intertwined with disrupting decision-making for batters, which can lead to weaker contact and increased probability of making outs. There are two key metrics that qualify the value of a baseball pitcher and reflect their ability to neutralize batting performance, namely, the pitcher's Fielding Independent Performance (FIP) and Wins Above Replacement (WAR) rating [1,2].When looking at these metrics, fastball velocity alone may not fully correlate with improvement. Equally important are a pitcher's ability to maintain velocity differentials between fastballs and change-ups, and improved pitch tunneling. The latter is the visual deception that occurs when the same pitch is thrown, yet the ball branches off in different directions due to ball speed and spin characteristics, which move the ball to the bottom of the strike zone [2–4]. Another apex quality that becomes increasingly important as pitchers develop and move through competitive rankings is the ability to throw strikes; this is termed pitch command, which is the ability to locate pitches in the strike zone. Collectively, the ability to deceive batters and throw pitches to locations that induce lower exit velocities and distance off the bat, while achieving fewer walks and hit batsmen, all raise the potential of FIP and WAR success [1,2].

Previous research has indicated that players can compensate biomechanically in a variety of ways and still maintain throwing velocity for both the change-up (CH) and fastball (FB) [3,5]. Athletes were forced to alter their stride strategy and, despite such gross changes in force production and momentum, velocities were unchanged and grip strength reduced [3,6]. What is unknown are the overall fatigue effects throughout the season that elevate joint stress and the potential risks of modifying pitching mechanics or throwing programs over the long term, such as weighted ball velocity enhancement programming. The quest to throw at higher velocities is more compelling in today's sport than at any other point in time. Generally, the selection criterion for high-level pitchers by Major League Baseball scouts is to identify amateur players who are at or above the current average velocity for the league, which motivates pitchers to engage in high-intensity velocity enhancement training [7–9]. Collegiate recruiting programs are following suit to motivate athletes to increase their throwing arm speed with "run and gun" deliveries without attention paid to accuracy, as athletes typically deliver the ball into a net or wall. It is believed that increasing arm speed with no emphasis on targeted throwing can alter the speed–accuracy trade off in commanding pitches; this can lead to greater accumulation of maximum effort pitches thrown, which can lead to more baserunners on base and reduce pitching success. Further, with increased pitch accumulation at maximum intent, pitchers elevate injury risk associated with overuse. This can be substantiated by previous research performed on velocity enhancement training, which showed 25% of the sample population terminated the study due to throwing arm injury [9].

Because of the injury risks associated with overuse at maximum throwing intensity, the need to improve the speed–accuracy trade off and the effect of velocity by altering speeds and added deception is warranted to improve not only performance, but also health, among competitive pitchers. Improved core function can improve consistency in the delivery, along with increased FB and CH pitching velocity and speed differentials, rotational deceleration, and co-contraction to stabilize the proximal body [10]. Elevated rotational trunk velocities have been shown to increase throwing velocity, while maintaining trunk position in the lateral plane can influence the medial release point position [11–13]. When the rotational control of the trunk impacts momentum exchange in combination with greater trunk lean, greater losses can be seen in functional forearm strength, which can lead to a loss of dynamic stability for the medial elbow, thereby raising Tommy John Surgery risks [6,12,14].

One way to improve trunk control is with more responsive core engagement, as seen through dynamic neuromuscular stabilization training, which is intimately tied to intra-abdominal pressure (IAP), to improve energy transfer, proximal stability, and distal segment joint power [10]. In connection with the positive performance contribution made by increased IAP, which can amplify throwing arm power and command and lessen medial elbow torque and forearm strength loss, a novel baseball belt has been innovated to heighten such effects in competition. The noted improvement in this case study shows that the IAP can offer a safe alternative to weighted ball training, raise the competitiveness and durability for baseball pitchers, and reduce the associated risks, e.g., current epidemiologic findings state that 5% of all pitchers will experience a throwing arm surgery [15]. High pitch totals can lead to overuse risk. A clear gap in the literature exists as it relates to the speed–accuracy tradeoff influenced by increased IAP and proximal core control that forms the basis of this case study. Therefore, the purpose of this study was to examine the pitching velocity, deception, and command impacts of wearing a baseball belt designed to increase IAP among high-level pitchers. It was hypothesized that improved dynamic stability offered through a baseball belt designed to raise IAP will increase fastball and change-up velocity, and increase the speed differential between pitches, while heightening accuracy, versus traditional belt wear in baseball.

2. Methods

Thirteen collegiate pitchers (height; 1.86 ± 0.06 m, weight; 88.5 ± 8.31 kg, age; 20.6 ± 1.39 years) signed an informed consent form to participate in this research study, which was approved by the Institutional Review Board at Arizona Christian University (IRB 21CFR56.108).

Pitchers went through a standardized lower-body dynamic warm-up routine before performing a self-selected throwing warm-up to ready the arm for competitive effort. Bullpens designed to encourage effort in competitive play were fully randomized across three conditions, with two conditions involving a specialized IAP belt (Core Technology Inc, Avon, OH, USA): (1) pitchers wearing their regular belt (REGB), (2) pitchers wearing the specialized IAP belt at regular belt length (IAPB), and (3) pitchers wearing the specialized IAP belt with a 2-inch cinch (IAP2) to create a maximum restraint. The IAP belt used in this study was interwoven and stretch-resistant, maintaining a 5 mm thickness compared to typical baseball belts, which are 1 mm in thickness. Both IAP and regular belts are worn across the waistline and can accommodate a variety of waist circumferences. Belts are secured by belt loops in baseball pants. However, the IAP is cut to the proximal body specification of the athlete by first measuring the athlete's waist circumference while in baseball pants to maintain the integrity and thickness of the belt in supporting the core region. The individual size specification promotes greater support when wearing baseball pants in raising IAP through co-contraction of the proximal muscles; this co-contraction can be elevated with cinching. In total, pitchers threw 159 pitches, including pre-inning warm-up pitches, spanning three bullpen sessions of 40 pitches that involved two innings of 20 pitches thrown in a sequence of 2 fastballs to 1 change up. Intermittent rest periods between pitches were set at 15 s, with a 5 min break between innings. To encourage high-level effort and competitive pressure, a handheld radar gun unit (Santa Rosa, CA, USA), capable of capturing velocities up to 130 mph, was integrated with an LED screen, which provided visual encouragement to throw at maximum intensity (Pocket Radar, Santa Rosa, CA, USA). A professional catcher indicated balls and strikes, which were confirmed on each pitch by the Principal Investigator prior to being analyzed. A minimum of 72 h rest was provided between bullpen sessions. Figure 1 illustrates the testing conditions for each simulated bullpen.

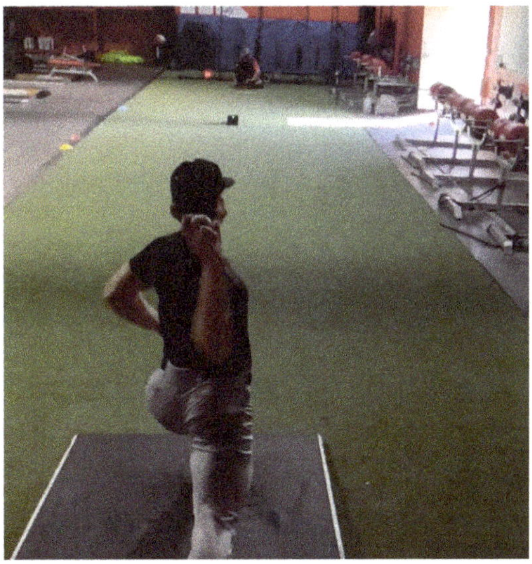

Figure 1. Visuals of equipment and set-up for game-simulated bullpensA regulation bullpen complete with an indoor mound was integrated in this study. A portable radar gun tethered to a LED screen captured pitching velocities, while a professional catcher determined balls and strikes, which were confirmed by the Principal Investigator for analyses.

Performance Analyses

Following testing sessions, all velocity and command data were manually entered into a spreadsheet to evaluate subject-specific analyses for performance tendencies in fastball and change-up velocities, command, and deception, which was calculated as the velocity difference between fastballs and change-up pitches. Data were aggregated in CSV format in Microsoft Excel (Redmond, WA, USA) and evaluated for subject-specific performance, as determined by the percentage of subjects experiencing benefit with the IAP belt.

3. Results

The exploratory case study revealed a positive individual effect on throwing arm strength when examining subject-specific responses, which can be seen in Tables 1–5. Each table represents the performance data associated with each belt condition and the percentage of athletes who had seen performance enhancement with use of the IAP belt.

Table 1. Subject-specific data indicating fastball velocity differences between belt conditions.

Player ID	REGB Avg (MPH)	IAPB Avg (MPH)	IAP2 Avg (MPH)
1	86.7	87.4	**87.7**
2	**75.7**	74.7	75.5
3	**79.3**	78.3	78.1
4	85.4	**85.5**	83.3
5	84.3	84.1	**86.1**
6	**81.0**	80.1	80.4
7	**85.5**	85.2	84.1
8	76.7	**78.6**	77.1
9	81.6	**81.7**	80.8
10	**84.0**	82.8	82.9
11	84.0	84.1	**84.5**
12	**84.4**	83.7	82.1
13	85.1	84.7	**85.3**

Table 2. Subject-specific data indicating change-up velocity differences between belt conditions.

Player ID	REGB Avg (MPH)	IAPB Avg (MPH)	IAP2 Avg (MPH)
1	**80.8**	79.5	80.6
2	**69.1**	67.6	69.0
3	**70.4**	**70.8**	68.8
4	**77.3**	76.7	75.2
5	73.1	74.2	**74.8**
6	**71.4**	70.8	70.7
7	74.3	**75.2**	74.9
8	70.8	**73.3**	72.0
9	74.0	74.1	**74.2**
10	73.4	73.1	**73.9**
11	**74.0**	73.9	72.8
12	**79.6**	78.1	77.8
13	81.0	81.8	**82.2**

Table 3. Subject-specific data indicating fastball command differences between belt conditions.

Player ID	REGB Avg (K%)	IAPB Avg (K%)	IAP2 Avg (K%)
1	66.7	**69.2**	68.0
2	**68.0**	66.7	38.5
3	55.6	55.6	**63.0**
4	63.0	51.9	**66.7**
5	61.5	**73.1**	51.9
6	**59.3**	55.6	55.6
7	48.1	59.3	**74.1**
8	63.0	**63.0**	59.3
9	77.8	**88.9**	63.0
10	**84.6**	81.5	66.7
11	**74.1**	59.3	40.7
12	38.5	**57.7**	44.4
13	**70.4**	63.0	66.7

Table 4. Subject-specific change-up command differences between belt conditions.

Player ID	REGB Avg (K%)	IAPB Avg (K%)	IAP2 Avg (K%)
1	**50.0**	23.1	33.3
2	**46.2**	**46.2**	41.7
3	**46.2**	23.1	30.8
4	30.8	46.2	**76.9**
5	30.8	38.5	**46.2**
6	**61.5**	23.1	**61.5**
7	**84.6**	46.2	61.5
8	**53.8**	38.5	**53.8**
9	61.5	**69.2**	30.8
10	53.8	**76.9**	53.8
11	38.5	38.5	**69.2**
12	38.5	**53.8**	38.5
13	30.8	**46.2**	38.5

Table 5. Subject-specific differences in fastball-change velocity ranges between belt conditions.

Player ID	REGB Avg (MPH Δ)	IAPB Avg (MPH Δ)	IAP2 Avg (MPH Δ)
1	5.9	**7.9**	7.1
2	6.6	**7.1**	6.5
3	8.9	7.5	**9.3**
4	8.1	**8.8**	8.1
5	11.2	9.9	**11.3**
6	9.6	9.3	**9.7**
7	**11.2**	10.0	9.2
8	**5.9**	5.3	5.1
9	7.6	**7.6**	6.6
10	**10.6**	9.7	9.0
11	10.0	10.2	**11.7**
12	4.8	**5.6**	4.3
13	**4.1**	2.9	3.1

Maximum fastball velocity for each subject in association with each belt condition. Bolded numbers indicate subjects' highest average velocity values across belt conditions. As shown, approximately 54% of subjects indicated greater fastball velocity using an intra-abdominal pressure belt, yet parametric statistics did not show statistically significant findings in relation to overall group means due to the case study sample being under-powered. Belt groups: Regular IAP Belt; IAPB, 2-Inch Cinch IAP Belt; IAP2, and Regular Belt; REGB.

Maximum change-up velocity for each subject in association with each belt condition. Bolded numbers indicate subjects' highest average velocity values across belt conditions. As shown, approximately 54% of subjects indicated greater change-up velocity using an intra-abdominal pressure belt, yet parametric statistics did not show statistically significant findings in relation to overall group means due to the case study sample being under-powered. Belt groups: Regular IAP Belt; IAPB, 2-Inch Cinch IAP Belt; IAP2, and Regular Belt; REGB.

Average fastball command for each subject in association with each belt condition. Bolded numbers indicate subjects' highest average strike-throwing percentages (K%) across belt conditions. As shown, approximately 62% of subjects indicated greater fastball command using an intra-abdominal pressure belt, yet parametric statistics did not show statistically significant findings in relation to overall group means due to the case study sample being under-powered. Belt groups: Regular IAP Belt; IAPB, 2-Inch Cinch IAP Belt; IAP2, and Regular Belt; REGB.

Average change-up command for each subject in association with each belt condition. Bolded numbers indicate subjects' highest average strike-throwing percentages (K%) across belt conditions. As shown, approximately 70% of subjects indicated greater fastball command (two excluded due to ties) using an intra-abdominal pressure belt, yet parametric statistics did not show statistically significant findings in relation to overall group means due to the case study sample being under-powered. Belt groups: Regular IAP Belt; IAPB, 2-Inch Cinch IAP Belt; IAP2, and Regular Belt; REGB

Average velocity differences between fastball and change-up pitches for each subject in association with each belt condition. Bolded numbers indicate subjects' highest level of deception as determined by greater average velocity differences (MPH Δ) across belt conditions. As shown, approximately 70% of subjects demonstrated greater deception, indicated by greater velocity differences between the fastball and change-up using an intra-abdominal pressure belt, yet parametric statistics did not show statistically significant findings in relation to overall group means due to the case study sample being under-powered. Belt groups: Regular IAP Belt; IAPB, 2-Inch Cinch IAP Belt; IAP2, and Regular Belt; REGB

4. Discussion

Baseball high-performance training has a spectrum of approaches for evaluating risk and rewards. As this relates to velocity enhancement training, several studies have indicated the increased loading risks associated with maximum-effort throwing, running at high speed, blocking the lead leg, and throwing as hard as possible into a wall or net [8,9,16]. Risk multiplies when throwing balls that are underweight, as throwing arm acceleration increases, and with larger players, the force potential can be greater than what they experience when pitching on a mound [8].

Major League Baseball has written numerous articles on the injury risks associated with the inception of the pitch clock, yet a consensus has been voiced by the readership and athletes alike that velocity enhancement training and the desire to throw at more than 100 mph are the culprits [17,18]. The conundrum of increased throwing-velocity performance with paralleled risk requires innovation in delivering methods and products to simultaneously maximize performance and health.

In this study, an IAP belt was introduced as a potential tool to raise and maintain velocity, establish more consistency, and add deception by establishing large differences in pitching speeds between pitchers' fastballs and change-ups. Our hypothesis was supported on a subject-specific level, as this case study presented greater benefits to velocity, command, and deception attributed to IAP belt use on a subject-specific level. One main postulate is that with increased IAP, the majority of pitchers were able to execute greater dynamic neuromuscular control to brace the lead leg, maintain trunk position, and sustain high throwing arm accelerations.

Dynamic neuromuscular control involves the execution of co-contracted bracing strategies in sport, and requires activating the diaphragm, intrinsic core musculature, and paraspinal muscle groups at the same time as increasing IAP in the abdominal cavity [10]. This coordinated bracing contraction adds to spinal column stiffness through rotation and is further augmented by compression of the stomach, an internal bladder, being held against the spine [10]. When it comes to trunk control, contralateral fascial lines are highly important for rotational athletes, as muscles and fascia are aligned in an "X" pattern and have been likened to a serape, an indigenous scarf that wraps around the body and forms a figure-eight pattern [19]. In essence, to increase rotational speed of the trunk, the athlete must optimize stretch-shortening responses between the lead hip and throwing shoulder [19]. Hip–shoulder separation between these two anatomical points is highly impacted by lead leg bracing and the rhomboids and posterior muscles of the throwing shoulder, as energy is transferred from the pelvis bi-directionally, going upward into the trunk and downward into the lead leg [19,20]. During the turn and to the terminal end-point of ball release, intra-abdominal pressure develops and rises sharply to the point of the highest shoulder compressive loads just after the ball leaves the hands, and therefore, athletes who can sustain highly responsive proximal bracing are likely to achieve consistent lower-body kinematics and ground reaction force applications, and reduce overloading the shoulder in its most vulnerable position at release [10,21].

Throwing athletes who have better dynamic stability tend to throw harder in overhand sport and are healthier [22]. This has been demonstrated in pitchers who display unilateral hip and lower-limb strength, an intersegmental interaction that is linked to athletes' proximal bracing capability [22–25]. As an analogy, a dynamic bracing strategy for the proximal chain in the pitching delivery is like cracking a whip. Intersegmental energy transfer hits an abrupt stopping point to generate as much speed as possible to the endpoint of the whip, which is analogous to the throwing hand in the kinetic chain [26]. Heightened IAP accelerates the whiplike action of throwing through optimizing momentum exchanges and maximizes the potential of the stretch-shortening cycle between maximum hip–shoulder separation between the lead hip and throwing shoulder [19,27,28]. As a result, it is possible to achieve higher throwing velocities with better trunk stability, and pitchers who maintain trunk positions that allow the shoulder to maintain a consistent release point can minimize elevations in elbow varus torque, a measure of medial elbow loading that can increase ulnar collateral ligament stress [12–14,22,29].

The theoretical mechanism for the IAP belt involved in this study is that the design furthers the bracing capacity for the athlete by providing a retaining wall for muscles to push into while the belt pushes back on the muscles to heighten the IAP. In a sense, this interaction between the external support of the IAP belt and intrinsic muscles is like wearing a powerlifting weight belt. Long-term health benefits arising from heightened IAP in powerlifting creates a potential parallel for IAP baseball belts, as powerlifters have been shown to have greater muscular power with minimal elevations in neuromuscular recruitment effort in barbell squatting [30]. Perhaps similar neuromuscular recruitment efficiency can be seen in rotational athletes such as baseball pitchers and hitters, thereby reducing overuse injury risks from managing muscular fatigue in the core region of the body, by maintaining paraspinal and oblique activation with gains in explosive rotational power [30]. As an extreme, the IAP belt was cinched two inches shorter than the pitchers' regular belt length and may have better regulated muscular recruitment efforts in stabilizing the proximal body to produce high velocities.

From the subject-specific data, the majority of pitchers in this study benefited from an IAP baseball belt versus their typical belt. The IAP belt allowed them to throw both their fastballs and change-ups at higher velocities, throw all pitches more accurately, and increase the velocity range between the fastball and change-up, which collectively would alter hitters' timing in recognizing pitches and coordinating a high-impact swing. Future work is needed to determine how altered bi-directional energy transfer in bracing from the pelvis, a direct result of less effective proximal stiffness, has the potential to be improved with a baseball belt designed to raise IAP. It was found that both extreme tightening and the regular belt length with the IAP belt provided individual benefits. Future work should emphasize a larger sample size and explore each individual belt setting to determine an optimum for IAP that aims to achieve improved subject-specific responses across velocity, command, and deception, as well as biomechanics looking at power dynamics.

5. Limitations

On a subject-specific level, this study indicated velocity, command, and deception benefits of wearing a specialized baseball belt designed to increase IAP. However, one must consider a few important limitations of this work in the interpretation of this case study's results. This case study was exploratory in nature, as this work was the first to explore an IAP apparatus that is functional in competitive settings and lacked the statistical power to determine the main effects between conditions. Future work should consider a larger-scale statistically powered investigation that can look at incremental changes in IAP through an incremental design, with the belt worn over multiple simulated bullpens to evaluate sustainable performance (minimal losses in velocity, command, and deception).

Outside covariates also proposed challenges in arriving at statistically significant group mean differences. Future research endeavors should incorporate controlled training regimens for athletes to mitigate the confounding effects of variable training schedules on the study outcomes. As a result, athletes in this study had varying workload and training schedules, which could have either undertrained or overtrained the athlete leading into the competitive bullpen simulations. A more stringent research design could have controlled for these confounders if implemented outside of the scholastic year, as athletes have greater control of their training and throwing programming. The study design did its best to encourage adrenaline; however, like other laboratory studies, the absence of real game conditions may have lowered contractile effort and could have produced differing results in actual game play. Given the stated limitations, this case study created a new avenue to evaluate velocity enhancement approaches that stabilize the speed–accuracy trade off (as speed increases, accuracy decreases) without the injury risks associated with throwing weighted baseballs to increase throwing arm acceleration and range of motion. As a result, increasing IAP in the pitching delivery with a specialized belt provides an opportunity to study a player-development technology that increases both performance and durability for competitive pitchers. Lastly, it is advisable to undertake long-term tracking studies to evaluate the prolonged use of the IAP belt and its effects on both the performance and health over extended periods to ensure longstanding efficacy for baseball players.

6. Conclusions

This exploratory case study found that a greater percentage of subjects wearing the intra-abdominal pressure belt saw an increase in throwing velocity, accuracy, and deception in bullpens that simulated competition. With further research, incremental tightening of the intra-abdominal pressure belt could identify optimal settings for each player to improve core engagement and proximal stiffness, with improved statistical performance.

Author Contributions: Conceptualization, R.L.C.; Methodology R.L.C.; Software and Data Analyses C.C.; Supervision, Project Administration, Investigation and Data Collection, R.L.C.; Writing Original Draft Preparation R.L.C. and C.C.; Review and Editing, R.L.C.; Funding Acquisition, R.L.C. All authors have read and agreed to the published version of the manuscript.

Funding: This research was funded by Core Technology USA Inc who manufactures the intra-abdominal pressure belt for baseball under the trade name, Core Energy Belt.

Institutional Review Board Statement: The study was conducted in accordance with the Declaration of Helsinki, and approved by the Arizona Christian University Institutional Review Board. (approval data: 29 June 2023).

Informed Consent Statement: Informed consent was obtained from all subjects involved in the study.

Data Availability Statement: De-identified data can be made available upon request to the corresponding author and permission granted from subjects involved in this study in release of their data.

Acknowledgments: A special thanks goes to Jamie Balivec, Richard Gannon III, and Brock Johnson for their dedicated work collecting data, assisting with warm-up procedures, and catching pitchers for the entire study. We would also like to thank Erin Carlson, Payton Deer, Grayson Hill, and Ximena Iniguez for their help in data entry and aggregation for this study. The investigators of this study would like to thank the Arizona Christian University baseball team for their participation in this work and the research sponsorship efforts of Core Technology USA Inc. for their dedication to making the game of baseball safer for all.

Conflicts of Interest: Funding for this work was provided through Core Technology USA Inc. a client of RC13 Baseball Consulting Services LLC (RC13 Sports), which is owned and operated by the corresponding author and performs sponsored research for innovative sports performance companies.

References

1. Conforti, C.M.; Crotin, R.L.; Oseguera, J. An analysis of playoff performance declines in Major League Baseball. *J. Strength Cond. Res.* **2021**, *35*, S36–S41. [CrossRef] [PubMed]
2. Conforti, C.M.; Crotin, R.L.; Oseguera, J. Major League Draft WARs: An analysis of wins Above re-placement in player selection. *J. Sports Anal.* **2022**, *8*, 77–84. [CrossRef]
3. Crotin, L.R.; Ramsey, K.D. Stride Length: A reactive response to prolonged exertion potentially effecting ball velocity among baseball pitchers. *Int. J. Perform. Anal. Sport.* **2015**, *15*, 254–267. [CrossRef]
4. Laby, D.M.; Kirschen, D.G.; Govindarajulu, U.; DeLand, P. The hand-eye coordination of professional baseball players: The relationship to batting. *Optom. Vis. Sci.* **2018**, *95*, 557–567. [CrossRef]
5. Dun, S.; Fleisig, G.S.; Loftice, J.; Kingsley, D.; Andrews, J.R. The relationship between age and baseball pitching kinematics in professional baseball pitchers. *J. Biomech.* **2007**, *40*, 265–270. [CrossRef]
6. Crotin, R.; Ramsey, D. Grip strength measurement in baseball pitchers: A Clinical examination to indicate stride length inefficiency. *Int. J. Sports Phys. Ther.* **2021**, *16*, 1330–1337. [CrossRef]
7. Caldwell, J.M.E.; Alexander, F.J.; Ahmad, C.S. Weighted-ball velocity enhancement programs for base-ball pitchers: A systematic review. *Orthop. J. Sports Med.* **2019**, *7*, 2325967118825469. [CrossRef]
8. Fleisig, G.S.; Diffendaffer, A.Z.; Aune, K.T.; Ivey, B.; Laughlin, W.A. Biomechanical analysis of weighted-ball exercises for baseball pitchers. *Sports Health* **2017**, *9*, 210–215. [CrossRef]
9. Reinold, M.M.; Macrina, L.C.; Fleisig, G.S.; Aune, K.; Andrews, J.R. Effect of a 6-week weighted baseball throwing program on pitch velocity, pitching arm biomechanics, passive range of motion, and injury rates. *Sports Health* **2018**, *10*, 327–333. [CrossRef]
10. Frank, C.; Kobesova, A.; Kolar, P. Dynamic neuromuscular stabilization & sports rehabilitation. *Int. J. Sports Phys. Ther.* **2013**, *8*, 62.
11. Cohen, A.D.; Garibay, E.J.; Solomito, M.J. The association among trunk rotation, ball velocity, and the elbow varus moment in collegiate-level baseball pitchers. *Am. J. Sports Med.* **2019**, *47*, 2816–2820. [CrossRef] [PubMed]
12. Matsuo, T.; Fleisig, G.S.; Zheng, N.; Andrews, J.R. Influence of shoulder abduction and lateral trunk tilt on peak elbow varus torque for college baseball pitchers during simulated pitching. *J. Appl. Biomech.* **2006**, *22*, 93–102. [CrossRef] [PubMed]
13. Oyama, S.; Yu, B.; Blackburn, J.T.; Padua, D.A.; Li, L.; Myers, J.B. Effect of excessive contralateral trunk tilt on pitching biomechanics and performance in high school baseball pitchers. *Am. J. Sports Med.* **2013**, *41*, 2430–2438. [CrossRef] [PubMed]
14. Whiteside, D.; Martini, D.N.; Lepley, A.S.; Zernicke, R.F.; Goulet, G.C. Predictors of ulnar collateral ligament reconstruction in major league baseball pitchers. *Am. J. Sports Med.* **2016**, *44*, 2202–2209. [CrossRef]
15. Shanley, E.; Thigpen, C.A.; Boes, N.; Bailey, L.; Arnold, A.; Bullock, G.; Kissenberth, M.J. Arm injury in youth baseball players: A 10-year cohort study. *J. Shoulder Elb. Surg.* **2023**, *32*, S106–S111. [CrossRef]
16. Bowman, E.N.; Camp, C.L.; Erickson, B.J.; Freehill, M.T.; Smith, M.V.; Madia, E.; Matthews, M.; Simister, S.; Wheelwright, C.; Ishikawa, H.; et al. Most high school baseball pitchers are using weighted ball throwing programs to increase ball velocity: Cross-sectional analysis of US high school pitchers. *JSES Rev. Rep. Tech.* **2023**, *3*, 137–141. [CrossRef]
17. Rogers, J. MLBPA Says Pitch Clock to Blame for Injuries; League Counters. The Associated Press. Available online: https://www.espn.com/mlb/story/_/id/39890102/mlbpa-says-shorter-pitch-clock-blame-pitcher-injuries (accessed on 6 April 2024).
18. The Associated Press. MLB Rejects Pitch Clock Injuries Theory, Says Spring Training or Early-Season Injuries More Likely. Available online: https://www.foxsports.com/stories/mlb/mlb-rejects-pitch-clock-injuries-theory-says-spring-training-early-season-injuries-more-likely (accessed on 23 May 2024).

19. Santana, J.C.; McGill, S.M.; Brown, L.E. Anterior and posterior serape: The rotational core. *Strength Cond. J.* **2015**, *37*, 8–13. [CrossRef]
20. Aguinaldo, A.; Nicholson, K. Lower body contributions to pelvis energy flow and pitch velocity in collegiate baseball players. *ISBS Proc. Arch.* **2021**, *39*, 137.
21. Keeley, D.W.; Oliver, G.D.; Dougherty, C.P.; Torry, M.R. Lower body predictors of glenohumeral com-pressive force in high school baseball pitchers. *J. Appl. Biomech.* **2015**, *31*, 181–188. [CrossRef]
22. Mathavan, B.S. Relationship between upper body anthropometric parameters and throwing performance of handball players. *Int J. Sci. Res. Publ.* **2012**, *2*, 2250–3153.
23. Chaudhari, A.M.W.; McKenzie, C.S.; Borchers, J.R.; Best, T.M. Lumbopelvic control and pitching performance of professional baseball pitchers. *J. Strength Cond. Res.* **2011**, *25*, 2127–2132. [CrossRef] [PubMed]
24. Laudner, K.; Wong, R.; Evans, D.; Meister, K. Lumbopelvic Control and the Development of Upper Extremity Injury in Professional Baseball Pitchers. *Am. J. Sports Med.* **2021**, *49*, 1059–1064. [CrossRef] [PubMed]
25. Laudner, K.G.; Wong, R.; Meister, K. The influence of lumbopelvic control on shoulder and elbow kinetics in elite baseball pitchers. *J. Shoulder Elb. Surg.* **2019**, *28*, 330–334. [CrossRef] [PubMed]
26. Howenstein, J.; Kipp, K.; Sabick, M.B. Energy flow analysis to investigate youth Pitching velocity and efficiency. *Med. Sci. Sports Exerc.* **2018**, *51*, 523–531. [CrossRef]
27. Ben Kibler, W. The role of the scapula in athletic shoulder function. *Am. J. Sports Med.* **1998**, *26*, 325–337. [CrossRef]
28. Yanai, T.; Crotin, R.; Du, T. Proximal to distal sequencing impacts on maximum shoulder joint angles and the risk of impingement in baseball pitching involving a scapular independent thoracohumeral model. *Scand. J. Med. Sci. Sports* **2023**, *33*, 1322–1334. [CrossRef]
29. Krishna, V.; Noronha, T.; Pathak, A.A. Association between core strength and dynamic balance of throwing hand in professional healthy cricket fast bowlers: A cross sectional study. *J. Bodyw. Mov. Ther.* **2024**, *39*, 156–161. [CrossRef]
30. Zink, A.J.; Whiting, W.C.; Vincent, W.J.; McLaine, A.J. The effects of a weight belt on trunk and leg muscle activity and joint kinematics during the squat exercise. *J. Strength Cond. Res.* **2001**, *15*, 235–240.

applied sciences

MDPI

Article

Notational Analysis of Men's Singles Pickleball: Game Patterns and Competitive Strategies

Iván Prieto-Lage [1,*], Xoana Reguera-López-de-la-Osa [2,*], Abel Juncal-López [1], Antonio José Silva-Pinto [1], Juan Carlos Argibay-González [1] and Alfonso Gutiérrez-Santiago [1]

[1] Observational Research Group, Faculty of Education and Sport, University of Vigo, 36005 Pontevedra, Spain; abeljuncal@gmail.com (A.J.-L.); toze-pinto@hotmail.com (A.J.S.-P.); juan.carlos.argibay@uvigo.es (J.C.A.-G.); ags@uvigo.es (A.G.-S.)

[2] Education, Physical Activity and Health Research Group (Gies10-DE3), Galicia Sur Health Research Institute (IIS Galicia Sur), SERGAS-UVIGO, 36208 Vigo, Spain

* Correspondence: ivanprieto@uvigo.es (I.P.-L.); xreguera@uvigo.es (X.R.-L.-d.-l.-O.)

Abstract: Background: Pickleball is an exponentially growing sport with a lack of notation-based studies. Consequently, this research aimed to conduct a match analysis in men's singles to enhance the understanding of the game and optimize training practices. Methods: Using observational methodology, a total of 1145 points were analyzed from the semifinal and final rounds of five Professional Pickleball Association Tour tournaments. Data were recorded with LINCE PLUS V.2.1.0 software using the OI-PICKLEBALL-S23 observational instrument. Descriptive statistical analyses were conducted with IBM-SPSS version 25.0, and gameplay patterns were detected using Theme 6.0 Edu. Statistical significance was set at $p < 0.05$. Results: The data indicated that service faults at the start of the game were minimal (2.4%). The server won fewer points than the returner in the overall set of analyzed points (46.6%). Most points were concluded in short rallies (1–4 shots; 43%) or medium-length rallies (5–8 shots; 44%), with the final shot predominantly occurring from striking zone 2, the area closest to the non-volley line (50.7%). Ground strokes (55.1%) and volleys (38.4%) were the most common final shots. Conclusions: The insights gained from this study can benefit high-performance players and coaches and provide a foundation for future notation-based research in pickleball.

Keywords: performance analysis; key performance indicators; match analysis; paddle sports

1. Introduction

Pickleball, a relatively new sport in the realm of racket sports, has experienced exponential growth since its creation in 1965 [1]. Conceived on Bainbridge Island, Washington, by Joel Pritchard, Bill Bell, and Barney McCallum, this sport merges elements of tennis, badminton, and table tennis. Initially designed as a recreational family activity, pickleball has significantly evolved, becoming a competitive sport with a growing global community [2]. Its popularity has particularly surged in the United States, where millions of people play it both recreationally and competitively [3]. This expansion has led the sport to other countries, consolidating its presence in various regions around the world. Its growth is partly attributed to the sport's dynamics, including its ease of technical learning due to the dimensions of the playing area and equipment, its strong social nature, affordable access for all, less demanding technical requirements compared to other sports, as well as physical demands that can be adapted to different ages and fitness levels [4].

Despite this rapid expansion and growing global acceptance, scientific research on pickleball has been limited to date. Most of the available publications have primarily focused on aspects related to health and leisure, especially highlighting the positive impact of the sport on older adults [5]. These studies have emphasized the physical and mental benefits associated with regular pickleball practice, such as improvements in coordination, balance, agility, and psychological well-being, particularly in older individuals [1,6,7]. Topics related to injuries [8,9] and the inclusion of pickleball as an alternative sport in physical education classes [10,11] have also been addressed. However, while these findings are valuable, they have left a significant gap in terms of notational analysis and competitive performance optimization, which are critical areas for the development of advanced training and gameplay strategies.

In contrast, sports like tennis and padel have been the subject of a wide range of notational studies that have allowed for a deep understanding of their game dynamics [12–17]. These studies have provided key data on service effectiveness, rally length, finishing zones, and other critical aspects of the game, which have enabled coaches and players to continuously improve their strategic approaches [18,19]. Even other racket sports, such as table tennis and badminton, though to a lesser extent, have been the subject of detailed analyses that have contributed to the evolution of their respective training and game tactics [20–23]. In the case of tennis, for example, it has been extensively documented how court surface influences rally dynamics and service success probability, guiding the development of specific strategies for each type of court [24,25].

Despite the similarities pickleball shares with these sports, the lack of exhaustive notational analysis has so far limited the understanding of its specific characteristics and the ability to systematically enhance performance. This highlights the need for research focused on unraveling the specific dynamics of pickleball, both in singles and doubles, to establish training strategies that optimize performance in competitive contexts.

This study aims to fill this research gap by conducting a detailed notational analysis of this sport, with the objective of generating precise and relevant data to guide high-performance training. Through this investigation, the goal is to establish a solid knowledge base on key game variables, such as rally length, common ending points, and shot directions that lead to winners or unforced errors. Additionally, the most characteristic playing patterns for winning points are identified, distinguishing between the server and the returner. This will enable a better understanding of game dynamics and help optimize training strategies. These data will provide a framework for continuous improvement in player preparation, something that has been challenging in the field of pickleball due to the scarcity of research.

Therefore, this study not only seeks to fill this knowledge gap but also aims to lay the groundwork for future research that continues to develop the competitive potential of pickleball. For all these reasons, the objective of this research is to analyze singles play in men's pickleball, identifying patterns of effectiveness based on rally type and the role of the server/returner. This study aims to offer a deeper understanding of the game, provide useful insights for optimizing training, and set a precedent for future investigations.

2. Methods

2.1. Design

This observational study aims to analyze the structure of play in men's singles pickleball. To achieve this, the observational methodology was utilized [26].

The observational design [27] employed is nomothetic, as it encompasses all points contested in the semifinals and finals during the 2023 season across five tournaments of the Professional Pickleball Association (PPA) Pro Tour of Pickleball (https://www.ppatour.com/ (accessed on 15 September 2023)) Additionally, the design is longitudinal (covering an entire season) and unidimensional (as the analysis does not account for the concurrency of behaviors).

2.2. Sample

The unit of analysis in this study was the points played in the observed pickleball matches. Specifically, five individual tournaments were analyzed (Las Vegas, Cincinnati, Kansas, Seattle, and Denver), resulting in the observation of 15 matches and a total sample of 1145 points. The selected tournaments represent the highest competitive level in this sport, bringing together only professional players from various countries around the world. The participants in this study were the players who reached at least the semifinal round in one of the five analyzed pickleball tournaments. Since this is an observational study conducted in a natural setting, using publicly available videos and not involving any form of experimentation, informed consent from the competitors was not required [28]. The study was approved by the Ethics Committee of the Faculty of Education and Sport Sciences (University of Vigo, application 07-280722).

2.3. Instruments

The observation instrument used was the OI-PICKLEBALL-S23 (observational instrument for analyzing pickleball during the 2023 season), a system of categories designed ad hoc to consider the various playing possibilities in pickleball. This instrument is based on tools previously developed for similar objectives in the field of tennis [18,19]. After designing and testing the observation instrument, its construct validity was assessed through its alignment with the theoretical framework [29] and through consultation with three experts in racket and/or paddle sports and observational methodology. The experts showed an agreement level with the instrument exceeding 95%.

The OI-PICKLEBALL-S23 consists of seven criteria that form a system of categories (see Table 1 and Figure 1) which meets the conditions of exhaustiveness and mutual exclusivity. Data recording was conducted using LINCE PLUS software, version 2.1.0 [30].

Table 1. Observational instrument OI-PICKLEBALL-S23.

Criteria	Code	Description
Service	FS	First service
	SF	Service fault
Rally length (the serve stroke is counted)	SH	Short rally (1–4 shots).
	MD	Medium rally (5–8 shots).
	LN	Long rally (9+ shots).
Strike zone (see Figure 1)	SZ1	Non-volley zone
	SZ2	Mid-court zone
	SZ3	Back court zone, including the baseline
	SZ4	Deep court zone, behind the baseline
	SZ	Service zone
Finish zone (see Figure 1)	FZ1	Left front zone
	FZ2	Right front zone
	FZ3	Left mid-court zone
	FZ4	Right mid-court zone
	FZ5	Left back court zone
	FZ6	Right back court zone
	NT	Net shot
	OUT	Shot out
Winner	SW	The point is won by the server
	RW	The point is won by the returner
Point ending	SWW	Server wins with a winner or a forced error
	SWUE	Server wins with an unforced error by the opponent
	RWW	Receiver wins with a winner or a forced error
	RWUE	Receiver wins with an unforced error by the opponent
Final stroke	ACE	Direct serve
	FH	Forehand
	BH	Backhand
	FHV	Forehand volley
	BHV	Backhand volley
	SM	Smash

Table 1. *Cont.*

Criteria	Code	Description
Final stroke	LB	Lob
	DS	Drop shot
	SC	Change of service due to an error in the service
	OT	Other type of stroke

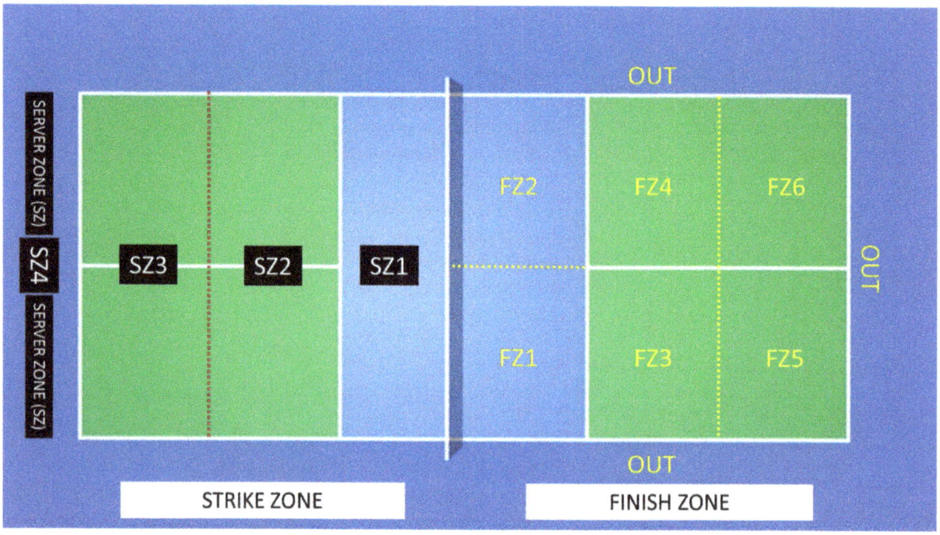

Figure 1. Court striking zones and finishing zones.

2.4. Procedure

Data collection was carried out by searching for, downloading, and viewing all the semifinals and finals of the five tournaments selected for the study. The videos, recorded in 1080p resolution (1920 × 1080), were analyzed on 27-inch monitors. Before conducting the data quality tests, which were performed by two experts in pickleball and observational methodology, specific training on the use of the observation instrument was provided. This training involved familiarization with the observation instrument and the LINCE PLUS recording software, version 2.1.0, through nine two-hour sessions over three weeks, using videos of men's pickleball matches from the 2022 season. The two expert observers are university professors with experience teaching in a research master's program, where they deliver a module on observational methodology in sports science. Both have numerous scientific publications on racket and paddle sports. Additionally, one of them is certified as a pickleball coach.

To ensure rigor in the data recording process [31], data quality was monitored by calculating intra-observer and inter-observer agreement using the Kappa coefficient [32], with the LINCE PLUS software, version 2.1.0. Both agreements were calculated on points that were not part of the final sample (n = 200; 1/10 of the final sample). The intra-observer Kappa was 0.96 for the first observer and 0.99 for the second, while the inter-observer Kappa was 0.98 (see Table 2). After the data quality tests, the second observer analyzed all the points in the study sample. Once all points were recorded, an Excel file was generated with the sequence of actions that occurred in each analyzed point. The versatility of this Excel file allowed for automatic transfer of the information to a file compatible with IBM-SPSS version 25 and THEME version 6 Edu, the software used for the various statistical analyses in the study.

Table 2. Degree of reliability of the study.

Criteria	Intra-Kappa Obs1-Obs1	Intra-Kappa Obs2-Obs2	Inter-Kappa Obs1-Obs2
Service	1	1	1
Rally length	0.98	0.99	0.98
Strike zone	0.96	0.97	0.96
Finish zone	0.97	0.99	0.98
Winner	0.99	0.99	0.97
Point ending	0.97	0.97	0.96
Final stroke	0.96	0.99	0.96
Mean reliability	0.98	0.99	0.97

2.5. *Data Analysis*

All descriptive statistical analyses were conducted using the Statistical Package for the Social Sciences version 25.0 (IBM-SPSS Inc., Chicago, IL, USA). Statistical significance was assumed for $p < 0.05$.

A descriptive analysis of the study variables was performed. The χ^2 test was used to assess differences within the categories of each employed criterion (χ^2 goodness-of-fit test). Additionally, this same test was applied, using crosstabs, to identify differences between the point-winning criterion and the method of winning the point with respect to the other analyzed variables (χ^2 test of independence). Furthermore, the effect size was calculated using Cramér's V to assess the strength of the associations observed, with the following interpretation: 0.00–0.10: very weak, 0.10–0.20: weak, 0.20–0.30: moderate, 0.30–0.40: relatively strong, 0.40–0.50: strong, and 0.50 or more: very strong. An analysis of adjusted residuals was also conducted to highlight significant deviations from the expected frequencies, providing further insight into the relationships between variables.

To identify playing patterns in pickleball, we utilized THEME 6 Edu software [33], a specialized statistical analysis tool designed for detecting temporal patterns in sequential data. Widely used in fields such as psychology, ethology, and sports analysis, THEME excels in identifying T-patterns—recurring temporal and/or sequential patterns that may not be immediately apparent. Its ability to analyze large data sets and detect patterns that do not follow rigid sequences makes it particularly valuable for studying complex or dynamic behaviors. T-pattern detection identifies recurrent patterns of behavioral events within a temporal sequence, based on statistical probabilities [34]. While THEME's primary strength lies in detecting temporal patterns, it also facilitates the identification of sequential structures through its order parameter function, adding depth to the analysis of behavioral and tactical dynamics. The following search criteria were applied: (a) the presence of at least three T-patterns in the observed sequence set; (b) a 90% redundancy reduction adjustment for similar T-pattern occurrences; and (c) a significance level of 0.005.

3. Results

Descriptive Analysis

Table 3 presents a descriptive analysis of the study, including the χ^2 goodness-of-fit test.

Significant statistical differences were found in the χ^2 test for each of the criteria analyzed.

In general terms, the start of the point predominantly occurred without a service fault (nearly 98%) and was followed by a medium-length rally (44%), although short rallies were also common (43%). It was more common for the returner to win the point (53%). Points mostly ended due to an unforced error (58%), with the server making the error more frequently (32.9%). In more than half of the points played (51%), the final shot was executed from striking zone 2. More than half of the final shots were hit out or into the net (58%). Winners were typically directed to finishing zone 4 (11%) or finishing zone 6

(9%). The most common final shot was a forehand (34%), followed by a backhand (22%), although numerous volleys were also observed (18% forehand and 21% backhand).

Table 3. Descriptive analysis of the investigation.

Criteria	Code	n	%	χ^2 Test	Criteria	Code	n	%	χ^2 Test
Service	FS	1118	97.6	χ^2 = 1039.547	Winner	RW	611	53.4	χ^2 = 5.178
	SF	27	2.4	$p < 0.001$		SW	534	46.6	$p < 0.023$
Rally length	LN	145	12.7	χ^2 = 220.215	Point ending	RWUE	377	32.9	χ^2 = 44.921
	MD	504	44.0	$p < 0.001$		RWW	234	20.4	$p < 0.001$
	SH	496	43.3			SWUE	291	25.4	
Strike zone	SZ1	12	1.0	χ^2 = 944.716		SWW	243	21.2	
	SZ2	581	50.7	$p < 0.001$	Final stroke	ACE	1	0.1	χ^2 = 1608.860
	SZ3	218	19.0			BH	248	21.7	$p < 0.001$
	SZ4	304	26.6			BHV	203	17.7	
	SZ	30	2.6			DS	7	0.6	
Finish zone	NT	316	27.6	χ^2 = 739.583		FH	394	34.4	
	OUT	348	30.4	$p < 0.001$		FHV	237	20.7	
	FZ1	27	2.4			LB	6	0.5	
	FZ2	20	1.7			OT	4	0.3	
	FZ3	109	9.5			SC	29	2.5	
	FZ4	126	11.0			SM	16	1.4	
	FZ5	93	8.1						
	FZ6	106	9.3						

On the other hand, significant differences (χ^2 = 38.200; p = 0.000) were observed when comparing the data concerning rally length based on the point winner (whether the server or the receiver wins the point). The effect size test indicated that the relationship was weak (V = 0.183). As shown in Figure 2a, the analysis of adjusted residuals reveals distinct patterns in point winning across different rally lengths. In short rallies (SH), servers won significantly more points than expected, with an adjusted residual of 6.2, indicating that this type of rally favors the server. Conversely, in medium rallies (MD), receivers gained more points than expected, reflected by an adjusted residual of 4.9, highlighting a significant advantage for them. In long rallies (LN), although receivers also won more points than anticipated, with an adjusted residual of 1.9, these differences did not reach statistical significance.

When crossing the variable point ending with rally length (Figure 2b), statistically significant differences are again observed (χ^2 = 106.774; p = 0.000). The effect size test indicated that the relationship was moderate (V = 0.216). In short rallies (SH), it was observed that servers predominantly won due to unforced errors by the opponent (SWUE), with an adjusted residual of 8.8. Overall, unforced errors (SWUE and RWUE) were more common than winners (SWW and RWW). In medium rallies (MD), the receiver won a greater number of points, primarily due to unforced errors (RWUE, with an adjusted residual of 0.8), but especially through winners (RWW), which had an adjusted residual of 5.6, showing a notable increase compared to short rallies. It is noteworthy that the server's unforced error (SWUE), which was the most recorded value in short rallies, became the least frequent in medium rallies, while the receiver's winners (RWW) increased. In long rallies (LN), a trend similar to that of medium rallies was maintained, though with a decrease in the number of recorded points.

When analyzing the data between winner/point ending and striking zones (Figure 2c,d), statistically significant differences were observed (χ^2 = 31.696; p = 0.000 and χ^2 = 437.636; p = 0.000, respectively). The effect size test indicated that the relationship was weak (V = 0.166) in the first case (none of the adjusted residuals exceeded the critical value of ±1.96) and relatively strong in the second (V = 0.357). Points won from striking zone 2, both on serve and return, were particularly noteworthy. From this mid-court zone, returners frequently won points with winners, while servers often benefitted from their opponents' unforced errors. In striking zones 3 (baseline area) and 4 (beyond the baseline), most points won by the returner resulted from unforced errors, whereas the server achieved numerous winners.

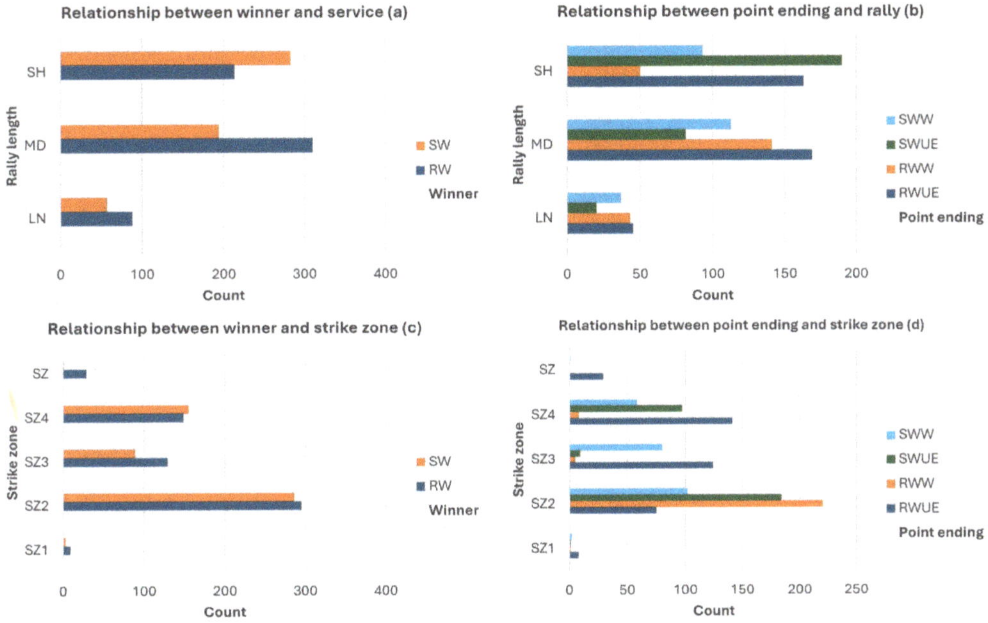

Figure 2. Relationship between research criteria (winner and service (**a**); point ending and rally length (**b**); winner and strike zone (**c**); point ending and strike zone (**d**). Note: SH: short rally, MD: medium rally, LN: long rally; SW: server wins, RW: receiver wins; SWW: server wins with a winner or a forced error, SWUE: server wins with an unforced error by the opponent, RWW: receiver wins with a winner or a forced error, RWUE: receiver wins with an unforced error by the opponent; SZ1: non-volley zone, SZ2: mid-court striking zone; SZ3: back court striking zone, including the baseline, SZ4: deep court striking zone, behind the baseline, SZ: service zone.

The analysis of the adjusted residuals reveals that striking zone 2 (SZ2) is crucial in scoring points during the match, particularly highlighting the winners from the receiver, which presented an adjusted residual of 14.8, as well as the errors from the receiver, with a residual of 4.9. This suggests that the receiver has a notable advantage in controlling the game in this zone. In striking zone 3 (SZ3), the server's errors were significantly higher than expected, with an adjusted residual of 8.4, while the winners from the receiver were less frequent, showing a residual of −7.4. This indicates that, although SZ3 favors the server, this advantage is primarily due to errors from the receiver rather than winning shots (6.0). On the other hand, in striking zone 4 (SZ4), both the server's errors (residual of 5.8) and the receiver's errors (residual of 3.0) exceeded expectations, while the winners from the receiver were significantly lower than expected, with an adjusted residual of −9.0.

Table 4 presents an analysis of play patterns that illustrates how points were concluded, taking into account the type of rally, the zone from which the final shot was executed, and the point ending.

The analysis reveals that, in short rallies, points were predominantly resolved with shots from striking zone 2 or striking zone 4. From striking zone 2, where the receiver was positioned in most cases, 67.1% of the points resulted in unforced errors and 33.7%

resulted in winners by that player. When the final shot came from striking zone 4, unforced errors were predominant for both the server and the receiver. In cases where a winner was recorded, it generally belonged to the server.

Table 4. Descriptive analysis of play patterns.

Play Pattern SZ2	*n*	%	Play Pattern SZ3	*n*	%	Play Pattern SZ4	*n*	%
SH	464	100						
SH-SZ2	140	30.2	SH-SZ3	96	20.7	SH-SZ4	228	49.1
SH-SZ2-SW	96	68.6	SH-SZ3-SW	46	47.9	SH-SZ4-SW	140	61.4
SH-SZ2-SW-SWW	2	1.4	SH-SZ3-SW-SWW	39	40.6	SH-SZ4-SW-SWW	51	22.4
SH-SZ2-SW-SWUE	94	67.1	SH-SZ3-SW-SWUE	7	7.3	SH-SZ4-SW-SWUE	89	39
SH-SZ2-RW	44	31.4	SH-SZ3-RW	52	54.2	SH-SZ4-RW	88	38.6
SH-SZ2-RW-RWW	43	30.7	SH-SZ3-RW-RWW	0	0	SH-SZ4-RW-RWW	7	3.1
SH-SZ2-RW-RWUE	1	0.7	SH-SZ3-RW-RWUE	52	54.2	SH-SZ4-RW-RWUE	81	35.5
MD	494	100						
MD-SZ2	331	67	MD-SZ3	105	21	MD-SZ4	58	12
MD-SZ2-SW	141	42.6	MD-SZ3-SW	38	36.2	MD-SZ4-SW	13	22.4
MD-SZ2-SW-SWW	69	20.8	MD-SZ3-SW-SWW	36	34.3	MD-SZ4-SW-SWW	7	12.1
MD-SZ2-SW-SWUE	72	21.7	MD-SZ3-SW-SWUE	2	1.9	MD-SZ4-SW-SWUE	6	10.3
MD-SZ2-RW	190	57.4	MD-SZ3-RW	67	63.8	MD-SZ4-RW	45	77.6
MD-SZ2-RW-RWW	135	40.7	MD-SZ3-RW-RWW	4	3.8	MD-SZ4-RW-RWW	1	1.7
MD-SZ2-RW-RWUE	55	16.6	MD-SZ3-RW-RWUE	63	60	MD-SZ4-RW-RWUE	44	75.9

Note: In this analysis, shots ending from striking zone 1 and long rallies have been excluded due to their low frequency, in order to simplify the data analysis. Note 2: SH: short rally, MD: medium rally; SW: server wins, RW: receiver wins; SWW: server wins with a winner or a forced error, SWUE: server wins with an unforced error by the opponent, RWW: receiver wins with a winner or a forced error, RWUE: receiver wins with an unforced error by the opponent; SZ2: mid-court striking zone; SZ3: back court striking zone, including the baseline, SZ4: deep court striking zone, behind the baseline.

In medium-length rallies, the final shot was most frequently executed from striking zone 2 (67%). The majority of points were won by the receiver (57.4%), often through winners (40.7%, representing 71% of the points won). The server also achieved a significant number of winners (21.7%, representing 51% of the points won). From striking zone 4, points were predominantly won by the receiver due to unforced errors from the opponent (75.9%).

Table 5 shows the T-pattern analysis carried out for this research. The data include only first-serve points, excluding those with service faults, and is organized by rally length and the player who wins the point.

Table 5. T-pattern analysis.

Search	Max.		T-Pattern	L	O	%
FS	1118	100%				
FS-SH	469	42%	(FS (SH SZ4))	3	228	48.6
			(FS (SH SZ2))	3	140	29.8
			((FS SH) (SZ4 FH))	4	179	38.1
			(((FS SH) (SZ2 SW)) SWUE)	5	94	20
FS-SH-SW	283	60.4%	((FS (SH SW)) (SWW FH))	5	80	28.2
			((FS (SH NT)) (SW SWUE))	5	85	30
			((FS (SH OUT)) (SW SWUE))	5	105	37.1
			((((FS SH) (SZ2 SW)) SWUE) BHV)	6	49	17.3
			(FS ((SH SZ4) (SW (SWUE FH))))	6	67	23.6
			((FS SH) ((SZ4 OUT) (SW (SWUE FH))))	7	44	15.5
FS-SH-RW	186	39.6%	((FS (SH RW)) (RWUE FH))	5	97	52.1
			(FS ((SH NT) (RW (RWUE FH))))	6	51	27.4
			(FS ((SH OUT) (RW (RWUE FH))))	6	46	24.7
			(FS ((SH SZ4) (RW (RWUE FH))))	6	61	32.7
			((((FS SH) (SZ2 RW)) RWW) FHV)	6	23	12.4
			((FS SH) ((SZ4 NT) (RW (RWUE FH))))	7	34	18.2

Table 5. *Cont.*

Search	Max.		T-Pattern	L	O	%
FS-MD	504	45.1%	((FS MD) (SZ2 FHV))	4	134	26.5
			(FS (MD SZ2))	3	331	65.6
			(FS (MD SZ3))	3	105	20.8
			(FS (MD BH))	3	130	25.8
			(FS (MD FH))	3	123	24.4
FS-MD-SW	194	38.5%	(FS (MD (SW SWW)))	4	113	58.2
			((FS MD) (SZ2 SW))	4	141	27.9
			((FS MD) (SZ2 (SW SWW)))	5	69	35.5
			((FS MD) (SZ3 (SW SWW)))	5	36	18.5
			((FS MD) (FZ4 (SW SWW)))	5	38	19.6
			((FS MD) (SZ2 (SW SWUE)))	5	72	37.1
			(((FS MD) (SZ2 FZ4)) (SW SWW))	6	26	13.4
			(FS ((MD SZ2) (SW (SWW FHV))))	6	31	15.9
			((FS MD) ((SZ2 FZ4) (SW (SWW FHV))))	7	12	6.2
FS-MD-RW	310	61.5%	(FS (MD (RW RWUE)))	4	169	54.5
			((FS MD) (SZ2 RW))	4	190	61.3
			((FS MD) (SZ2 (RW RWW)))	5	135	43.5
			(FS ((MD SZ2) (RW (RWW FHV))))	6	72	23.2
			(((FS MD) (SZ2 FZ4)) (RW RWW))	6	38	12.2
			(((FS MD) (SZ2 FZ3)) (RW RWW))	6	31	10
			(((FS MD) (SZ2 FZ6)) (RW RWW))	6	31	10
			((FS MD) (SZ3 (RW RWUE)))	5	63	20.3
			((FS (MD RW)) (RWUE BH))	5	75	24.1
			((FS (MD RW)) (RWUE FH))	5	61	19.7
FS-LN	145	13%	(FS (LN SZ2))	3	110	75.9
			(FS (LN (SZ2 BHV)))	4	36	24.8
			(FS (LN (SZ2 FHV)))	4	34	23.4
FS-LN-SW	57	39.3%	((FS LN) (SZ2 SW))	4	49	85.9
			(FS (LN (SW SWW)))	4	37	64.9
			((FS LN) (SZ2 (SW SWW)))	5	31	54.3
			(((FS LN) (SZ2 SW)) (SWW FHV))	6	14	24.5
FS-LN-RW	88	60.7%	(FS (LN (RW RWUE)))	4	45	51.1
			((FS LN) (SZ2 RW))	4	61	69.3
			((FS LN) (SZ2 (RW RWW)))	5	42	28.9
			((FS LN) (SZ2 (RW RWW)))	5	42	47.7
			(((FS LN) (SZ2 FZ3)) (RW RWW))	6	14	15.9
			(((FS LN) (SZ2 RW)) (RWW BHV))	6	16	18.1
			(((FS LN) (SZ2 RW)) (RWW FHV))	6	13	14.7

Note: Max refers to the maximum possible frequency of points with this sequence; L indicates the pattern length; O represents the occurrence of that sequence. Note 2: FS: first service; SH: short rally, MD: medium rally, LN: long rally; SW: server wins, RW: receiver wins; SWW: server wins with a winner or a forced error, SWUE: server wins with an unforced error by the opponent, RWW: receiver wins with a winner or a forced error, RWUE: receiver wins with an unforced error by the opponent; SZ2: mid-court striking zone; SZ3: back court striking zone, including the baseline, SZ4: deep court striking zone, behind the baseline; FZ3: finishing zone left mid-court zone, FZ4: finishing zone right mid-court zone, FZ6: finishing zone right back court zone; FH: forehand, BH: backhand, FHV: forehand volley, BHV: backhand volley; OUT: shot out, NT: net shot.

To facilitate the understanding of a T-pattern, let us take the fifth pattern presented in the Table 5 as an example: (FS (SH SW)) (SWW FH)). This T-pattern indicates that, after executing a successful first serve (FS), the server tends to win the point quickly (SW) in short rallies (SH), finishing with a winner (SWW) through a forehand shot (FH). This pattern, which spans 5 categories, occurred 80 times, representing 28.2% of the points won in short rallies by the server, which accounts for 17% of all short rally points and 7% of all points played. The recurrence of this pattern suggests that the server is very effective in short-duration points and typically finishes them offensively with their forehand.

In short rallies, which accounted for 42% of the total points recorded, the server won a significantly higher percentage of points compared to the returner (60.4% versus 39.6%). Most of these points were finished from striking zone 4, representing nearly half of the cases, with a clear predominance of forehand shots (38.1%), often followed by an unforced error (14% from the returner and 13% from the server). Additionally, a considerable number of points concluded with a shot from striking zone 2 (29.8%).

Up to 14% of all points in this type of rally were won by the server due to an unforced error from the returner following a forehand shot from striking zone 4, representing 23.6% of the points won by the server. Nearly 70% of the points won by the server resulted from unforced errors by the returner, with most of the winners being achieved through a forehand shot.

On the other hand, approximately 5% of all points in this type of rally were decided by a forehand volley winner from the returner, accounting for 33% of the points won by this player. Additionally, more than half of the points won by the returner (52.1%) were the result of unforced errors from the opponent via a forehand shot.

In medium-length rallies, which accounted for 45.1% of the points analyzed, the returner won 61.5% of these points. Notably, 65.6% of these rallies ended with a shot from striking zone 2, while nearly 20.8% concluded with a shot from striking zone 3. A forehand volley was the decisive shot in 26.5% of the points, representing 40.5% of all points that concluded from striking zone 2. The number of points concluded with a forehand and backhand in this type of rally were relatively similar, accounting for 24.4% and 26.5% of the points, respectively.

Among the points won by the server, 58.2% were achieved through winners, which comprised 22.4% of the total points. In contrast, the returner primarily won points due to unforced errors, accounting for 66.5% of their points won and 33.5% of the total points. The majority of the server's winners were executed from striking zone 2 (35.5%), with finishing zone 4 being a common area for finishing shots. The most frequent winning pattern for the server involved a shot from striking zone 2 directed toward finishing zone 4, often concluding with a forehand volley, which represented 6.2% of all points won by the server.

For the returner, it is notable that 43.5% of their points were won through winners from striking zone 2, with 14.2% of these points concluding with a forehand volley. These points were hit toward finishing zones 3, 4, and 6 in similar proportions. Points won due to unforced errors were predominantly preceded by an opponent's shot from striking zone 3 (20.3% of all points won), often involving a backhand stroke.

Long rallies were the least frequent, accounting for only 13% of the analyzed points. Of these, 60.7% were won by the returning player. Approximately half of the points ended with a volley, with 23.4% being forehand volleys and 24.8% backhand volleys. The server won 64.9% of their points through winners, most of which were generated from striking zone 2. Regarding the returning player, the points they won were almost equally divided between unforced errors from the opponent and their own winners. Striking zone 2 stood out as the main zone from which to hit winners, with volleys predominating as the final shot. The majority of winners were directed toward finishing zone 3.

4. Discussion

The objective of this study was to conduct a notational analysis of pickleball to generate accurate and relevant data that can contribute to optimizing high-performance training in this sport. The research provided significant findings on various key variables, such as rally duration, the most common final shot zones, and ball trajectories associated with winners or forced errors. Additionally, detailed statistics were gathered on the probability of winning a point, distinguishing between the server and the receiver.

Previous research in other racquet and paddle sports has demonstrated that the serve is a fundamental component of the game. When comparing pickleball to sports such as tennis or padel, it has been observed that the ball is put into play with the first serve at a high percentage, close to 97%, far exceeding the values recorded in tennis [35,36] and more similar to those in padel [14,17]. This percentage is more akin to sports like badminton, where, as in pickleball, there is no option for a second serve. However, it has been found that the serve in pickleball is significantly less effective compared to other racquet and paddle sports [17,37], particularly in relation to tennis [18]. In fact, among the more than 1100 points observed, only one ace was recorded. Despite the fact that players serve underhand in this sport, training with various spins and trajectories could enhance the chances of winning points. This variability in serves could be an area to optimize during practice, as it would allow players to develop more effective strategies and better adapt to different game situations.

Regarding rally length, the study data showed that the proportion of points ending in short rallies (between one and four shots) and medium rallies (between five and eight shots) was quite similar, at approximately 43% in both cases. Long rallies, those with nine or more shots, were relatively infrequent. When compared to other sports, it could be said that the structure of play is more similar to padel, where rallies of fewer than 12 shots (including short, medium, and long rallies in this study) are common and occur at a similar rate [17,38,39], in contrast to tennis, where short rallies clearly predominate, especially on fast surfaces such as hard courts and grass [18,35,40,41]. Given the rarity of long rallies in men's singles pickleball, players are encouraged to quickly adapt to situations and play proactively, fostering a more offensive and aggressive style.

In terms of court striking zones from where the final shot is executed, pickleball showed greater similarity to padel than to tennis. Previous research in padel has revealed that up to 40% of final shots are made from the middle zone of the court, with similar percentages from the zone near the net [17,42]. In contrast, in tennis, final shots from the baseline dominate across all surfaces, highlighting a significant difference in point dynamics between these sports [18]. These data suggest that, in this sport, as in padel, mastering both the net and forehand and backhand volleys is crucial [43]. This contrasts with tennis, where these shots are less frequent due to the predominance of baseline rallies through groundstrokes [18,44]. It is important to note that in pickleball there is a zone close to the net that, for regulatory reasons, cannot be used as a zone from which the final shot is executed. This reinforces the idea that controlling the area near the net is fundamental, similar to padel. A clear difference between padel and pickleball in this respect is that in the latter, the smash is hardly used, whereas in padel, it is a decisive stroke [17,42]. In any case, the high percentage of unforced errors committed by the receiver near the net during short rallies suggests that the tactic of advancing toward the net may not be as effective as previously considered. This aspect requires further exhaustive analysis in future research.

According to the data obtained from the study, the receiving player won slightly more than half of the points played (54%). This finding contrasts markedly with padel and, especially, with tennis, where the serve tends to clearly favor the server. Previous studies have shown that, in padel, the probability of winning a point on serve is approximately 60% [17,45], while in tennis, it ranges between 65% and 70%, depending on the surface [18,46]. The rule in pickleball that requires the ball to bounce before being returned on the first shot by the server after the serve could explain this difference. Therefore, coaches have a significant opportunity to improve performance by focusing on optimizing the serve and the first return following the serve, to increase the chances of winning the point.

Regarding point endings, it was observed that nearly 60% of the points ended with an unforced error, predominantly committed by the server. These values are more similar to those in tennis [18,47] than in padel, where recent research indicates that approximately 40% of points are decided by unforced errors [17]. Although in tennis the data are also close to the findings of this study, in that sport, unforced errors are more common from the receiving player.

Regarding the stroke used to finish points in this study, it was observed that forehands and backhands predominated, along with a significant number of volleys, both forehand and backhand. These characteristics show clear similarities to padel, where, in addition to these shots, finishes with smashes are also common [48]. However, in pickleball, the smash was less frequent. In contrast, tennis presents a different profile, with a lower proportion of volleys as final shots, since points in this sport are typically resolved with shots from the baseline. Thus, while pickleball and padel share a more dynamic and offensive approach to point endings, tennis is characterized by baseline play, with a predominance of forehand and backhand strokes. The data reveal that in men's singles pickleball, simply mastering groundstrokes from the back of the court is not enough to win matches, nor is being skilled only at volleying near the net. Both areas of play are essential, and success requires a well-rounded game that integrates proficiency from both positions.

The sequential analysis of the study has revealed patterns of play and point-winning chances that a descriptive analysis could have overlooked or misinterpreted. This type of analysis, recently implemented in other racquet sports [13,17], has proven useful. For example, although the receiver generally wins more points overall, this trend does not hold in short rallies, where the server wins a greater proportion of points. This indicates that the serve can be a decisive factor in point development, especially when resolved in the first few shots. Although it may seem that the receiver has the initiative in the point, similar to the dynamic in volleyball, this theory is not entirely accurate, since if the server manages to shorten the rally, the possibility of success tilts in their favor. As expected, certain zones of the court are more favorable for winning points, but the study reveals that it is crucial to combine this information with the type of rally to obtain precise performance data. This integrated approach allows coaches to optimize match tactics, adapting the game not only based on the striking zone but also according to the dynamics of the rallies.

4.1. Practical Implications

The data presented in the research provide a more detailed understanding of the internal dynamics of the game and are crucial for designing specific tasks to optimize training and improve performance. For instance, although it is believed that being close to the net facilitates scoring points in this sport, it has been observed that the returner frequently makes errors in the area near the no-volley zone during short rallies. This suggests that coaches should focus on improving this aspect of the game.

While servers win more points in short rallies, the difference is relatively small. This indicates that there is still room for improvement in this area, as it has not been conclusively demonstrated that serving significantly benefits the returner.

Focusing on striking zones 2 and 4, which are critical for finishing points, is also essential. Since a significant number of points are resolved with shots from near the no-volley zone, it is important for players to practice precise shot execution in these areas. Additionally, considering that striking zone 4 is crucial for servers, training should include exercises to explore how to capitalize on these zones for both offensive and defensive plays.

The analysis highlights the importance of both forehand and backhand volleys and groundstrokes. Therefore, players should engage in exercises that emphasize these shots equally, ensuring they can execute them effectively in various situations, especially during short and medium-length rallies.

Moreover, given the significant role of unforced errors in determining point outcomes, training should include practices aimed at reducing these errors, particularly in striking zone 2. Players need to work on maintaining control and composure in this critical area to minimize the likelihood of making unforced errors.

Finally, it is important to tailor training sessions to the duration of rallies. For short rallies, the focus should be on aggressive play and quick strategies to finish points. In medium and long rallies, the emphasis should shift to consistency, patience, and strategic shot placement to outmaneuver the opponent.

4.2. Limitations and Future Perspectives

For this study, data from the semifinals and finals of five tournaments from the 2023 professional pickleball circuit were collected. Despite the number of points recorded and analyzed, the results obtained might have varied if points from earlier rounds or additional tournaments had been included. Competitive stress associated with final rounds or even physical fatigue may have influenced the resulting data.

In this study, player rankings, the state of the scoreboard, and player handedness were not considered. These factors could be examined in future research.

For future studies, it is suggested to conduct a temporal analysis of the effort-pause time between points and to compare results with the female category or different doubles categories. Given that pickleball is an expanding sport, it would be beneficial to compare these findings with future seasons to observe the evolution of the game and the changes that may occur.

5. Conclusions

The research provides significant findings regarding successful patterns of rallies/play in pickleball. Although this sport shares some similarities with padel and tennis, it has distinctive characteristics that require specific and differentiated training compared to other racket and paddle sports. In general, most rallies in men's singles end within eight shots. Returners win more points than servers, although in shorter rallies the advantage tends to favor the server. Most points conclude near the no-volley zone, indicating that players actively seek to approach the net due to the competitive advantage this position offers. The most frequently used finishing shots are the forehand and backhand, but when the point ends near the net, forehand and backhand volleys prevail, while the use of smashes and drop shots is minimal.

These findings can contribute to a better understanding of the game, helping athletes improve their decision-making during competition. Additionally, they provide valuable information for designing specific drills and training sessions, especially considering the lack of previous studies on this sport.

Author Contributions: Conceptualization, I.P.-L., A.J.S.-P., A.J.-L., X.R.-L.-d.-l.-O. and A.G.-S.; methodology, I.P.-L., J.C.A.-G., X.R.-L.-d.-l.-O. and A.G.-S.; software, I.P.-L., A.J.-L. and A.G.-S.; validation, J.C.A.-G., A.J.-L. and X.R.-L.-d.-l.-O.; formal analysis, I.P.-L. and A.G.-S.; investigation, I.P.-L., J.C.A.-G., A.J.S.-P., A.J.-L., X.R.-L.-d.-l.-O. and A.G.-S.; resources, I.P.-L., A.J.S.-P., J.C.A.-G., A.J.-L. and X.R.-L.-d.-l.-O.; data curation, I.P.-L., A.J.S.-P., J.C.A.-G. and A.G.-S.; writing—original draft, I.P.-L., A.J.-L., A.J.S.-P. and A.G.-S.; writing—review and editing, I.P.-L., X.R.-L.-d.-l.-O. and A.G.-S.; visualization, A.J.S.-P., J.C.A.-G. and A.J.-L.; supervision, I.P.-L., A.J.S.-P. and A.G.-S.; project administration, I.P.-L., J.C.A.-G., X.R.-L.-d.-l.-O. and A.G.-S.; funding acquisition, I.P.-L. and A.G.-S. All authors have read and agreed to the published version of the manuscript.

Funding: This study was funded by the Ministerio de Cultura y Deporte (https://www.culturaydeporte.gob.es/portada.html (accessed on 20 June 2024)), Consejo Superior de Deportes (https://www.csd.gob.es/es (accessed on 20 June 2024)) and European Union (https://european-union.europa.eu/index_es (accessed on 20 June 2024)) under Project "Integración entre datos observacionales y datos provenientes de sensores externos: Evolución del software LINCE PLUS y desarrollo de la aplicación móvil para la optimización del deporte y la actividad física beneficiosa para la salud (2023)" EXP_74847 to A.G.-S and I.P.-L.

Institutional Review Board Statement: The study was approved by the ethics committee of the Faculty of Education and Sport Science (University of Vigo, application 08-280722).

Informed Consent Statement: Not applicable.

Data Availability Statement: The raw data supporting the conclusions of this article will be made available by the authors on request.

Acknowledgments: This publication was made possible thanks to the research stays during the years 2023 and 2024 at the Instituto Politécnico de Viana do Castelo [IPVC]—Escola Superior de Desporto e Lazer.

Conflicts of Interest: The authors declare no conflicts of interest.

References

1. Terrell, S.L.; Ficquette, P. Exploring Training Strategies to Optimize Court Performance in Older Pickleball Athletes. Available online: https://journals.lww.com/10.1519/SSC.0000000000000703 (accessed on 15 August 2024).
2. USA Pickleball. History of the Game. Available online: https://usapickleball.org/what-is-pickleball/history-of-the-game/ (accessed on 26 August 2024).
3. Ryu, J.; Yang, H.; Kim, A.C.H.; Kim, K.M.; Heo, J. Understanding pickleball as a new leisure pursuit among older adults. *Educ. Gerontol.* **2018**, *44*, 128–138. [CrossRef]
4. Buzzelli, A.A.; Draper, J.A. Examining the Motivation and Perceived Benefits of Pickleball Participation in Older Adults. *J. Aging Phys. Act.* **2020**, *28*, 180–186. [CrossRef] [PubMed]
5. Heo, J.; Ryu, J.; Yang, H.; Kim, A.C.H.; Rhee, Y. Importance of playing pickleball for older adults' subjective well-being: A serious leisure perspective. *J. Posit. Psychol.* **2018**, *13*, 67–77. [CrossRef]
6. Cerezuela, J.-L.; Lirola, M.-J.; Cangas, A.J. Pickleball and mental health in adults: A systematic review. *Front. Psychol.* **2023**, *14*, 1137047. [CrossRef] [PubMed]
7. Casper, J.M.; Bocarro, J.N.; Drake, N.R. Physical Activity Associated with Older Adult Pickleball Participation: A Pilot Study. *Recreat. Sports J.* **2023**, *47*, 49–56. [CrossRef]
8. Forrester, M.B. Pickleball-Related Injuries Treated in Emergency Departments. *J. Emerg. Med.* **2020**, *58*, 275–279. [CrossRef] [PubMed]
9. Weiss, H.; Dougherty, J.; DiMaggio, C. Non-fatal senior pickleball and tennis-related injuries treated in United States emergency departments, 2010–2019. *Inj. Epidemiol.* **2021**, *8*, 34. [CrossRef]
10. Barranca-Martínez, J.M.; Hernández-Beltrán, V.; Gamonales, J.M. Pickleball: Deporte alternativo para el área de Educación Física. *Lect. Educ. Fís. Deport.* **2023**, *28*, 146–160. [CrossRef]
11. Kim, I.; Oh, D.; Kim, M.; Cho, K. Teaching Pickleball with In-Depth Content Knowledge in Middle School Physical Education. *J. Phys. Educ. Recreat. Danc.* **2020**, *91*, 29–38. [CrossRef]
12. Sánchez-Pay, A.; Ortega-Soto, J.A.; Sánchez-Alcaraz, B.J. Notational analysis in female grand slam tennis competitions. *Kinesiology* **2021**, *53*, 154–161. [CrossRef]
13. Gutiérrez-Santiago, A.; Cidre-Fuentes, P.; Orío-García, E.; Silva-Pinto, A.J.; Reguera-López-de-la-Osa, X.; Prieto-Lage, I. Women's Singles Tennis Match Analysis and Probability of Winning a Point. *Appl. Sci.* **2024**, *14*, 6761. [CrossRef]
14. Sánchez-Alcaraz, B.J.; Muñoz, D.; Pradas, F.; Ramón-Llin, J.; Cañas, J.; Sánchez-Pay, A. Analysis of serve and serve-return strategies in elite male and female padel. *Appl. Sci.* **2020**, *10*, 6693. [CrossRef]
15. Escudero-Tena, A.; Sánchez-Alcaraz, B.J.; García-Rubio, J.; Ibáñez, S.J. Analysis of Game Performance Indicators during 2015–2019 World Padel Tour Seasons and Their Influence on Match Outcome. *Int. J. Environ. Res. Public Health* **2021**, *18*, 4904. [CrossRef] [PubMed]
16. Escudero-Tena, A.; Muñoz, D.; Sánchez-Alcaraz, B.J.; García-Rubio, J.; Ibáñez, S.J. Analysis of Errors and Winners in Men's and Women's Professional Padel. *Appl. Sci.* **2022**, *12*, 8125. [CrossRef]
17. Prieto-Lage, I.; Reguera-López-de-la-Osa, X.; Durán-Rodríguez, N.; Silva-Pinto, A.J.; Argibay-González, J.C.; Gutiérrez-Santiago, A. Assessing the Probability of Winning a Point in Men's Padel: A Comprehensive Analysis. *Appl. Sci.* **2024**, *14*, 6642. [CrossRef]
18. Prieto-Lage, I.; Paramés-González, A.; Torres-Santos, D.; Argibay-González, J.C.; Reguera-López-de-la-Osa, X.; GutiérrezSantiago, A. Match analysis and probability of winning a point in elite men's singles tennis. *PLoS ONE* **2023**, *18*, e0286076. [CrossRef]
19. Prieto-Lage, I.; Paramés-González, A.; Argibay-González, J.C.; Reguera-López-de-la-Osa, X.; Ordóñez-Álvarez, S.; Gutiérrez Santiago, A. Match Analysis in Women's Tennis on Clay, Grass and Hard Courts. *Int. J. Environ. Res. Public Health* **2022**, *19*, 7955. [CrossRef]
20. Abdullahi, Y.; Coetzee, B. Notational singles match analysis of male badminton players who participated in the African Badminton Championships. *Int. J. Perform. Anal. Sport* **2017**, *17*, 1–16. [CrossRef]
21. Abian-Vicen, J.; Castanedo, A.; Abian, P.; Sampedro, J. Temporal and notational comparison of badminton matches between men's singles and women's singles. *Int. J. Perform. Anal. Sport* **2013**, *13*, 310–320. [CrossRef]
22. Fadhil Abdullah, M.; Janep, M.; Shahrul Azzfar, M.; Abd Karim, Z.; Rahmat, A.; Md Nadzalan, A. Playing Pattern Analysis of Men's Single Badminton Matches. *Int. J. Eng. Technol.* **2018**, *7*, 168. [CrossRef]
23. Malagoli Lanzoni, I.; Di Michele, R.; Merni, F. A notational analysis of shot characteristics in top-level table tennis players. *Eur. J. Sport Sci.* **2014**, *14*, 309–317. [CrossRef] [PubMed]
24. Doğan, İ.; Revan, S.; Arikan, Ş. Analysis of tennis competitions on different court surface. *Turk. J. Sport Exerc.* **2021**, *23*, 60–66. [CrossRef]
25. Vaverka, F.; Nykodym, J.; Hendl, J.; Zhanel, J.; Zahradnik, D. Association between serve speed and court surface in tennis. *Int. J. Perform. Anal. Sport* **2018**, *18*, 262–272. [CrossRef]
26. Anguera, M.T.; Blanco-Villaseñor, A.; Losada, J.L.; Portell, M. Guidelines for designing and conducting a study that applies observational methodology. *Anu. Psicol.* **2018**, *48*, 9–17. [CrossRef]
27. Anguera, M.T.; Blanco-Villaseñor, A.; Hernández-Mendo, A.; Losada-López, J.L. Observational designs: Their suitability and application in sports psychology. *Cuad. Psicol. Deport.* **2011**, *11*, 63–76.
28. American Psychological Association Ethical principles of psychologists and code of conduct. *Am. Psychol.* **2002**, *57*, 1060–1073. [CrossRef]

29. González-Prado, C.; Iglesias, X.; Anguera, M.T. Detección de regularidades en taekwondo de alto nivel. *Cuad. Psicol. Deport.* **2015**, *15*, 99–110. [CrossRef]
30. Soto, A.; Camerino, O.; Iglesias, X.; Anguera, M.T.; Castañer, M. LINCE PLUS: Research Software for Behavior Video Analysis. *Apunt. Educ. Física i Esports* **2019**, *137*, 149–153. [CrossRef]
31. Blanco-Villaseñor, A.; Anguera, M.T. Evaluación de la calidad en el registro del comportamiento: Aplicación a deportes de equipo. In *Métodos Numéricos en Ciencias Sociales*; Oñate, E., García-Sicilia, F., Ramallo, L., Eds.; Centro Internacional de Métodos Numéricos en Ingeniería: Barcelona, Spain, 2000; pp. 30–48.
32. Cohen, J. Weighted kappa: Nominal scale agreement with provision for scaled disagreement of partial credit. *Psychol. Bull.* **1968**, *70*, 213–220. [CrossRef]
33. Magnusson, M.S. Discovering hidden time patterns in behavior: T-patterns and their detection. *Behav. Res. Methods Instrum. Comput.* **2000**, *32*, 93–110. [CrossRef]
34. Magnusson, M.S. Why Search for Hidden Repeated Temporal Behavior Patterns: T-Pattern Analysis with Theme. *Int. J. Clin. Pharmacol. Pharmacother.* **2017**, *2*, 10–15344. [CrossRef] [PubMed]
35. Fitzpatrick, A.; Stone, J.A.; Choppin, S.; Kelley, J. Important performance characteristics in elite clay and grass court tennis match-play. *Int. J. Perform. Anal. Sport* **2019**, *19*, 942–952. [CrossRef]
36. Fernández-García, Á.I.; Blanca-Torres, J.C.; Hernández-García, R.; Torres-Luque, G. Analysis of the statistical variables related to the service in high performance male tennis in junior and absolute category. *Cultura_Ciencia_Deporte* **2019**, *14*, 289–295.
37. Ramón-Llin, J.; Guzmán, J.F.; Llana, S.; Martínez-Gallego, R.; James, N.; Vučković, G. The Effect of the Return of Serve on the Server Pair's Movement Parameters and Rally Outcome in Padel Using Cluster Analysis. *Front. Psychol.* **2019**, *10*, 1194. [CrossRef]
38. Courel-Ibáñez, J.; Sánchez-Alcaraz Martínez, B.J.; Cañas, J. Game performance and length of rally in professional padel players. *J. Hum. Kinet.* **2017**, *55*, 161–169. [CrossRef]
39. Sánchez-Alcaraz, B.J.; Jiménez, V.; Muñoz, D.; Ramón-Llin, J. External training load differences between male and female professional padel. *J. Sport Health Res.* **2021**, *13*, 445–454.
40. Fitzpatrick, A.; Stone, J.A.; Choppin, S.; Kelley, J. A simple new method for identifying performance characteristics associated with success in elite tennis. *Int. J. Sports Sci. Coach.* **2019**, *14*, 43–50. [CrossRef]
41. Carboch, J.; Placha, K.; Sklenarik, M. Rally pace and match characteristics of male and female tennis matches at the Australian Open 2017. *J. Hum. Sport Exerc.* **2018**, *13*, 743–751. [CrossRef]
42. Mellado-Arbelo, Ó.; Baiget Vidal, E.; Usón, M.V. Analysis of game actions in professional male padel. *Cultura_Ciencia_Deporte* **2019**, *14*, 191–201. [CrossRef]
43. Sánchez-Alcaraz, B.J.; Jiménez, V.; Muñoz, D.; Ramón-Llin, J. Effectiveness and Distribution of Attacking Strokes to Finish the Point in Professional Padel. *Rev. Int. Med. Cienc. Act. Fís. Deport.* **2022**, *22*, 635–648. [CrossRef]
44. Zhou, Y.; Zong, S.; Cao, R.; Gómez, M.Á.; Chen, C.; Cui, Y. Using network science to analyze tennis stroke patterns. *Chaos Solitons Fractals* **2023**, *170*, 113305. [CrossRef]
45. Ramón-Llin, J.; Guzmán, J.; Martínez-Gallego, R.; Muñoz, D.; Sánchez-Pay, A.; Sánchez-Alcaraz, B.J. Analysis of the situation on the court of the players in the serve and itsrelationship with the direction, the side of the court and the result of the pointin high-level padel. *Retos* **2021**, *41*, 399–405. [CrossRef]
46. Reid, M.; McMurtrie, D.; Crespo, M. The relationship between match statistics and top 100 ranking in professional men's tennis. *Int. J. Perform. Anal. Sport* **2010**, *10*, 131–138. [CrossRef]
47. Sánchez-Pay, A.; Palao, J.M.; Torres-Luque, G.; Sanz-Rivas, D. Differences in set statistics between wheelchair and conventional tennis on different types of surfaces and by gender. *Int. J. Perform. Anal. Sport* **2015**, *15*, 1177–1188. [CrossRef]
48. Ramón-Llin, J.; Guzmán, J.; Martínez-Gallego, R.; Muñoz, D.; Sánchez-Pay, A.; Sánchez-Alcaraz, B.J. Stroke Analysis in Padel According to Match Outcome and Game Side on Court. *Int. J. Environ. Res. Public Health* **2020**, *17*, 7838. [CrossRef]

applied sciences

MDPI

Article

The Effectiveness of Exercise Programs on Balance, Functional Ability, Quality of Life, and Depression in Progressive Supranuclear Palsy: A Case Study

Panagiotis Papamichail [1], Michail Michalas [1], Dimitris Krokos [1], Maria Balamoutsou [1], Panagiota Karkoula [2], Epameinondas Lyros [1], Vasiliki Sakellari [3,]* and Anna Christakou [3,4]

[1] Department of Physiotherapy, School of Health Sciences, University of Peloponnese, 23100 Sparta, Greece; p.papamic@gmail.com (P.P.); michailmichalas12@gmail.com (M.M.); dimitriskkrokos@gmail.com (D.K.); mariabalamoutsou2@gmail.com (M.B.); lyrosep@yahoo.gr (E.L.)

[2] Physiotherapy Clinic "Fisiokinisis", 23100 Sparta, Greece; fusiokinisis@outlook.com.gr

[3] Department of Physiotherapy, School of Health Studies, University of West Attica, 12243 Athens, Greece; a.christakou@go.uop.gr

[4] Lab Biomechanics, Department of Physiotherapy, School of Health Sciences, University of Peloponnese, 23100 Sparta, Greece

* Correspondence: vsakellari@uniwa.gr

Abstract: Progressive supranuclear palsy is a form of atypical Parkinsonism. People living with Progressive Supranuclear Palsy have various symptoms, such as movement and cognitive disorders, which mainly affect balance and functional ability with an increased risk of falls, dexterity, and dementia. The role of exercise at the early stage of progressive supranuclear palsy remains unclear. The aim of the present study was to examine the effectiveness of an exercise program at the early stage of progressive supranuclear palsy. A patient with a diagnosis of progressive supranuclear palsy within the past year followed a supervised 12-week exercise program (two times per week) by a physiotherapist, with a session lasting about 40 min at a private physiotherapy clinic. Functional status, balance, quality of life, anxiety, and depression were assessed four times with valid instruments and tests. The results from the timed-up-and-go test demonstrated an improvement in performance (MCID value = 3.4). Improvements were observed in the scores of the Parkinson's Disease Questionnaire-39 (MCID value = 0.6). Finally, an improvement was reported in the score of the anxiety factor of the hospital anxiety and depression scale (MCID value = 1.5). Physiotherapy appears to improve functional capacity, quality of life, and mental health. Further research is needed to confirm these results with a large sample size in combination with other complementary therapies such as mental imagery.

Keywords: physiotherapy; Parkinson's disease; PSP; exercise; balance; functional ability; quality of life; depression; anxiety

1. Introduction

Progressive supranuclear palsy (PSP) is the most frequent form of atypical Parkinsonism, with a prevalence of 5–6 cases per 100,000 patients [1,2]. People living with PSP have various symptoms, such as movement disorders mainly affecting balance, functional inability with an increased risk of falls, and dexterity. Also, they demonstrate facial and cervical dystonia and oculomotor disorders [3,4]. Cognitive impairment, dementia, and depression are also associated with the overall progression of PSP [5,6]. Finally, they also often present with other comorbidities, such as cardiovascular, neurological, muscular, and urological disorders [7].

Early-stage PSP often manifests as behavioral changes, such as irritability and agitation, as well as subtle motor impairments, such as postural instability and falls, gait instability, and gaze abnormalities [8], which may affect an individual's quality of life and functional independence. This early phase of the disease may present a critical window of opportunity for interventions that could potentially maintain or even improve functional abilities.

Few studies have investigated the role of exercise in PSP. Exercise is defined as a repetitive, planned, structured activity aimed at improving and maintaining muscle strength, function, and fitness [9]. Exercise interventions have been shown to play a crucial role in improving balance and gait in patients with PSP. A pilot study reported improvements on balance performance after a therapeutic exercise program in PSP patients within a short duration of 4 weeks [10]. Similarly, other studies have reported that a structured physical therapy program is thought to be beneficial for individuals living with PSP [11–13]. Moreover, a case report showed the effectiveness of long-term locomotor training, stretching and strengthening exercises in enhancing balance, slowing the rate of gait decline, preventing wheelchair dependence, and reducing falls in a patient with mixed PSP and corticobasal degeneration features [14]. Due to the initial symptoms of PSP resembling those of idiopathic Parkinson's Disease (PD), physiotherapists often implement rehabilitation programs similar to those targeted at PD, focusing on increasing strength [15–17] and balance [18,19]. Commonly applied aerobic exercises for PD patients, such as cycling and dancing, may have potential applications for PSP as well [20,21]. However, the existing research is limited, and there is a need for further exploration of exercise-based approaches tailored to individuals with early-stage PSP.

The results of the present study provide a unique contribution to the field by examining the effects of a supervised exercise program on balance, functional ability, quality of life, and depression in an individual with early-stage of PSP. This approach contrasts with previous studies, which have predominantly focused on exercise interventions for individuals with moderate-to-advanced stages of the disease [10,22,23]. In contrast, the existing literature has tended to focus on single outcome measures, limiting the ability to capture the multifaceted impact of the disease and the diverse effects of exercise interventions [10].

Furthermore, the detailed description of an exercise program, encompassing warm-up, main exercises, and recovery components, provides valuable information for clinicians and researchers seeking to replicate or adapt successful exercise strategies for individuals with an early-stage PSP. This level of programmatic detail is often lacking in the current literature, hindering the translation of research findings into clinical practice.

By addressing these gaps in the existing literature, the results of the present study have the potential to inform the development of more effective, stage-appropriate exercise interventions for individuals with early-stage PSP, ultimately contributing to improved clinical outcomes and enhanced quality of life for this clinical population. Also, this study aimed to bridge the gap between the scarce literature available and clinical practice and to describe the effectiveness of a structured exercise program.

2. Materials and Methods

2.1. Participants

The inclusion criteria of the sample were as follows: (a) diagnosed with early-stage PSP, (b) understanding spoken and written language, (c) ambulatory, (d) no other serious health problems in the last month, and (e) willingness to take part in the study.

The exclusion criteria were: (a) moderate and severe stage PSP; (b) severe psychiatric problems; (c) serious health issues (e.g., medically significant cardiac or respiratory disease); and (d) inability to walk.

Three participants met the inclusion criteria, but finally one of them agreed to take part in the present study. The participant was a 78-year-old male diagnosed with PSP one year prior to the assessment. He demonstrated mild symmetrical limb Parkinsonism, voice change, and vertical gaze restriction, as well as balance problems, but has not yet used a walking aid. Other medical problems included arterial pressure and chronic obstructive pulmonary disease. Other demographic data are depicted in Table 1. A signed form was completed after being informed about the study's procedure. This study received approval from the Ethics Committee of the University of Peloponnese (661/11-1-2023).

Table 1. Characteristics of the participant.

Characteristics	
Gender	Male
Age (years)	78
Duration of illness (years)	1
Height (cm)	176
Body mass (kg)	90
BMI [1] kg/m^2	29.1

Abbreviations: [1] BMI: body mass index.

2.2. Measures and Instruments

Personal data were collected in the baseline assessment. Outcome measures were evaluated at four time points: (a) prior to the intervention (1st baseline assessment—E1), (b) at the 4th week of the intervention program—E2, (c) at the 8th week of the intervention program—E3, and (d) at the end of the exercise program at 12 weeks—E4. The outcome measures included:

1. Balance

The timed-up-and-go (TUG) test examines mobility and balance in elderly people. The time required for the participant to stand up from the chair, walk a distance of three meters, turn, walk back to the chair, and sit in it is recorded. For the execution, the physiotherapist uses a chair (with back and arms), a tape measure, a tape, and a watch or stopwatch. From the chair, we measure and mark a distance of three meters. As soon as the patient is seated, the timing stops. The time required to perform the test is approximately 10–35 s. The test has good reliability for Parkinson's disease [24].

2. Functional ability

The five times sit-to-stand test (FTSST) assesses the functional ability of the lower limbs. It is simple and short and designed for elderly people. The test begins with the participant sitting with their back on the chair, feet shoulder-width apart and arms crossed at chest level. The participant stands up using only the lower limbs and returns to the sitting position without touching the back of the chair 5 times as fast as possible. The test has good reliability in patients with Parkinson's Disease [25].

3. Quality of life

The Parkinson's disease questionnaire (PDQ-39) consists of 39 questions covering eight factors of patient's health. The score ranges from 0–4. A higher score indicates a worse quality of life. It has good internal consistency (Cronbach $\alpha = 0.71$–0.94) [26,27].

4. Depression

The hospital anxiety and depression scale (HADS) consists of 14 questions, examining anxiety and depression, 7 questions each, through a 4-point Likert-type scale from 0 (not at all) to 3 (happens to me all the time/often). The total score ranges from 0 to 21 for each factor. Higher scores also indicate increased levels of anxiety-depression. The classification for each factor separately is: 8–10 (mild), 11–14 (moderate), and 15–21 (severe). A score below 8 indicates no clinical findings of anxiety-depression. The scale shows high internal consistency (Cronbach $\alpha = 0.884$; anxiety factor 0.829, depression factor 0.840). Also, it has high test–retest reliability (ICC = 0.944) [28].

2.3. Procedure

The participant followed a 12-week intervention exercise program supervised by an experienced physiotherapist. The exercise program had a frequency of 2 times/week with 30–40 min duration per session. The customized exercises for this clinical population included three phases: the warm-up, the main part of the program, and the recovery (Table 2). The warm-up exercises, lasting 5–10 min, aimed to promote circulation and prepare the body for the rest of the program. The participant mobilized his joints and stretched his muscles. The main part of the program consisted of muscle-strengthening exercises, endurance exercises, balance exercises, upper and lower extremity exercises, trunk twists, fast and slow-tempo exercises, and movements with a sudden change of direction [29]. This phase, lasting 20–25 min, included moderate to high aerobic exercise based on the rating of perceived exertion scale (RPE) [30]. Specifics regarding the number of repetitions or sets for each exercise were incorporated for optimal effectiveness. The recovery phase, lasting 5–10 min, included stretching of the core muscles and relaxing exercises [31]. Another physiotherapist undertook the assessment of balance, functional ability, quality of life, and depression 4 times: at the beginning, during, and at the end of the exercise program, using the instruments described above.

Table 2. Description of the exercise program.

Variables	Warm Up	Main Program	Recovery
Duration	5–10 min	20–25 min	5–10 min
Exercises	Walking on the spot while simultaneously swinging the arms alternately	Rhythmic alternating movement of the lower limbs, with one limb always in contact with the ground	Cat–cow from a sitting position
	Neck turns	Light running	Vakrasana from a sitting position *
	Side bending of the head	Monopod support	Konasana *
	Shoulder lift	Jumping jack	Konasana from a sitting position
	Chest muscle stretching *	Big sideways steps	Vakrasana
	Hamstring stretch	Superman exercise *	Konasana 2 *
	Quadriceps stretch	Leg kicks	
		Hips sideways	

* Described in the Supplementary Materials (Appendix: Description of exercises).

2.4. Statistical Analysis

Descriptive statistics, including mean and standard deviation, were calculated for the four assessments of the study. The study used the minimal clinically important differences (MCID) values. As MCID is defined as the smallest difference in score in any domain or outcome that patients can perceive as beneficial or harmful, it would possibly require a change in their health care approach. This analysis aimed to determine if there were any clinical changes in the treatment outcome resulting from the implementation of the exercise program. A literature review was conducted to acknowledge the MCIDv for the present study's instruments. MCIDv is defined as the value of the MCID, which was used in the comparison with the reported differences (pre–post) of the participant's assessments. There have been no studies reporting the MCIDv for the instruments used in populations with PSP. However, the MCIDv for the PDQ-39 and its factors were found from Peto et al. [32], in which they followed a distribution-based approach to estimate them. The MCIDv for the FTSTS were found in studies regarding vestibular disorders [33,34], for the TUG in studies regarding postoperative patients with degenerative discopathy [35], and for the HADS and its factors (HADS-A and HADS-D) in populations with cardiovascular disease [36]. Then a comparison was made between the MCIDv and the reported differences (pre–post) of the participant's assessments. The MCIDv served as a threshold, identifying a reported difference (pre–post) as clinically important if its value exceeded the MCID [37].

3. Results

The participant demonstrated a high level of adherence, missing only one session throughout the entire 12-week intervention period, and that absence was due to personal reasons. The TUG and the FTSST were employed to assess participants' balance and functional ability, respectively. The HADS was used to assess depression and anxiety, and PQD-39 was used to evaluate the quality of life of the participant.

The MCIDv for TUG revealed an improvement in performance between E2−E1. However, threshold-based comparisons between MCID and reported differences in E3−E2 and E4−E3 showed no further differences since the difference value was lower than the MCIDv (Table 3), indicating a plateau in improvement over time.

Table 3. Differences between the four assessments on functional ability, balance, quality of life, and depression of the participant.

	Baseline E1	4 Weeks E2	8 Weeks E3	12 Weeks E4	MCID ∣E2 − E1∣	MCID ∣E3 − E2∣	MCID ∣E4 − E3∣	MCID Value
PDQ-39	5.12	7.5	5	5625	2.38 *	2.5 *	0.625 *	0.6
PDQ-39-Mobility	50	65	52.5	45	15 *	12.5 *	7.5 *	1.5
PDQ-39-ADL	29.1	29.1	20	20.8	-	9.1 *	0.8 *	0.7
PDQ-39-Emotional well-being	25	29.1	33.3	25	4.1 *	4.2 *	8.3 *	0.3
PDQ-39-Stigma	12.5	43.7	0	31.2	31.2 *	-	31.2 *	0.8
PDQ-39-Social support	0	8.3	0	16.6	8.3 *	-	16.6 *	1.2
PDQ-39-Cognition	18.7	37.5	6.2	31.25	18.8 *	31.3 *	25.05 *	0.4
PDQ-39-Communication	0	8.3	8.3	8.3	8.3 *	-	-	0.8
PDQ-39-Bodily discomfort	25	41.6	33.3	25	16.6 *	7.3 *	8.3 *	1.3
TUG	18	14	16	14	4 *	2	2	3.4
FTSST	17	14	21	17	3 *	7 *	4 *	2.3
HADS	20	22	14	16	2 *	7 *	2 *	1.7
HADS-Anxiety	14	10	10	11	4 *	-	1	1.5
HADS-Depression	6	12	4	5	6 *	8 *	1 *	0.5

Abbreviations: PDQ-39: The Parkinson's Disease Questionnaire-39; ADL: activities of daily living; TUG: timed-up-and-go; FTSST: five times sit-to-stand test; HADS: hospital anxiety and depression scale. * $p < 0.05$.

The statistical analysis for FTSST demonstrated an initial improvement in performance speed, followed by a subsequent deterioration. Ultimately, the final performance was similar to the baseline (Table 3).

The PQD-39 was used to assess the quality of life. The overall score had changed in all the MCID comparisons of the questionnaire, i.e., mobility, emotional well-being, cognition and bodily discomfort. The ADL dimension did not show a difference at the comparison between E1 and E2. The communication dimension did not show a difference at the comparison between E3−E2 and E4−E3 (Table 3).

HADS was used to examine the participant's anxiety and depression. The comparison between MCIDv and reported differences in E3−E2 and E4−E3 of the HADS-A revealed no change; only in E2−E1 appeared a reduction of anxiety. However, at the end of the program, differences were observed in the HADS-total score and in the HADS-D factor (Table 3).

4. Discussion

The purpose of the present study was to investigate the impact of an exercise program on balance, functional ability, quality of life, anxiety, and depression in an individual at an early stage of PSP. The results revealed some improvements in functional status and quality of life, as well as some reductions in anxiety and depression symptoms. However, the exercise program appeared to not have influenced balance.

The current case study found that a 12-week exercise program may not contribute to an improvement in balance; thus, more research with a larger group sample is needed.

This finding appears to be in contrast with some previous research on the effects of exercise interventions in individuals with PSP. Several case studies and small trials, included in a systematic review [38], did report improvements in balance and functional mobility following exercise interventions [10,18,39,40]. The exercise programs' duration and frequency of these four aforementioned studies were from 4 weeks to 3 years and from three to five times per week, respectively. The authors concluded that exercise therapy may help maintain or improve physical function, including balance, in people with PSP. However, the findings of the current case study are not entirely surprising, as the progressive nature of PSP presents significant challenges for rehabilitation. It is possible that the 12-week exercise program at the early stage of the PSP was not intensive or long-lasting enough to overcome the underlying neurological deficits contributing to the participant's balance difficulties. Additionally, the single-case design of the current study limits the generalizability of the findings. Individual responses to exercise can vary greatly, especially in a complex neurodegenerative condition like PSP. Larger-scale studies with more participants would be needed to better understand the role of exercise in managing balance problems in this population.

The findings of this case study reported some improvements in functional ability after a 12-week exercise program. This finding is generally consistent with the existing literature on the benefits of exercise for individuals with PSP [14,40–42]. Steffen et al. [14] reported that a physiotherapy intervention including locomotor training and exercise programs improved balance, slowed the rate of gait decline, decreased wheelchair dependence, and decreased falls in a patient with mixed PSP. Similarly, Suteerawattananon et al. [40] showed improved gait, fall reduction, and enhanced balance following physical therapy in a person with PSP [40]. A systematic review by Slade et al. [38], aiming to assess the efficacy of exercise and physical activity interventions in the PSP, concluded that exercise training may be beneficial [42]. A series of three case reports examined the effects of physical therapy and exercise interventions for patients with PSP reporting improvements in physical functional status [39]. Other studies demonstrate that exercise programs targeting muscle strengthening, balance, and mobility could improve functional outcomes and quality of life in this population [23,43–46]. The mechanisms by which exercise may benefit functional ability in PSP likely involve improvements in muscular strength, postural control, and mobility—all of which are typically impaired in this neurodegenerative disorder [46,47].

The study's findings may indicate improvements in participant scores in HADS-D due to an exercise intervention in individuals with PSP. Regarding the effect of exercise on depression in people with PSP, this study is unique and innovative as there are no other studies studying this topic; however, these findings are supported by a body of evidence exploring the mechanisms by which physical activity can influence psychological well-being in chronic neurologic disorders [48–50]. A systematic review reported that exercise programs targeting balance, gait, and physical functioning often resulted in improvements in measures of depression and quality of life [50]. These positive changes may be attributed to psychological mechanisms that influence the participant's self-image [51]. Exercise plays a role in removing the patient from negative thoughts enhancing self-esteem through the theory of self-efficacy and self-mastery [52]. From a neurobiological perspective, exercise has been shown to increase the production and release of neurotransmitters such as serotonin, dopamine, and endorphins, which can have mood-enhancing effects and contribute to the reduction of anxiety and depressive symptoms [53,54]. Additionally, physical activity can modulate the hypothalamic–pituitary–adrenal (HPA) axis, leading to decreased cortisol levels and improved regulation of the stress response system, which is often dysregulated in mood disorders [55]. Furthermore, exercise has been associated with increased hippocampal volume, enhanced neurogenesis, and improved connectivity in brain regions involved in emotional regulation, such as the prefrontal cortex and limbic system, all of which can contribute to the observed psychological benefits [56,57].

This study found an improvement in the quality of life of the participant. This result is in agreement with the limited existing research on the potential benefits of exercise for quality of life in individuals with PSP. A systematic review [58] provided preliminary evidence that exercise programs may improve quality of life in different studies with a small sample of PSP patients [23,43,59,60]. The current case study builds upon these findings, demonstrating that a 12-week exercise intervention targeting muscular strength, endurance, balance, and flexibility can lead to meaningful improvements in self-reported quality of life for an individual with early stage PSP.

Exercise has been demonstrated to influence a variety of neurobiological mechanisms that can have profound impacts on neurological health and function. One of the key processes is neuroplasticity, which refers to the brain's ability to reorganize and adapt its connections and function in response to changes in behavior, environment, or neural processes [61]. Turning to the specific case of PSP, these exercise-induced neurobiological changes could have therapeutic implications. PSP is a rare and debilitating neurodegenerative disorder characterized by progressive impairment of balance, gait, eye movements, and cognitive function [62]. The neurodegeneration in PSP is thought to involve excessive oxidative stress, mitochondrial dysfunction, and impaired neuroplasticity [6,63]. By enhancing neuroplasticity, promoting neurogenesis, and bolstering antioxidant defenses, exercise may help offset the neurological decline associated with PSP and potentially improve functional outcomes and quality of life for patients [64].

The exercise program, which included aerobic exercise in its main part, may prove effective in improving motor condition and functional ability. It targeted the most basic motor symptoms, resulting in some improvements. In the early stages of idiopathic Parkinson's disease, high-intensity interval training and progressive resistive strength training combined with movement strategies and education have been found to be effective for both motor symptoms such as gait and balance and falls rates [65,66]. The rehabilitation program followed by PSP patients often is similar to that of idiopathic Parkinson's disease's because initial symptoms or difficulty with function and activity limitations can appear similar [11,67]. As PSP progresses, the exercise programs often need to be adjusted to account for the changing functional abilities of the patient.

However, as the disease advances and balance, gait, and physical function decline, more targeted exercise strategies may be required. Restorative exercise approaches, such as those incorporating core stabilization, postural control, and compensatory movement patterns, might be beneficial. Additionally, exercise programs may need to be adapted to the specific stage of the disease. In the later stages of PSP, when mobility is severely impaired, exercises focusing on maintenance of range of motion, seated exercises, and activities to promote respiratory function may be more appropriate.

One limitation of the present study was the challenge in reaching general conclusions. Also, the use of TUG as the only tool to assess balance is a limitation of this study. However, the study's strength and differentiation was the use of MCIDv in the PSP population. To the best of our knowledge, no other study has demonstrated MCIDv in this clinical population until now. It is essential to acknowledge that MCIDv for various assessments, such as the FTSST in vestibular system disorders [33,34], the TUG in postoperative patients with degenerative disc disease [35], and the HADS in cardiovascular disease [36], have been reported in different contexts. Future research using larger sample sizes should be conducted to assess the effect of exercise programs, particularly at early stages, on PSP with more specific measurement tools like the progressive supranuclear palsy quality of life scale.

5. Conclusions

Participants with PSP commonly experience cognitive, emotional, and functional challenges. Therapeutic interventions for PSP often incorporate exercise programs. This study demonstrated that such exercise programs may have positive effects, improving patients' functional status, quality of life, anxiety, and depression at the early stage of PSP. While additional research is warranted to validate and strengthen the findings of the present study, those suggest that an exercise program may help mitigate the debilitating effects of this neurodegenerative disorder on patient wellbeing and daily functioning.

Supplementary Materials: The following supporting information can be downloaded at: https://www.mdpi.com/article/10.3390/app14188368/s1, Appendix: Description of exercises.

Author Contributions: Conceptualization, P.P. and A.C.; methodology, P.P., P.K. and A.C.; software, P.P. and D.K.; validation, E.L., V.S., P.K. and A.C.; formal analysis, M.M.; investigation, P.P., M.M. and M.B.; resources, P.P., D.K., M.M. and M.B.; data curation, D.K. and P.P.; writing—original draft preparation, P.P. and M.M.; writing—review and editing, A.C., E.L. and V.S.; visualization, P.P. and A.C.; supervision, A.C.; project administration, A.C. and V.S. All authors have read and agreed to the published version of the manuscript.

Funding: This research received no external funding.

Institutional Review Board Statement: The study was conducted in accordance with the Declaration of Helsinki and approved by the Ethics Committee of the School of Health Studies at the University of Peloponnese (661/11-1-2023).

Informed Consent Statement: Informed consent was obtained from all subjects involved in the study. Written informed consent was obtained from the patient to publish this paper.

Data Availability Statement: The data are available upon request from the corresponding author.

Acknowledgments: We would like to thank our participants for taking part in the present study.

Conflicts of Interest: The authors declare no conflicts of interest.

References

1. Ali, F.; Josephs, K. The Diagnosis of Progressive Supranuclear Palsy: Current Opinions and Challenges. *Expert. Rev. Neurother.* **2018**, *18*, 603–616. [CrossRef]
2. Stamelou, M.; Quinn, N.P.; Bhatia, K.P. "Atypical" Atypical Parkinsonism: New Genetic Conditions Presenting with Features of Progressive Supranuclear Palsy, Corticobasal Degeneration, or Multiple System Atrophy-a Diagnostic Guide. *Mov. Disord.* **2013**, *28*, 1184–1199. [CrossRef]
3. Glasmacher, S.A.; Leigh, P.N.; Saha, R.A. Predictors of Survival in Progressive Supranuclear Palsy and Multiple System Atrophy: A Systematic Review and Meta-Analysis. *J. Neurol. Neurosurg. Psychiatry* **2017**, *88*, 402–411. [CrossRef] [PubMed]
4. Lamb, R.; Rohrer, J.D.; Lees, A.J.; Morris, H.R. Progressive Supranuclear Palsy and Corticobasal Degeneration: Pathophysiology and Treatment Options. *Curr. Treat. Options Neurol.* **2016**, *18*, 42. [CrossRef] [PubMed]
5. Bluett, B.; Litvan, I. Pathophysiology, Genetics, Clinical Features, Diagnosis and Therapeutic Trials in Progressive Supranuclear Palsy. *Expert. Opin. Orphan Drugs* **2015**, *3*, 253–265. [CrossRef]
6. Boxer, A.L.; Yu, J.-T.; Golbe, L.I.; Litvan, I.; Lang, A.E.; Höglinger, G.U. Advances in Progressive Supranuclear Palsy: New Diagnostic Criteria, Biomarkers, and Therapeutic Approaches. *Lancet Neurol.* **2017**, *16*, 552–563. [CrossRef]
7. Zella, M.A.S.; Bartig, D.; Herrmann, L.; Respondek, G.; Höglinger, G.; Gold, R.; Woitalla, D.; Krogias, C.; Tönges, L. Hospitalization Rates and Comorbidities in Patients with Progressive Supranuclear Palsy in Germany from 2010 to 2017. *J. Clin. Med.* **2020**, *9*, 2454. [CrossRef]
8. Han, H.J.; Kim, H.; Park, J.-H.; Shin, H.-W.; Kim, G.U.; Kim, D.S.; Lee, E.J.; Oh, H.E.; Park, S.-H.; Kim, Y.J. Behavioral Changes as the Earliest Clinical Manifestation of Progressive Supranuclear Palsy. *J. Clin. Neurol.* **2010**, *6*, 148–151. [CrossRef]
9. Ellis, T.; Rochester, L. Mobilizing Parkinson's Disease: The Future of Exercise. *J. Parkinsons Dis.* **2018**, *8*, S95–S100. [CrossRef]
10. Matsuda, N.; Takamatsu, Y.; Aiba, I. Effect of Therapeutic Exercise on the Balance of Patients with Progressive Supranuclear Palsy: A Pilot Study. *Front. Neurol.* **2022**, *13*, 955893. [CrossRef]
11. Intiso, D.; Bartolo, M.; Santamato, A.; Di Rienzo, F. The Role of Rehabilitation in Patients with Progressive Supranuclear Palsy: A Narrative Review. *PM&R* **2018**, *10*, 636–645. [CrossRef]
12. Tilley, E.; White, S.; Peters, M.; Koblar, S.A.; McLoughlin, J. The Effectiveness of Allied Health Therapy in the Symptomatic Management of Progressive Supranuclear Palsy: A Systematic Review. *Protoc. JBI Database Syst. Rev. Implement. Rep.* **2014**, *12*, 119–137. [CrossRef]
13. Tilley, E.; McLoughlin, J.; Koblar, S.A.; Doeltgen, S.H.; Stern, C.; White, S.; Peters, M.D.J. Effectiveness of Allied Health Therapy in the Symptomatic Management of Progressive Supranuclear Palsy: A Systematic Review. *JBI Database Syst. Rev. Implement. Rep.* **2016**, *14*, 148–195. [CrossRef]
14. Steffen, T.M.; Boeve, B.F.; Mollinger-Riemann, L.A.; Petersen, C.M. Long-Term Locomotor Training for Gait and Balance in a Patient with Mixed Progressive Supranuclear Palsy and Corticobasal Degeneration. *Phys. Ther.* **2007**, *87*, 1078–1087. [CrossRef] [PubMed]

15. Canning, C.G.; Sherrington, C.; Lord, S.R.; Close, J.C.T.; Heritier, S.; Heller, G.Z.; Howard, K.; Allen, N.E.; Latt, M.D.; Murray, S.M.; et al. Exercise for Falls Prevention in Parkinson Disease: A Randomized Controlled Trial. *Neurology* **2015**, *84*, 304–312 [CrossRef] [PubMed]
16. Vieira de Moraes Filho, A.; Chaves, S.N.; Martins, W.R.; Tolentino, G.P.; de Cássia Pereira Pinto Homem, R.; Landim de Farias, G.; Fischer, B.L.; Oliveira, J.A.; Pereira, S.K.A.; Vidal, S.E.; et al. Progressive Resistance Training Improves Bradykinesia, Motor Symptoms and Functional Performance in Patients with Parkinson's Disease. *Clin. Interv. Aging* **2020**, *15*, 87–95. [CrossRef]
17. Gamborg, M.; Hvid, L.G.; Thrue, C.; Johansson, S.; Franzén, E.; Dalgas, U.; Langeskov-Christensen, M. Muscle Strength and Power in People with Parkinson Disease: A Systematic Review and Meta-Analysis. *J. Neurol. Phys. Ther.* **2023**, *47*, 3–15. [CrossRef]
18. Silva-Batista, C.; Corcos, D.M.; Kanegusuku, H.; Piemonte, M.E.P.; Gobbi, L.T.B.; de Lima-Pardini, A.C.; de Mello, M.T.; Forjaz, C.L.M.; Ugrinowitsch, C. Balance and Fear of Falling in Subjects with Parkinson's Disease Is Improved after Exercises with Motor Complexity. *Gait Posture* **2018**, *61*, 90–97. [CrossRef]
19. Giardini, M.; Nardone, A.; Godi, M.; Guglielmetti, S.; Arcolin, I.; Pisano, F.; Schieppati, M. Instrumental or Physical-Exercise Rehabilitation of Balance Improves Both Balance and Gait in Parkinson's Disease. *Neural Plast.* **2018**, *2018*, 5614242. [CrossRef]
20. Rocha, P.A.; Slade, S.C.; McClelland, J.; Morris, M.E. Dance Is More than Therapy: Qualitative Analysis on Therapeutic Dancing Classes for Parkinson's. *Complement Ther. Med.* **2017**, *34*, 1–9. [CrossRef]
21. Shanahan, J.; Morris, M.E.; Bhriain, O.N.; Volpe, D.; Lynch, T.; Clifford, A.M. Dancing for Parkinson Disease: A Randomized Trial of Irish Set Dancing Compared with Usual Care. *Arch. Phys. Med. Rehabil.* **2017**, *98*, 1744–1751. [CrossRef] [PubMed]
22. Zampieri, C.; Di Fabio, R.P. Balance and Eye Movement Training to Improve Gait in People with Progressive Supranuclear Palsy: Quasi-Randomized Clinical Trial. *Phys. Ther.* **2008**, *88*, 1460–1473. [CrossRef] [PubMed]
23. Clerici, I.; Ferrazzoli, D.; Maestri, R.; Bossio, F.; Zivi, I.; Canesi, M.; Pezzoli, G.; Frazzitta, G. Rehabilitation in Progressive Supranuclear Palsy: Effectiveness of Two Multidisciplinary Treatments. *PLoS ONE* **2017**, *12*, e0170927. [CrossRef] [PubMed]
24. Luque-Casado, A.; Novo-Ponte, S.; Sánchez-Molina, J.A.; Sevilla-Sánchez, M.; Santos-García, D.; Fernández-Del-Olmo, M. Test-Retest Reliability of the Timed Up and Go Test in Subjects with Parkinson's Disease: Implications for Longitudinal Assessments *J. Parkinsons Dis.* **2021**, *11*, 2047–2055. [CrossRef]
25. Duncan, R.P.; Leddy, A.L.; Earhart, G.M. Five Times Sit-to-Stand Test Performance in Parkinson's Disease. *Arch. Phys. Med. Rehabil.* **2011**, *92*, 1431–1436. [CrossRef]
26. Peto, V.; Jenkinson, C.; Fitzpatrick, R.; Greenhall, R. The Development and Validation of a Short Measure of Functioning and Well Being for Individuals with Parkinson's Disease. *Qual. Life Res.* **1995**, *4*, 241–248. [CrossRef]
27. Katsarou, Z.; Bostantjopoulou, S.; Peto, V.; Alevriadou, A.; Kiosseoglou, G. Quality of Life in Parkinson's Disease: Greek Translation and Validation of the Parkinson's Disease Questionnaire (PDQ-39). *Qual. Life Res.* **2001**, *10*, 159–163. [CrossRef]
28. Michopoulos, I.; Douzenis, A.; Kalkavoura, C.; Christodoulou, C.; Michalopoulou, P.; Kalemi, G.; Fineti, K.; Patapis, P.; Protopapas, K.; Lykouras, L. Hospital Anxiety and Depression Scale (HADS): Validation in a Greek General Hospital Sample. *Ann. Gen. Psychiatry* **2008**, *7*, 4. [CrossRef]
29. King, L.A.; Horak, F.B. Delaying Mobility Disability in People with Parkinson Disease Using a Sensorimotor Agility Exercise Program. *Phys. Ther.* **2009**, *89*, 384–393. [CrossRef]
30. Ferguson, B. *ACSM's Guidelines for Exercise Testing and Prescription*, 9th ed.; Lippincott Williams & Wilkins: Philadelphia, PA, USA, 2014; Volume 58, p. 328.
31. Kwok, J.Y.Y.; Kwan, J.C.Y.; Auyeung, M.; Mok, V.C.T.; Lau, C.K.Y.; Choi, K.C.; Chan, H.Y.L. Effects of Mindfulness Yoga vs Stretching and Resistance Training Exercises on Anxiety and Depression for People with Parkinson Disease: A Randomized Clinical Trial. *JAMA Neurol.* **2019**, *76*, 755–763. [CrossRef]
32. Peto, V.; Jenkinson, C.; Fitzpatrick, R. Determining Minimally Important Differences for the PDQ-39 Parkinson's Disease Questionnaire. *Age Ageing* **2001**, *30*, 299–302. [CrossRef] [PubMed]
33. Godi, M.; Franchignoni, F.; Caligari, M.; Giordano, A.; Turcato, A.M.; Nardone, A. Comparison of Reliability, Validity, and Responsiveness of the Mini-BESTest and Berg Balance Scale in Patients with Balance Disorders. *Phys. Ther.* **2013**, *93*, 158–167 [CrossRef] [PubMed]
34. Meretta, B.M.; Whitney, S.L.; Marchetti, G.F.; Sparto, P.J.; Muirhead, R.J. The Five Times Sit to Stand Test: Responsiveness to Change and Concurrent Validity in Adults Undergoing Vestibular Rehabilitation. *J. Vestib. Res.* **2006**, *16*, 233–243. [CrossRef]
35. Gautschi, O.P.; Stienen, M.N.; Corniola, M.V.; Joswig, H.; Schaller, K.; Hildebrandt, G.; Smoll, N.R. Assessment of the Minimum Clinically Important Difference in the Timed Up and Go Test After Surgery for Lumbar Degenerative Disc Disease. *Neurosurgery* **2017**, *80*, 380–385. [CrossRef] [PubMed]
36. Lemay, K.R.; Tulloch, H.E.; Pipe, A.L.; Reed, J.L. Establishing the Minimal Clinically Important Difference for the Hospital Anxiety and Depression Scale in Patients with Cardiovascular Disease. *J. Cardiopulm. Rehabil. Prev.* **2019**, *39*, E6–E11. [CrossRef] [PubMed]
37. Mouelhi, Y.; Jouve, E.; Castelli, C.; Gentile, S. How Is the Minimal Clinically Important Difference Established in Health-Related Quality of Life Instruments? Review of Anchors and Methods. *Health Qual. Life Pote* **2020**, *18*, 136. [CrossRef]
38. Slade, S.C.; Finkelstein, D.I.; McGinley, J.L.; Morris, M.E. Exercise and Physical Activity for People with Progressive Supranuclear Palsy: A Systematic Review. *Clin. Rehabil.* **2020**, *34*, 23–33. [CrossRef] [PubMed]

9. Mateus, M.; Castro Caldas, A. Physiotherapy Case Reports on Three People with Progressive Supranuclear Palsy. *Front. Aging Neurosci.* **2023**, *15*, 1294293. [CrossRef]
0. Suteerawattananon, M.; MacNeill, B.; Protas, E.J. Supported Treadmill Training for Gait and Balance in a Patient with Progressive Supranuclear Palsy. *Phys. Ther.* **2002**, *82*, 485–495. [CrossRef]
1. Shen, X.; Wong-Yu, I.S.K.; Mak, M.K.Y. Effects of Exercise on Falls, Balance, and Gait Ability in Parkinson's Disease: A Meta-Analysis. *Neurorehabil. Neural Repair* **2016**, *30*, 512–527. [CrossRef]
2. Shetty, A.; Krishnaprasad, K.M. Progressive Supranuclear Palsy-a Mirror Image of Parkinson's Disease, A Literature Review of Rehabilitation Strategies. *JPRI* **2021**, *57A*, 449–458. [CrossRef]
3. Wittwer, J.E.; Winbolt, M.; Morris, M.E. A Home-Based, Music-Cued Movement Program Is Feasible and May Improve Gait in Progressive Supranuclear Palsy. *Front. Neurol.* **2019**, *10*, 116. [CrossRef] [PubMed]
4. Dale, M.L.; Silva-Batista, C.; de Almeida, F.O.; Horak, F.B. Balance and Gait in Progressive Supranuclear Palsy: A Narrative Review of Objective Metrics and Exercise Interventions. *Front. Neurol.* **2023**, *14*, 1212185. [CrossRef] [PubMed]
5. Morris, M.E.; Slade, S.C.; Bruce, C.; McGinley, J.L.; Bloem, B.R. Enablers to Exercise Participation in Progressive Supranuclear Palsy: Health Professional Perspectives. *Front. Neurol.* **2020**, *11*, 635341. [CrossRef]
6. Litvan, I.; Bhatia, K.P.; Burn, D.J.; Goetz, C.G.; Lang, A.E.; McKeith, I.; Quinn, N.; Sethi, K.D.; Shults, C.; Wenning, G.K.; et al. Movement Disorders Society Scientific Issues Committee Report: SIC Task Force Appraisal of Clinical Diagnostic Criteria for Parkinsonian Disorders. *Mov. Disord.* **2003**, *18*, 467–486. [CrossRef]
7. Bloem, B.R. Postural Instability in Parkinson's Disease. *Clin. Neurol. Neurosurg.* **1992**, *94*, S41–S45. [CrossRef]
8. Dauwan, M.; Begemann, M.J.H.; Slot, M.I.E.; Lee, E.H.M.; Scheltens, P.; Sommer, I.E.C. Physical Exercise Improves Quality of Life, Depressive Symptoms, and Cognition across Chronic Brain Disorders: A Transdiagnostic Systematic Review and Meta-Analysis of Randomized Controlled Trials. *J. Neurol.* **2021**, *268*, 1222–1246. [CrossRef]
9. Cheon, S.-M.; Chae, B.-K.; Sung, H.-R.; Lee, G.C.; Kim, J.W. The Efficacy of Exercise Programs for Parkinson's Disease: Tai Chi versus Combined Exercise. *J. Clin. Neurol.* **2013**, *9*, 237–243. [CrossRef]
0. Adamson, B.C.; Ensari, I.; Motl, R.W. Effect of Exercise on Depressive Symptoms in Adults with Neurologic Disorders: A Systematic Review and Meta-Analysis. *Arch. Phys. Med. Rehabil.* **2015**, *96*, 1329–1338. [CrossRef]
1. Silva, J.M.; Klatsky, J. Body Image and Physical Activity. In *Recreation for the Disabled Child*; Routledge: London, UK, 1985; ISBN 9780203056325.
2. Mikkelsen, K.; Stojanovska, L.; Polenakovic, M.; Bosevski, M.; Apostolopoulos, V. Exercise and Mental Health. *Maturitas* **2017**, *106*, 48–56. [CrossRef]
3. Rethorst, C.D.; Wipfli, B.M.; Landers, D.M. The Antidepressive Effects of Exercise: A Meta-Analysis of Randomized Trials. *Sports Med.* **2009**, *39*, 491–511. [CrossRef] [PubMed]
4. Dishman, R.K.; Berthoud, H.-R.; Booth, F.W.; Cotman, C.W.; Edgerton, V.R.; Fleshner, M.R.; Gandevia, S.C.; Gomez-Pinilla, F.; Greenwood, B.N.; Hillman, C.H.; et al. Neurobiology of Exercise. *Obesity* **2006**, *14*, 345–356. [CrossRef] [PubMed]
5. Hamer, M.; Endrighi, R.; Poole, L. Physical Activity, Stress Reduction, and Mood: Insight into Immunological Mechanisms. *Methods Mol. Biol.* **2012**, *934*, 89–102. [CrossRef] [PubMed]
6. Schuch, F.B.; Deslandes, A.C.; Stubbs, B.; Gosmann, N.P.; da Silva, C.T.B.; de Fleck, M.P. A Neurobiological Effects of Exercise on Major Depressive Disorder: A Systematic Review. *Neurosci. Biobehav. Rev.* **2016**, *61*, 1–11. [CrossRef]
7. Firth, J.; Solmi, M.; Wootton, R.E.; Vancampfort, D.; Schuch, F.B.; Hoare, E.; Gilbody, S.; Torous, J.; Teasdale, S.B.; Jackson, S.E.; et al. A Meta-Review of "Lifestyle Psychiatry": The Role of Exercise, Smoking, Diet and Sleep in the Prevention and Treatment of Mental Disorders. *World Psychiatry* **2020**, *19*, 360–380. [CrossRef]
8. Slade, S.C.; Underwood, M.; McGinley, J.L.; Morris, M.E. Exercise and Progressive Supranuclear Palsy: The Need for Explicit Exercise Reporting. *BMC Neurol.* **2019**, *19*, 305. [CrossRef]
9. Nicolai, S.; Mirelman, A.; Herman, T.; Zijlstra, A.; Mancini, M.; Becker, C.; Lindemann, U.; Berg, D.; Maetzler, W. Improvement of Balance after Audio-Biofeedback. A 6-Week Intervention Study in Patients with Progressive Supranuclear Palsy. *Z. Gerontol. Geriatr.* **2010**, *43*, 224–228. [CrossRef]
0. Sale, P.; Stocchi, F.; Galafate, D.; De Pandis, M.F.; Le Pera, D.; Sova, I.; Galli, M.; Foti, C.; Franceschini, M. Effects of Robot Assisted Gait Training in Progressive Supranuclear Palsy (PSP): A Preliminary Report. *Front. Hum. Neurosci.* **2014**, *8*, 207. [CrossRef]
1. Kolb, B.; Gibb, R. Searching for the Principles of Brain Plasticity and Behavior. *Cortex* **2014**, *58*, 251–260. [CrossRef]
2. Williams, D.R.; Litvan, I. Parkinsonian Syndromes. *Continuum* **2013**, *19*, 1189–1212. [CrossRef]
3. Apetauerova, D.; Scala, S.A.; Hamill, R.W.; Simon, D.K.; Pathak, S.; Ruthazer, R.; Standaert, D.G.; Yacoubian, T.A. CoQ10 in Progressive Supranuclear Palsy. *Neurol. Neuroimmunol. Neuroinflamm* **2016**, *3*, e266. [CrossRef] [PubMed]
4. Frazzitta, G.; Maestri, R.; Ghilardi, M.F.; Riboldazzi, G.; Perini, M.; Bertotti, G.; Boveri, N.; Buttini, S.; Lombino, F.L.; Uccellini, D.; et al. Intensive Rehabilitation Increases BDNF Serum Levels in Parkinsonian Patients: A Randomized Study. *Neurorehabil Neural Repair.* **2014**, *28*, 163–168. [CrossRef] [PubMed]
5. Schenkman, M.; Moore, C.G.; Kohrt, W.M.; Hall, D.A.; Delitto, A.; Comella, C.L.; Josbeno, D.A.; Christiansen, C.L.; Berman, B.D.; Kluger, B.M.; et al. Effect of High-Intensity Treadmill Exercise on Motor Symptoms in Patients With De Novo Parkinson Disease: A Phase 2 Randomized Clinical Trial. *JAMA Neurol.* **2018**, *75*, 219–226. [CrossRef]

66. Morris, M.E.; Menz, H.B.; McGinley, J.L.; Watts, J.J.; Huxham, F.E.; Murphy, A.T.; Danoudis, M.E.; Iansek, R. A Randomized Controlled Trial to Reduce Falls in People with Parkinson's Disease. *Neurorehabil Neural Repair.* **2015**, *29*, 777–785. [CrossRef]
67. Ashok, C.; Anitha, A.; Keerthi, P. Physiotherapy management for progressive Supranuclear palsy. *Int. J. Physiother. Res.* **2013**, 2 41–45.

applied sciences

MDPI

Article

Effects of Exercise and Pomegranate–Black Carrot Juice Interventions on Mineral Metabolism and Fatty Acids

Kenan Bozbay [1], Vedat Çinar [2], Taner Akbulut [2], Isa Aydemir [3], Yavuz Yasul [4], Kursat Yusuf Aytac [5], Ahmet Ozkaya [6], Luca Russo [7,*], Andrea Fusco [8,†] and Gian Mario Migliaccio [9,†]

1 Institute of Health Sciences, Faculty Sport Science, Firat University, Elazig 23119, Turkey; kenanbozbay21@gmail.com
2 Department of Physical Education and Sport, Faculty Sport Science, Firat University, Elazig 23119, Turkey; vcinar@firat.edu.tr (V.Ç.); takbulut@firat.edu.tr (T.A.)
3 Department of Physical Education and Sport, Faculty of Education, Hakkari University, Hakkari 30100, Turkey; aydemirisa23@gmail.com
4 Bafra Vocational School, Ondokuz Mayıs University, Samsun 55400, Turkey; yavuz.yasul@omu.edu.tr
5 Department of Physical Education and Sport, Faculty Sport Science, Adiyaman University, Adiyaman 0200, Turkey; kyaytac@adiyaman.edu.tr
6 Department of Chemistry and Chemical Processing Techniques, Vocational School of Technical Sciences, Adiyaman University, Adiyaman 0200, Turkey; aozkaya@adiyaman.edu.tr
7 eCampus University, 22060 Novedrate, Italy
8 Department of Medicine and Aging Sciences, University "G. d'Annunzio" of Chieti-Pescara, 66100 Chieti, Italy; andrea.fusco@unich.it
9 Department of Human Sciences and Promotion of the Quality of Life, San Raffaele Rome Open University, 00166 Rome, Italy; gianmario.migliaccio@uniroma5.it
* Correspondence: luca.russo2@uniecampus.it
† These authors contributed equally to this work.

Abstract: In this study, the effects of exercise applied to sedentary individuals and the use of pomegranate–black carrot juice on minerals, fatty acids and some biochemical parameters were examined. Twenty healthy sedentary men participated in this study. This research consisted of three stages. Blood samples were taken from the participants before this study (Baseline), after the participants exercised (60 min/day) for 10 days ($Exercise_{only}$), after the participants were given pomegranate–black carrot juice mixture (100 mL/100 mL) along with exercise (60 min/day) for 10 days ($Exercise_{+supp}$). While AST and ALT levels increased in the $Exercise_{only}$ phase, they showed a relative decrease in the $Exercise_{+supp}$ phase. It was determined that Mg level in the $Exercise_{only}$ phase decreased compared to the Baseline and the $Exercise_{+supp}$ phase. It was determined that the Zn level in the $Exercise_{+supp}$ phase increased compared to the Zn level in the $Exercise_{only}$ phase. It was determined that 6:0, 12:0 and 14:0 fatty acid levels increased in the $Exercise_{only}$ phase compared to the Baseline. A decrease was detected in the $Exercise_{only}$ phase compared to the Baseline 18:2n6c, 18:3n6 and 18:3n3 fatty acid levels. It can be said that exercise and the use of pomegranate–black carrot juice mixture in sedentary individuals have supportive and corrective effects on serum mineral, fatty acids and some biochemical parameters.

Keywords: exercise; pomegranate–black carrot juice; minerals; lipid metabolism

1. Introduction

Athletes often turn to micronutrient supplements to improve their performance, improve immune function, or correct mineral and vitamin deficiencies [1]. In addition, athletes consume antioxidant-containing foods to minimize oxidative stress that may occur due to exercise as well as to increase their performance [2]. One of the important antioxidant sources that can reduce the harmful effects of oxidative stress is fruits and vegetables [3]. Fruits and vegetables have a very rich content of vitamins, minerals, fiber and antioxidants [4].

It has been stated that pomegranate (*Punica granatum* L.) fruit, which has many healing properties for health, prevents or helps treat various disease risk markers (such as oxidative stress, hyperglycemia, high cholesterol and inflammatory activities) [5]. It has been reported that regular consumption of pomegranate juice or pomegranate juice concentrate (PJC) is associated with a decrease in blood pressure, improvement in blood lipid levels and reduction in oxidative stress [6,7]. Fuster-Mũnoz et al. (2016) reported that pomegranate juice supplementation had a positive effect on the modulation of fat and protein damage in endurance-based athletes [8]. The reason for this healing feature of pomegranate is due to the various phytochemicals it contains, which are responsible for its strong antioxidant and anti-inflammatory potential [9]. It is emphasized that black carrot (*Dacus carota* L.), which has another antioxidant property and is a source of polyphenols, including phenolic acids, has significant effects on improving health [10]. These, like pomegranate, increase antioxidant activity [11] and also lead to improvements in lipid peroxidation and cardiovascular risk markers [12]. Additionally, a recent study reported that the combined application of pomegranate–black carrot juice with exercise reduced the level of oxidative stress [13]. It is stated that exercise causes an increase in oxidative enzymes and microinjuries in skeletal muscle [14]. Additionally, some studies have reported that Aspartate Aminotransferase (AST) and Alanine Aminotransferase (ALT) enzymes increase, depending on the type and intensity of exercise [15–17]. However, there is no clear consensus in the literature as to which form of exercise can change these parameters and to what extent.

One of the macronutrients that is important for the human body is lipids [18]. Since the lipid profile changes depending on physical activity, it is very important to understand the working mechanism of lipid metabolism for both athletes and sedentary individuals [19]. In a study conducted by Bengin et al., it was reported that exercise and diet application can regulate one's lipid profile, ghrelin, and leptin levels, and increased irisin with exercise can activate lipid metabolism and support positive changes in lean mass [20]. Fatty acids (FAs) are also an important energy source during exercise [21–23]. FAs are considered a basic component of the erythrocyte membrane. In addition, exercise and nutrition are two factors that affect their structure and function [24]. In a study conducted by Corsetto et al., it was reported that physical activity application combined with a standard diet program caused a significant decrease in linoleic acid (C18:2) and omega-6 PUFAs and an increase in stearic acid (C18:0) and oleic acid (C18:1) concentrations [25]. FAs are an important energy source for skeletal muscle contraction, especially during light–moderate intensity and long-term exercise [26]. It has been stated that FAs and lipid intermediates derived from them may play a role in the regulation of skeletal muscle mass and function [27].

Consuming antioxidant-containing foods can reduce exercise-induced muscle damage and oxidative stress markers. For this reason, the hypothesis that the beneficial effects of pomegranate–black carrot juice, known for its rich antioxidant content, may have positive effects on mineral metabolism, fatty acids and some biochemical parameters was tested in this study.

In light of all this information, this study aimed to examine the effects of pomegranate–black carrot juice mixture applied together with exercise on mineral metabolism, fatty acids and some biochemical parameters in sedentary individuals.

2. Materials and Methods

Before starting this research, ethical approval was received from Fırat University/Non-Interventional Research Ethics Committee, dated 25 April 2019, meeting number 07 and decision number 15. A total of 20 healthy male students studying at Fırat University, not doing sports regularly, living in dormitories affiliated with the credit dormitories institution, subject to the same nutrition program and having no obstacle to doing sports voluntarily participated in this study (age: mean $\pm$ s.d. = 21.1 $\pm$ 2.3 years, height: mean $\pm$ s.d. = 175.6 $\pm$ 2.9 cm, body weight: mean $\pm$ s.d. = 75.2 $\pm$ 3.1 kg). Before this study, an analysis was conducted using G*Power (Version 3.1) to determine the statistical power and the required minimum sample size. Based on the research findings of Ammar et al. [28], this analysis indicated that with a Type I error rate (alpha) of 0.05, a test power (1-beta) of 0.80 and an effect size of 1.439, a minimum sample size of 9 participants was necessary to detect a significant difference under a two-tailed alternative hypothesis (H1). However, to obtain stronger and more reliable results, this study was conducted with 20 participants. Exclusion criteria from this study were (1) not following the exercise program and not consuming pomegranate–black carrot juice throughout this study and (2) refusing to donate blood and experiencing any injury during this study. This study was designed as a non-randomized, single-blind and crossover research design model. This research consisted of three stages. Serum samples were obtained from blood samples taken from the participants at each stage (three different stages).

2.1. Research Design

The research design consists of three different phases. It is shown in the figure (Figure 1).

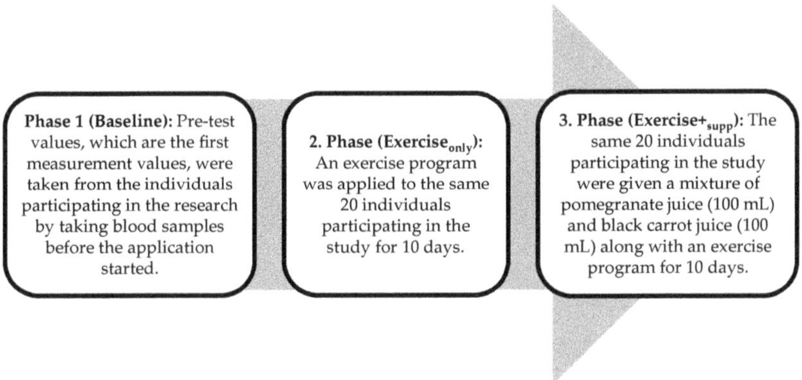

Figure 1. General research protocol.

2.2. Exercise Protocol

This research was carried out at Fırat University/Multi-Purpose Sports Hall, and before starting this research, a comprehensive explanation was given to the participants about the exercise program to be implemented with expert trainers. The participants completed long-term aerobic flat running (5000 m) over 10 days. Then, they completed 3 × 10 sit-ups and 3 × 10 push-ups and performed cool-down exercises. Exercises were performed every day between 16.00 and 17.00 to avoid circadian variations as with other study protocols [29–31]. Participants completed flat running exercises at a standard pace of 65–70% of their maximum heart rate (HR) (50–55% VO_2max). Maximum HR was calculated according to the Karvonen formula (220-Age-DN × Exercise intensity + DN). To control running speeds, HR during exercise was monitored simultaneously with a telemetric HR monitor (S610i, Polar Electro Oy, Kempele, Finland).

2.3. Giving Pomegranate–Black Carrot Juices

The pomegranate fruit taken daily was cleaned by washing with distilled water, and the juice was obtained in a juicer after the pomegranates were separated from their peels. Black carrot juice was also obtained using the same method. Pomegranate–black carrot juice was given to the participants daily, 45 min before starting each exercise program (for 10 days) in the second stage [13]. No additional chemical products were added to the natural pomegranate–black carrot juice. In the literature, the content of pomegranate juice was determined as 490.75 mg/kg of phenolic acid, 137.1 mg/L of anthocyanin, 175 mg/100 g of ellagic acid, 63 mg/kg of total flavonoids and 1530 mg/kg of total antioxidants [32]. In black carrot juice, anthocyanins were found to be 837 mg/100 g, total phenolics 7.98–291.48 mg/100 g, flavonoids 3.00–111.70 mg/100 g, flavonols 51.6 mg/100 g and falcarinol 1.55 mg/100 g [33].

2.4. Analysis of Biochemical Parameters

2.4.1. Obtaining Serum Samples

When each stage of this research was completed, venous blood samples were taken from the participants' arms with a heparin syringe that can draw 5 mL of blood. In order to make blood collection easier after exercise, an intraket was inserted into the participants before exercise. Serum samples were obtained by centrifuging the blood samples at 4000 rpm for 10 min under appropriate conditions. The analysis of the serums was performed by the photometric method on the ARCHITECT Cİ 16,200 TM analyzer in the biochemistry laboratory of Fırat University Faculty of Medicine. AST, ALT, TG and cholesterol measurements were made of the serum samples in a short time.

2.4.2. Analysis of Serum Mineral Levels

Of the samples, 0.5 g was taken and transferred to the DAP60-K PTFE containers of the microwave dissolving system and 4 Ml HNO_3 (65% *w*/*v*), and 1 mL $HClO_4$ (60% *v*/*w*) was added. After thawing, the dissolved samples were transferred to 20 mL volumetric flasks and made up a final volume of 0.1 M HNO_3. Additionally, blank samples were prepared and thawed in the same manner. Stock solutions of the analyzed Copper (Cu), Magnesium (Mg), Manganese (Mn), Iron (Fe) and Zinc (Zn) minerals were prepared and calibrated on the device. Finally, the obtained solutions were analyzed using the ICP-MS device [34].

2.4.3. Analysis of Serum Fatty Acid Levels

Of the serum samples, 0.5 mL was taken and homogenized in a hexane/isopropanol (3:2 *v*/*v*) mixture. Lipid extracts were centrifuged at 5000 rpm for 5 min. Afterwards, the solvents were removed at 40 °C [35]. Fatty acids in lipid extracts were treated with 2% sulfuric acid (*v*/*v*) in methanol and converted into methyl esters. Fatty acids present in lipid extracts were analyzed using gas chromatography. Three repeat measurements were made for each sample. The results obtained were expressed as the total percentage of each fatty acid among the total fatty acids, and the calculations were carried out using the GC Solutions 2.42 program.

2.5. Statistical Analysis

The data were analyzed using SPSS version 22.0 (SPSS Inc., Chicago, IL, USA). The data are reported as mean and standard deviation. Data normality was verified using the Shapiro–Wilk test. The assumptions of sphericity were assessed by Mauchly's test. Whenever an assumption was violated, a Greenhouse–Geisser correction was applied on the degree of freedom if the epsilon (ε) value was <0.75 and a Huynh–Feldt correction was applied if ε was >0.75. A one-way analysis of variance for repeated measures was used to compare the variables related to different exercise forms. When a difference was found, a Bonferroni post hoc test was applied. Partial eta squared ($\eta_p{}^2$) was used to evaluate effect sizes. The alpha level was set at 0.05 for all the tests.

3. Results

When looking at Table 1, while an increase was observed in the AST and ALT levels of the $\text{Exercise}_{\text{only}}$ phase compared to the AST and ALT levels of the Baseline phase ($p < 0.05$), a relative decrease was detected in the AST and ALT levels of the $\text{Exercise}_{\text{+supp}}$ phase ($p > 0.05$). The $\text{Exercise}_{\text{+supp}}$ phase AST and ALT levels decreased compared to $\text{Exercise}_{\text{only}}$ phase AST and ALT levels ($p < 0.05$). No statistical difference was observed between cholesterol levels of all stages ($p > 0.05$). A decrease was detected in the TG level in the $\text{Exercise}_{\text{only}}$ and $\text{Exercise+}_{\text{supp}}$ phases compared to the TG level in the Baseline phase ($p < 0.05$).

Table 1. Serum biochemistry levels.

Stages	AST (U/L)	ALT (U/L)	CHOLESTEROL (mg/dL)	TG (mg/dL)
Baseline	26.66 ± 1.40	25.33 ± 1.23	144.22 ± 4.58	91.01 ± 4.86
Exercise$_{only}$	29.22 ± 0.98 ^{a}	28.88 ± 1.26 ^{a}	138.66 ± 5.28	67.77 ± 5.32 ^{a}
Exercise$_{+supp}$	24.77 ± 0.52 ^{x}	24.66 ± 1.45 ^{x}	136.33 ± 5.29	68.55 ± 5.02 ^{a}
	η_p^2: 0.33	η_p^2: 0.32	η_p^2: 0.02	η_p^2: 0.65

Comparison of other stages according to the Baseline stage; a: $p < 0.05$. Comparison of Exercise$_{only}$ and Exercise+$_{supp}$ phases; x: $p < 0.05$; η_p^2: partial eta squared.

When looking at Table 2, it was observed that there was no statistical difference between Cu levels at all stages ($p > 0.05$). It was determined that the Exercise$_{only}$ phase Mg level decreased compared to the Baseline phase and Exercise$_{+supp}$ phase Mg level ($p < 0.05$). It was determined that there was no statistical difference between Mn levels at all stages ($p > 0.05$). It was determined that Fe levels in the Exercise$_{only}$ phase and Exercise$_{+supp}$ phase decreased significantly compared to the Fe level in the Baseline phase ($p < 0.001$). A decrease in Zn level was observed in the Exercise$_{only}$ phase ($p < 0.001$) and Exercise$_{+supp}$ phase ($p < 0.01$) compared to the Zn level in the Baseline phase. It was determined that the Zn level in the Exercise$_{+supp}$ phase increased compared to the Zn level in the Exercise$_{only}$ phase ($p < 0.001$).

Table 2. Serum mineral levels (ppb).

Stages	Cu	Mg	Mn	Fe	Zn
Baseline	748.55 ± 21.03	18,626.31 ± 206.01	5.70 ± 0.25	2883.90 ± 123.88	1270.26 ± 22.08
Exercise$_{only}$	776.47 ± 19.92	17,798.75 ± 171.65 ^{a}	4.85 ± 0.24	1680.52 ± 62.34 ^{c}	885.84 ± 24.97 ^{c}
Exercise$_{+supp}$	797.64 ± 18.47	18,689.53 ± 337.32 ^{x}	4.69 ± 0.26	1591.20 ± 63.24 ^{c}	1090.22 ± 18.30 ^{bz}
	η_p^2: 0.02	η_p^2: 0.04	η_p^2: 0.34	η_p^2: 0.90	η_p^2: 0.39

Comparison of other stages according to the Baseline stage. a: $p < 0.05$; b: $p < 0.01$; c: $p < 0.001$. Comparison of Exercise$_{only}$ and Exercise+$_{supp}$ phases. x: $p < 0.05$; z: $p < 0.001$; η_p^2: partial eta squared.

When looking at Table 3, it was determined that the ∑SFA level in the Exercise$_{only}$ and Exercise$_{+supp}$ phases was higher than the ∑SFA level in the Baseline phase ($p < 0.05$). It was observed that ∑PUFA and ∑USFA levels in Exercise$_{only}$ and Exercise$_{+supp}$ phases decreased compared to Baseline phase ∑PUFA and ∑USFA levels ($p > 0.05$, $p < 0.01$). In the Exercise$_{only}$ phase, 6:0, 12:0 and 14:0 fatty acid levels were found to increase compared to the Baseline phase ($p < 0.05$). Exercise$_{only}$ and Exercise$_{+supp}$ phase 16:1 fatty acid levels decreased compared to of the Baseline phase fatty acid levels ($p < 0.05$, $p < 0.01$). It was observed that the 18:0 level in the Exercise$_{only}$ and Exercise$_{+supp}$ phases increased compared to the Baseline phase ($p < 0.05$). A decrease was detected in the Exercise$_{only}$ phase compared to the Baseline phase 18:2n6c, 18:3n6 and 18:3n3 fatty acid levels ($p < 0.05$; $p < 0.01$). It was determined that the level of 18:2n6c in the Exercise$_{+supp}$ phase increased compared to the Exercise$_{only}$ phase ($p < 0.05$). It was observed that the 20:5n3 level in the Exercise$_{only}$ phase decreased compared to the Baseline phase ($p < 0.001$).

Table 3. Serum fatty acid levels (%).

		Stages			
Fatty Acids		**Baseline**	**Exercise$_{only}$**	**Exercise$_{+supp}$**	η_p^2
Caproic acid	(6:0)	0.173 ± 0.017	0.232 ± 0.007 ^{a}	0.208 ± 0.006	0.98
Lauric acid	(12:0)	0.054 ± 0.012	0.130 ± 0.028 ^{a}	0.090 ± 0.014	0.97
Myristic acid	(14:0)	0.321 ± 0.031	0.383 ± 0.023 ^{a}	0.339 ± 0.032	0.37

Table 3. *Cont.*

Fatty Acids		Stages Baseline	$Exercise_{only}$	$Exercise_{+supp}$	η_p^2
Pentadeconic acid	(15:0)	0.126 ± 0.009	0.134 ± 0.015	0.155 ± 0.012	0.30
Palmitic acid	(16:0)	22.484 ± 0.498	24.159 ± 0.279	22.808 ± 0.535	0.08
Heptadeconic acid	(17:0)	0.342 ± 0.012	0.331 ± 0.021	0.317 ± 0.014	0.03
Stearic acid	(18:0)	26.090 ± 0.520	29.845 ± 0.327 [a]	29.882 ± 0.833 [a]	0.23
Arachidic acid	(20:0)	0.361 ± 0.017	0.409 ± 0.015	0.444 ± 0.019 [a]	0.20
Behenic acid	(22:0)	0.339 ± 0.031	0.399 ± 0.017	0.378 ± 0.028	0.32
Trichosanoic acid	(23:0)	0.077 ± 0.008	0.112 ± 0.008	0.121 ± 0.033	0.70
Lingoseric acid	(24:0)	0.285 ± 0.038	0.339 ± 0.020	0.302 ± 0.020	0.36
Total saturated fatty acid level	(∑SFA)	50.652 ± 1.551	56.473 ± 2.014 [a]	55.044 ± 1.706 [a]	0.17
Pentadecanoic acid	(15:1)	0.657 ± 0.024	0.815 ± 0.024 [b]	0.793 ± 0.019 [b]	0.45
Palmitoleic acid	(16:1)	1.241 ± 0.065	1.035 ± 0.029 [a]	0.828 ± 0.012 [b]	0.42
Oleic acid	(18:1n9c)	8.665 ± 0.241	7.802 ± 0.219	8.195 ± 0.395	0.16
Eicosenoic acid	(20:1n9c)	0.135 ± 0.009	0.132 ± 0.008	0.139 ± 0.005	0.04
Nervonic acid	(24:1)	0.262 ± 0.015	0.320 ± 0.015	0.304 ± 0.017	0.41
Total monounsaturated fatty acid level	(∑MUFA)	10.96 ± 0.542	10.104 ± 0.437	10.259 ± 0.611	0.10
Linoleic acid	(18:2n6c)	23.153 ± 0.113	20.637 ± 0.149 [a]	22.174 ± 0.120 [x]	0.19
Linoleadic acid	(18:2n6t)	0.033 ± 0.002	0.045 ± 0.002 [a]	0.038 ± 0.002	0.66
Gamma-linolenic acid	(18:3n6)	0.115 ± 0.014	0.069 ± 0.008 [b]	0.070 ± 0.006 [b]	0.88
Alpha-linolenic acid	(18:3n3)	0.172 ± 0.082	0.097 ± 0.013 [b]	0.118 ± 0.011 [b]	0.90
Eicosatrienoic acid	(20:3n6)	2.034 ± 0.191	1.750 ± 0.159 [a]	1.750 ± 0.166 [a]	0.30
Eicosapentaenoic acid	(20:5n3)	0.242 ± 0.026	0.116 ± 0.023 [c]	0.169 ± 0.017 [a]	0.95
Docosahexaenoic acid	(22:6n3)	2.520 ± 0.066	1.517 ± 0.025 [a]	1.548 ± 0.037 [a]	0.88
Eicosadienoic acid	(20:2n6)	0.292 ± 0.018	0.278 ± 0.019	0.255 ± 0.020	0.11
Eicosatetraenoic acid	(20:4n6)	9.827 ± 0.265	8.914 ± 0.299	8.575 ± 0.431	0.15
Total polyunsaturated fatty acid level	(∑PUFA)	38.388 ± 1.478	33.423 ± 1.130 [b]	34.697 ± 1.342 [a]	0.26
Total unsaturated fatty acid level	(∑USFA)	49.348 ± 1.854	43.527 ± 1.566 [b]	44.956 ± 1.415 [a]	0.22

Comparison of other stages according to the Baseline stage. a: $p < 0.05$; b: $p < 0.01$; c: $p < 0.001$. Comparison of $Exercise_{only}$ and $Exercise_{+supp}$ phases. x: $p < 0.05$; η_p^2: partial eta squared.

4. Discussion

This study aimed to examine the effects of an exercise program applied to sedentary individuals and the use of pomegranate–black carrot juice mixture on serum mineral and fatty acid levels and some biochemical parameters.

In this study, when the changes in serum biochemistry levels were evaluated (Table 1), no statistical difference was observed between cholesterol levels of all stages. A decrease in TG levels in the $Exercise_{only}$ and $Exercise_{+supp}$ phases was detected compared to the TG level in the Baseline phase. In addition, while an increase was observed in the $Exercise_{only}$ phase compared to the AST and ALT levels of the Baseline phase, a relative decrease was detected in the AST and ALT levels of the $Exercise_{+supp}$ phase. Considering the studies conducted in this context, it has been reported that aerobic exercise significantly reduces low-density lipoprotein cholesterol (LDL-C), very low-density lipoprotein cholesterol (VLDL-C) and TG, while improving high-density lipoprotein cholesterol (HDL-C) [36]. It has been reported in different studies that regular exercise has positive effects on LDL-C,

TG and HDL-C [37,38]. Although the mechanisms underlying the effect of exercise on the lipid profile are not clear, it is stated that exercise increases the ability of skeletal muscles to use lipids instead of glycogen, thus reducing plasma lipid levels [39]. It has been reported that AST and ALT levels increased significantly at the end of the run compared to before the run in three different long-distance runs and ultramarathon runners [40,41]. In a study conducted on pomegranate juice, it was reported that an 8-week combined application (aerobic training and pomegranate juice intake) significantly reduced AST, ALT and Gamma Glutamyl Transferase (GGT) enzymes compared to the aerobic training group alone and the pomegranate juice group alone [42]. This effect of pomegranate juice is thought to be due to its ability to reduce the activity of AST, ALT and GGT enzymes, possibly by reducing blood glucose, increasing the glycation of antioxidant enzymes and the level of reactive oxygen species (ROS) [43]. In line with the findings obtained in this study, the changes in serum AST and ALT are similar to the research findings in the literature. We think that the decrease in AST and ALT levels in the $\text{Exercise}_{+\text{supp}}$ phase back to the levels in the Baseline phase is due to the effect of the pomegranate–black carrot juice mixture.

In this study, when the changes in serum mineral levels were evaluated (Table 2) and compared to the Baseline phase, Mg, Mn, Fe and Zn levels decreased in the $\text{Exercise}_{\text{only}}$ phase, while only the Cu level increased. An increase in Cu, Mg and Zn levels was observed in the $\text{Exercise}_{+\text{supp}}$ phase compared to the $\text{Exercise}_{\text{only}}$ phase. Minerals and trace elements are micronutrients that play a role in hundreds of biological processes, and their deficiency can negatively affect athletic performance [44]. Considering the studies conducted in this context, it has been reported that Mg intake has a positive effect on exercise performance and different muscle strength measurements [45–48]. It has been stated that exercise performance is negatively affected by Mg deficiency [49,50]. Additionally, when studies on Zn are examined, it has been observed that serum Zn levels decrease after exercise compared to before exercise in different physical effort tests defined as aerobic endurance and muscle strength [51–53]. It has been reported that Zn deficiency causes decreases in physical performance and is associated with higher oxidative stress [54,55]. When we look at the studies on Mg and Zn in the literature, it is seen that the intake of these minerals has effects on exercise performance. When the findings of this research are evaluated, it is thought that the Mg and Zn levels decreased in the $\text{Exercise}_{\text{only}}$ phase and increased again in the $\text{Exercise}_{+\text{supp}}$ phase due to the minerals contained in the pomegranate–black carrot juice mixture.

When changes in serum fatty acid levels are evaluated (Table 3) in the $\text{Exercise}_{\text{only}}$ phase, serum-saturated fatty acids of 6:0, 12:0, 14:0 and 18:0 fatty acids were found to be statistically higher than the Baseline phase. Additionally, a relative increase in the 16:0 fatty acid level was observed. It was observed that the levels of serum fatty acids 16:1, 18:2n6c, 18:3n6, 18:3n3, 20:3n6, 20:5n3 and 22:6n3 in the $\text{Exercise}_{\text{only}}$ phase decreased compared to the Baseline phase. In addition, it was observed that 18:1n9c, 18:2n6c and 20:4n6 fatty acids, which are important unsaturated fatty acids, decreased in the $\text{Exercise}_{\text{only}}$ phase compared to the Baseline phase. It was observed that 18:2n6c fatty acid, which decreased with the effect of the pomegranate–black carrot juice mixture, increased during the $\text{Exercise}_{+\text{supp}}$ phase. Relative improvements in serum fatty acid levels were detected with the effect of the pomegranate–black carrot juice mixture. 16:0 and 18:0 fatty acids are used as substrates by the stearyl-CoA desaturase (Δ-9-desaturase) enzyme. Fatty acids are formed from 16:0 to 16:1 and from 18:0 to 18:1. Stearyl-CoA desaturase enzyme is a very important enzyme for the biochemistry of the cell. It also plays a role in protecting the membrane structure of the cell. Nutrition and hormones are effective in the activity of this enzyme [56]. In this study, while the 18:0 level increases in the $\text{Exercise}_{\text{only}}$ phase, we think that the decrease in the 18:1n9c level is due to decreases in the activity of the stearyl-CoA desaturase enzyme. Looking at the studies conducted in this context, Lyudinina et al. (2018) reported that after 1.3 km and 15 km races in cross-country skiing athletes, there was no change in long-chain fatty acid levels compared to the athletes' initial values, while a significant increase was observed in the levels of C10:0, C12:0 and C14:0 has been reported [57]. Gollasch et al.

(2019) found that an acute maximal exercise resulted in relatively high plasma levels of free fatty acids C16:0, C16:1, C18:0, C18:1 cis and C18:2, while there was no change in the fatty acid level in erythrocytes. It has been stated that the levels of, C12:0, C14:1, C18:3n-6, C20:4n-3 and C22:1 are relatively low [58]. Xu et al. (2021) found that the 4-week combinatorial group (including exercise and dietary restriction) had significant changes in body composition compared to the control group. Significant changes in SFAs, MUFAs and especially a decrease in the levels of C14:0, C15:0, C18:0, C20:0, C22:0, C16:1n-7, C18:1n-9 and C20:1n-9 were also reported [59]. When studies on the effect of exercise (acute or chronic) on fatty acid levels are examined, it has been observed that exercise can change these levels. There are similarities between the research findings in the literature and the findings of this study.

5. Limitations

This study has some limitations. First, the individuals participating in this study were selected only from sedentary men and the sample size was limited. Second, there was no purification between the stages and this study was conducted on a single sample group.

As a result, with the findings of this research, it was determined that pomegranate–black carrot juice mixture showed positive corrective effects on serum AST, ALT, Zn, Mg and some fatty acid levels from stress caused by exercise in sedentary individuals. It is thought that further research is needed in both sedentary individuals and athlete groups to support these research findings and explain the potential mechanisms underlying our findings.

Author Contributions: Conceptualization, K.B., V.Ç. and A.O.; methodology, K.B., V.Ç. and T.A.; validation, K.B., I.A. and K.Y.A.; formal analysis, T.A. and Y.Y.; investigation, V.Ç. and K.Y.A.; data curation, K.B., I.A. and T.A.; writing—original draft preparation, K.B., A.O. and V.Ç.; writing—review and editing, K.B., V.Ç., T.A., L.R., A.F. and G.M.M.; visualization, L.R., A.F. and G.M.M.; supervision, L.R. and A.F.; project administration, G.M.M. All authors have read and agreed to the published version of the manuscript.

Funding: This study was supported by the Fırat University Scientific Research Projects Coordination Unit (FÜBAP, project number: BSY.19.05).

Institutional Review Board Statement: Before starting this research, ethical approval was received from Fırat University/Non-Interventional Research Ethics Committee, dated 25 April 2019, meeting number 07 and decision number 15.

Informed Consent Statement: Informed consent was obtained from all subjects involved in this study.

Data Availability Statement: The data presented in this study are available on request from the corresponding authors.

Conflicts of Interest: The authors declare no conflicts of interest.

References

1. Beck, K.L.; von Hurst, P.R.; O'Brien, W.J.; Badenhorst, C.E. Micronutrients and athletic performance: A review. *Food Chem. Toxicol.* **2021**, *158*, 112618. [CrossRef] [PubMed]
2. Mason, S.A.; Trewin, A.J.; Parker, L.; Wadley, G.D. Antioxidant supplements and endurance exercise: Current evidence and mechanistic insights. *Redox Biol.* **2020**, *35*, 101471. [CrossRef] [PubMed]
3. Rao, A.V.; Rao, L.G. Carotenoids and human health. *Pharmacol. Res.* **2007**, *55*, 207–216. [CrossRef] [PubMed]
4. Mojikon, F.D.; Kasimin, M.E.; Molujin, A.M.; Gansau, J.A.; Jawan, R. Probiotication of Nutritious Fruit and Vegetable Juices: An Alternative to Dairy-Based Probiotic Functional Products. *Nutrients* **2022**, *14*, 3457. [CrossRef] [PubMed]
5. Dżugan, M.; Wesołowska, M.; Zaguła, G.; Puchalski, C. The comparison of the physicochemical parameters and antioxidant activity of homemade and commercial pomegranate juices. *Acta Sci. Pol. Technol. Aliment.* **2018**, *17*, 59–68. [CrossRef] [PubMed]
6. Barati Boldaji, R.; Akhlaghi, M.; Sagheb, M.M.; Esmaeilinezhad, Z. Pomegranate juice improves cardiometabolic risk factors, biomarkers of oxidative stress and inflammation in hemodialysis patients: A randomized crossover trial. *J. Sci. Food Agric.* **2020**, *100*, 846–854. [CrossRef]
7. Asgary, S.; Karimi, R.; Pour, P.M.; Heydarpour, F.; Mostafaei, S.; Farzaei, M.H.; Moradi, S.; Aneva, I.Y. Is Consumption of Pomegranate Supplementation Effective on Oxidative Stress Biomarkers Including MDA, ox-LDL, POX 1, GPX, TAC, and TBRAS? A Systematic Review and Meta-Analysis of Randomized Controlled Trials. *Curr. Probl. Cardiol.* **2023**, *48*, 101198. [CrossRef]

8. Fuster-Muñoz, E.; Roche, E.; Funes, L.; Martínez-Peinado, P.; Sempere, J.M.; Vicente-Salar, N. Effects of pomegranate juice in circulating parameters, cytokines, and oxidative stress markers in endurance-based athletes: A randomized controlled trial. *Nutrition* **2016**, *32*, 539–545. [CrossRef]
9. Vučić, V.; Grabež, M.; Trchounian, A.; Arsić, A. Composition and Potential Health Benefits of Pomegranate: A Review. *Curr. Pharm. Des.* **2019**, *25*, 1817–1827. [CrossRef]
10. Kamiloglu, S.; Camp, J.V.; Capanoglu, E. Black carrot polyphenols: Effect of processing, storage and digestion- an overview. *Phytochem. Rev.* **2018**, *17*, 379–395. [CrossRef]
11. Sharma, K.D.; Karki, S.; Thakur, N.S.; Attri, S. Chemical composition, functional properties and processing of carrot—A review. *J. Food Sci. Technol.* **2012**, *49*, 22–32. [CrossRef]
12. Raczyk, M.; Kruszewski, B.; Zachariasz, E. Effect of Tomato, Beetroot and Carrot Juice Addition on Physicochemical, Antioxidant and Texture Properties of Wheat Bread. *Antioxidants* **2022**, *3*, 2178. [CrossRef]
13. Aytac, K.Y.; Ozkaya, A.; Oztekin, A.; Cinar, V.; Akbulut, T.; Demirbag, R.; Comaklı, V.; Bozbay, K. The Effect of Pomegranate-Black Carrot Juice on Serum and Erythrocytes of Sedentary Subjects Exposed to Exhausting Exercise. *J. Chem.* **2023**, *2023*, 9489018. [CrossRef]
14. Hazar, M.; Otag, A.; Otag, I.; Sezen, M.; Sever, O. Effect of increasing maximal aerobic exercise on serum muscles enzymes in professional field hockey players. *Glob. J. Health Sci.* **2014**, *7*, 69–74. [CrossRef] [PubMed]
15. Pettersson, J.; Hindorf, U.; Persson, P.; Bengtsson, T.; Malmqvist, U.; Werkström, V.; Ekelund, M. Muscular exercise can cause highly pathological liver function tests in healthy men. *Br. J. Clin. Pharmacol.* **2008**, *65*, 253–259. [CrossRef] [PubMed]
16. Lippi, G.; Schena, F.; Salvagno, G.L.; Montagnana, M.; Gelati, M.; Tarperi, C.; Banfi, G.; Guidi, G.C. Acute variation of biochemical markers of muscle damage following a 21-km, half-marathon run. *Scand. J. Clin. Lab. Investig.* **2008**, *68*, 667–672. [CrossRef] [PubMed]
17. Pal, S.; Chaki, B.; Chattopadhyay, S.; Bandyopadhyay, A. High-Intensity Exercise Induced Oxidative Stress and Skeletal Muscle Damage in Postpubertal Boys and Girls: A Comparative Study. *J. Strength. Cond. Res.* **2018**, *32*, 1045–1052. [CrossRef] [PubMed]
18. Ratnayake, W.M.; Galli, C. Fat and fatty acid terminology, methods of analysis and fat digestion and metabolism: A background review paper. *Ann. Nutr. Metab.* **2009**, *55*, 8–43. [CrossRef]
19. Muscella, A.; Stefàno, E.; Lunetti, P.; Capobianco, L.; Marsigliante, S. The Regulation of Fat Metabolism During Aerobic Exercise. *Biomolecules* **2020**, *10*, 1699. [CrossRef] [PubMed]
20. Bengin, E.; Kırtepe, A.; Çınar, V.; Akbulut, T.; Russo, L.; Aydemir, İ.; Migliaccio, G.M. Leptin, Ghrelin, Irisin, Asprosin and Subfatin Changes in Obese Women: Effect of Exercise and Different Nutrition Types. *Medicina* **2024**, *60*, 1118. [CrossRef] [PubMed]
21. Gemmink, A.; Schrauwen, P.; Hesselink, M.K.C. Exercising your fat (metabolism) into shape: A muscle-centred view. *Diabetologia* **2020**, *63*, 1453–1463. [CrossRef]
22. Akbulut, T.; Cinar, V.; Aydin, S.; Yardim, M. The role of different exercises in irisin, heat shock protein 70 and some biochemical parameters. *J. Med. Biochem.* **2022**, *41*, 149–155. [CrossRef]
23. Jeppesen, J.; Kiens, B. Regulation and limitations to fatty acid oxidation during exercise. *J. Physiol.* **2012**, *590*, 1059–1068. [CrossRef]
24. Alves Vas, F.J.; Grijota Pérez, F.J.; Toro-Román, V.; Sánchez, I.B.; Maynar Mariño, M.; Barrientos Vicho, G. Changes in the Fatty Acid Profile in Erythrocytes in High-Level Endurance Runners during a Sports Season. *Nutrients* **2024**, *16*, 1895. [CrossRef]
25. Corsetto, P.A.; Montorfano, G.; Klersy, C.; Massimino, L.; Infantino, V.; Iannello, G.; Anna Faliva, M.; Lukaski, H.; Perna, S.; Alalwan, T.A.; et al. Fatty Acid Profile and Antioxidant Status Fingerprint in Sarcopenic Elderly Patients: Role of Diet and Exercise. *Nutrients* **2019**, *11*, 2569. [CrossRef]
26. Martin, W.H. Effects of acute and chronic exercise on fat metabolism. *Exerc. Sport Sci. Rev.* **1996**, *24*, 203–231. Available online: https://pubmed.ncbi.nlm.nih.gov/8744251/ (accessed on 3 January 2024). [CrossRef]
27. Lipina, C.; Hundal, H.S. Lipid modulation of skeletal muscle mass and function. *J. Cachexia Sarcopenia Muscle* **2017**, *8*, 190–201. [CrossRef]
28. Ammar, A.; Turki, M.; Hammouda, O.; Chtourou, H.; Trabelsi, K.; Bouaziz, M.; Abdelkarim, O.; Hoekelmann, A.; Ayadi, F.; Souissi, N.; et al. Effects of Pomegranate Juice Supplementation on Oxidative Stress Biomarkers Following Weightlifting Exercise. *Nutrients* **2017**, *9*, 819. [CrossRef]
29. Migliaccio, G.M.; Di Filippo, G.; Russo, L.; Orgiana, T.; Ardigò, L.P.; Casal, M.Z.; Peyré-Tartaruga, L.A.; Padulo, J. Effects of Mental Fatigue on Reaction Time in Sportsmen. *Int. J. Environ. Res. Public. Health* **2022**, *19*, 14360. [CrossRef]
30. Racil, G.; Russo, L.; Migliaccio, G.M.; Signorelli, P.; Larion, A.; Padulo, J.; Jlid, M.C. High-Intensity Interval Training in Female Adolescents with Moderate or Severe Obesity. *Children* **2023**, *10*, 1495. [CrossRef]
31. Racil, G.; Chelly, M.-S.; Coquart, J.; Padulo, J.; Teodor, D.F.; Russo, L. Long- and Short-Term High-Intensity Interval Training on Lipid Profile and Cardiovascular Disorders in Obese Male Adolescents. *Children* **2023**, *10*, 1180. [CrossRef]
32. Annaç, E.; Uçkun, M.; Özkaya, A.; Yoloğlu, E.; Pekmez, H.; Bulmuş, Ö.; Aydın, A. The protective effects of pomegranate juice on lead acetate-induced neurotoxicity in the male rat: A histomorphometric and biochemical study. *J. Food Biochem.* **2022**, *46*, e13881. [CrossRef]
33. Akhtar, S.; Rauf, A.; Imran, M.; Qamar, M.; Riaz, M.; Mubarak, M.S. Black carrot (*Daucus carota* L.), dietary and health promoting perspectives of its polyphenols: A review. *Trends Food Sci. Technol.* **2017**, *66*, 36–47. [CrossRef]

34. Ciftci, H.; Ozkaya, A.; Kariptas, E. Determination of fatty acids, vitamins and trace elements in Pistacia terebinthus coffee. *J. Food Agric. Environ.* **2009**, *7*, 72–74. Available online: https://openaccess.ahievran.edu.tr/xmlui/handle/20.500.12513/2605 (accessed on 3 January 2024).
35. Hara, A.; Radin, N.S. Lipid extraction of tissues with a low-toxicity solvent. *Anal. Biochem.* **1978**, *90*, 420–426. [CrossRef]
36. Gordon, B.; Chen, S.; Durstine, J.L. The effects of exercise training on the traditional lipid profile and beyond. *Curr. Sports Med Rep.* **2014**, *13*, 253–259. [CrossRef]
37. Trejo-Gutierrez, J.F.; Fletcher, G. Impact of exercise on blood lipids and lipoproteins. *J. Clin. Lipidol.* **2007**, *1*, 175–181. [CrossRef]
38. Afşin, A.; Bozyılan, E.; Asoğlu, R.; Hoşoğlu, Y.; Dündar, A. Effects of regular exercise on inflammatory biomarkers and lipid parameters in soccer players. *J. Immunoassay Immunochem.* **2021**, *42*, 467–477. [CrossRef]
39. Earnest, C.P.; Artero, E.G.; Sui, X.; Lee, D.C.; Church, T.S.; Blair, S.N. Maximal estimated cardiorespiratory fitness, cardiometabolic risk factors, and metabolic syndrome in the aerobics center longitudinal study. *Mayo Clin. Proc.* **2013**, *88*, 259–270. [CrossRef]
40. Shin, K.A.; Park, K.D.; Ahn, J.; Park, Y.; Kim, Y.J. Comparison of Changes in Biochemical Markers for Skeletal Muscles, Hepatic Metabolism, and Renal Function after Three Types of Long-distance Running: Observational Study. *Medicine* **2016**, *95*, e3657 [CrossRef]
41. Tirabassi, J.N.; Olewinski, L.; Khodaee, M. Variation of Traditional Biomarkers of Liver Injury After an Ultramarathon at Altitude *Sports Health.* **2018**, *10*, 361–365. [CrossRef]
42. Nemati, S.; Tadibi, V.; Hoseini, R. Pomegranate juice intake enhances the effects of aerobic training on insulin resistance and liver enzymes in type 2 diabetic men: A single-blind controlled trial. *BMC Nutr.* **2022**, *8*, 48. [CrossRef] [PubMed]
43. Olvera-Sandoval, C.; Fabela-Illescas, H.E.; Fernández-Martínez, E.; Ortiz-Rodríguez, M.A.; Cariño-Cortés, R.; Ariza-Ortega, J.A.; Hernández-González, J.C.; Olivo, D.; Valadez-Vega, C.; Belefant-Miller, H.; et al. Potential Mechanisms of the Improvement of Glucose Homeostasis in Type 2 Diabetes by Pomegranate Juice. *Antioxidants* **2022**, *11*, 553. [CrossRef]
44. Volpe, S.L. Micronutrient requirements for athletes. *Clin. Sports Med.* **2007**, *26*, 119–130. [CrossRef] [PubMed]
45. Cheng, S.M.; Yang, L.L.; Chen, S.H.; Hsu, M.H.; Chen, I.J.; Cheng, F.C. Magnesium sulfate enhances exercise performance and manipulates dynamic changes in peripheral glucose utilization. *Eur. J. Appl. Physiol.* **2010**, *108*, 363–369. [CrossRef] [PubMed]
46. Gedmantaite, A.; Celis-Morales, C.A.; Ho, F.; Pell, J.P.; Ratkevicius, A.; Gray, S.R. Associations between diet and handgrip strength: A cross-sectional study from UK Biobank. *Mech. Ageing Dev.* **2020**, *189*, 111269. [CrossRef]
47. Setaro, L.; Santos-Silva, P.R.; Nakano, E.Y.; Sales, C.H.; Nunes, N.; Greve, J.M.; Colli, C. Magnesium status and the physical performance of volleyball players: Effects of magnesium supplementation. *J. Sports Sci.* **2014**, *32*, 438–445. [CrossRef]
48. Dominguez, L.J.; Barbagallo, M.; Lauretani, F.; Bandinelli, S.; Bos, A.; Corsi, A.M.; Simonsick, E.M.; Ferrucci, L. Magnesium and muscle performance in older persons: The InCHIANTI study. *Am. J. Clin. Nutr.* **2006**, *84*, 419–426. [CrossRef]
49. Bohl, C.H.; Volpe, S.L. Magnesium and exercise. *Crit. Rev. Food Sci. Nutr.* **2002**, *42*, 533–563. [CrossRef]
50. Lukaski, H.C.; Nielsen, F.H. Dietary magnesium depletion affects metabolic responses during submaximal exercise in post-menopausal women. *J. Nutr.* **2002**, *132*, 930–935. [CrossRef]
51. Chu, A.; Petocz, P.; Samman, S. Plasma/Serum Zinc Status During Aerobic Exercise Recovery: A Systematic Review and Meta-Analysis. *Sports Med.* **2017**, *47*, 127–134. [CrossRef]
52. Granell, J. Zinc and copper changes in serum and urine after aerobic endurance and muscular strength exercise. *J. Sports Med Phys. Fitness.* **2014**, *54*, 232–237. Available online: https://europepmc.org/article/med/24509996 (accessed on 3 January 2024) [PubMed]
53. Maynar, M.; Muñoz, D.; Alves, J.; Barrientos, G.; Grijota, F.J.; Robles, M.C.; Llerena, F. Influence of an Acute Exercise Until Exhaustion on Serum and Urinary Concentrations of Molybdenum, Selenium, and Zinc in Athletes. *Biol. Trace Elem. Res.* **2018**, *186*, 361–369. [CrossRef] [PubMed]
54. Lukaski, H.C. Low dietary zinc decreases erythrocyte carbonic anhydrase activities and impairs cardiorespiratory function in men during exercise. *Am. J. Clin. Nutr.* **2005**, *81*, 1045–1051. [CrossRef] [PubMed]
55. Song, Y.; Leonard, S.W.; Traber, M.G.; Ho, E. Zinc deficiency affects DNA damage, oxidative stress, antioxidant defenses, and DNA repair in rats. *J. Nutr.* **2009**, *139*, 1626–1631. [CrossRef]
56. Ntambi, J.M. Regulation of stearoyl-CoA desaturase by polyunsaturated fatty acids and cholesterol. *J. Lipid Res.* **1999**, *40* 1549–1558. [CrossRef]
57. Lyudinina, A.Y.; Ivankova, G.E.; Bojko, E.R. Priority use of medium-chain fatty acids during high-intensity exercise in cross-country skiers. *J. Int. Soc. Sports Nutr.* **2018**, *15*, 57. [CrossRef]
58. Gollasch, B.; Dogan, I.; Rothe, M.; Gollasch, M.; Luft, F.C. Maximal exercise and erythrocyte fatty-acid status: A lipidomics study *Physiol. Rep.* **2019**, *7*, e14040. [CrossRef]
59. Xu, L.; Zou, X.; Gao, Z.; Mao, C.; Su, H.; Li, C.; Chen, N. Improved fatty acid profile reduces body fat and arterial stiffness in obese adolescents upon combinatorial intervention with exercise and dietary restriction. *J. Exerc. Sci. Fit.* **2021**, *19*, 234–240. [CrossRef]

applied sciences

MDPI

Article

Perceptions and Practices of Accredited Tennis Coaches When Teaching Foundational Grip Development

Nicholas A. Busuttil [1,2,3], Alexandra H. Roberts [2], Marcus Dunn [4,5], Minh Hyunh [2] and Kane J. Middleton [2,*]

1 Institute for Health and Sport, Victoria University, Melbourne, VIC 3011, Australia; nick.busuttil@vu.edu.au
2 Sport, Performance, and Nutrition Research Group, School of Allied Health, Human Services and Sport, La Trobe University, 1 Kingsbury Drive, Bundoora, Melbourne, VIC 3083, Australia; alexhroberts17@gmail.com (A.H.R.); m.huynh@latrobe.edu.au (M.H.)
3 Performance Science, Research and Innovation, The Movement Institute, Melbourne, VIC 3042, Australia
4 School of Energy, Geoscience, Infrastructure and Society, Heriot-Watt University, Edinburgh EH14 4AS, UK; marcus.dunn@hw.ac.uk
5 Centre for Sports Engineering Research, Sheffield Hallam University, Sheffield S9 3TY, UK
* Correspondence: k.middleton@latrobe.edu.au

Abstract: This study aimed to understand how tennis coaches perceive and approach the development of grip positions, a foundational skill in tennis. Professionally accredited coaches, classed as less (n = 140) or more (n = 86) experienced, participated in an online survey where they provided their perspectives on the importance of developing grip positions and their opinions on using physically constraining tools for coaching. Irrespective of coach experience level, the findings revealed that technique development and grip position training were ranked as the two most important components in foundational tennis skill development. The Semi-western grip for forehand (less: 68%; more: 65%), a combination of Continental and Eastern grips for double-handed backhand (less: 59%; more: 48.8%), and the Continental grip for serves (both: 94%) were identified as the most commonly taught positions for different shots. Perceived barriers to developing grip positions were out of habit (less: 62%; more: 56%), discomfort (less: 58%; more: 50%), and lack of confidence (less: 44%; more: 21%). Notably, 65% of coaches expressed an openness to incorporating physically constraining tools to enhance grip-specific skill development. Overall, this study serves as a foundational resource, guiding coaches in optimising their strategies for foundational tennis development, prompting further research in this area.

Keywords: coaching; pedagogy; tennis; grip positions

1. Introduction

Individuals require the parallel development of effective shot mechanics, motor coordination, physical conditioning, and tactical development for sport-specific skills. In tennis, sport-specific skills include, but are not limited to the serve, groundstrokes (forehand and backhand) and volleys [1]. One skill that is highly important to racket- and club-based sports is the use of different grip positions, as they provide a fundamental contribution to effective techniques [1,2]. Grip positions in tennis orientate the hand around the racket's handle to execute a stroke. Each grip position (e.g., Continental, Western, Semi-Western, Eastern) has different implications for both performance and injury [3–5], which have been shown to affect upper limb, racket, and ball kinematics in the forehand and double-handed backhand tennis strokes [3,6,7]. Specifically, the Eastern grip position has been featured with increased horizontal racket head velocity across the forehand and backhand, suggesting an improvement in hitting performance [3,7], whereas the Continental and Western grip positions are featured with increased ulnar deviation [3,6], a rotation which if excessive is suggested to increase extensor carpi ulnaris-based injuries [5,6]. These differences are also evident in golf, where grip positions have been associated with changes in ulnar deviation and clubhead velocity [2,8], suggesting that grip positions have a fundamental contribution to shot performance.

During the early years of foundational tennis development, grip positions inherently evolve through methodology by coaches that encourage discovery. Traditionally, these grip positions were predominantly trained during the initial stages of tennis development, with specific positions selected and taught by coaches [9]. Common skill development methods used by coaches include skill decomposition, optimal technique demonstration, utilising feedback strategies, and skill isolation from the performance environment [10–12]. An additional method that coaches employ is the utilisation of physically constraining tools (PCTs). These are devices that physically constrain and/or guide an athlete's movement [13] and are used to facilitate skill development. PCTs may be considered traditional tools in coaching, fixing movement to predefined movement planes and positions. Past research has reported that training with a PCT improves shot accuracy during a golf drive compared with training without a PCT [13]; however, such devices do not provide practicality and possibly remove learners from a representative performance environment. To date, there is a limited understanding of the use of PCTs, with a recent scoping review reporting zero studies on the efficacy of PCTs for grip-specific skill development [14]. Grip positions and their effects on performance and injury has been a growing body of research [3,5–8,14]; however, little is known about coaches' considerations when developing grip positions. Understanding the considerations of accredited tennis coaches when developing grip positions may provide essential information for best-practice recommendations in aiding foundational tennis development.

Grip positions of established tennis players have been documented in relation to performance [15] and injury association [5]; however, limited research details the perceptions and related practices of accredited tennis coaches when teaching grip positions during foundational tennis development. The experiential knowledge of expert coaches has previously been suggested to provide complementary information to support the empirical understanding of performance in sports and to guide future research questions [16,17]. Exploring the perceptions and practices of accredited tennis coaches provides the opportunity to understand the current insights across experience levels, and initially understand the practical considerations about grip positions to develop practitioner-led research.

The purpose of this exploratory study was to understand the current perceptions and practices of accredited tennis coaches regarding the development of grip positions, and their opinions on using PCTs to assist development. It was hypothesised that more experienced coaches would have similar priorities during foundational tennis development compared with less experienced coaches. It was also hypothesised that only a limited number of coaches, irrespective of experience level, would not use a physically constraining tool for grip-specific skill development.

2. Materials and Methods

2.1. Study Design

The following study was an online questionnaire that was approved by the La Trobe University Human Ethics Committee (#HEC20336).

2.1.1. Questionnaire Development

An online questionnaire was developed comprising questions related to important factors in tennis stroke development, grip positions, and perceptions of the use of PCTs for grip positions. The questionnaire was piloted in the form of cognitive interviews [18–20] with eight professional tennis coaches who were not included in the final sample. The purpose of cognitive interviewing is to pre-test and validate questionnaires, which is a valuable process when surveying specific groups to ensure that meaning of concepts and terms are shared between the researcher(s) and participants, and to help reduce participant questionnaire non-completion [18]. Based on feedback, changes were made to improve the clarity of instructions within the online form to create the final online version of the questionnaire.

The questionnaire was divided into three categories. Section one asked for background information, including the participants' demographics, tennis coaching experience and qualifications, educational qualifications, and athlete demographics/ability level. Section two asked for information about participants' current practices when teaching grip positions, and probed both student adherence to and difficulties with these positions. Section three asked for the participant's opinions on the use of PCTs for grip-specific skill development in tennis. Participants were asked for their opinion on the utility and efficacy of PCTs to help athletes learn and transfer new grip positions into match-play and their likelihood of using a PCT in their coaching should it be readily available.

2.1.2. Procedure

An a priori goodness-of-fit test for contingency tables was conducted using G*Power (V 3.1.9.7, Keil, Germany). With an effect size (w) of 0.3, an α error probability of 0.05, 80% power, and 2 degrees of freedom, a sample size of 108 participants would be required ($\chi^2 = 5.99$, $\lambda = 9.72$). Participants completed a 15 min, anonymous online questionnaire in REDCap (Research Electronic Data Capture, Fort Lauderdale, FL, USA; [21]). The data collection period was from 1 October 2020 to 30 March 2021. Prior to beginning the questionnaire, participants were provided with relevant study information, a consent form via email, and an optional link to the questionnaire. As this was an optional link, consent was implied when the participant chose to begin the questionnaire. The questionnaire was distributed via email to national tennis organisations, inviting their member coaches to participate, as well as through the personal social media channels of the researchers. Snowball sampling [22] was also used, encouraging coaches to forward the questionnaire to their colleagues. Participants were above 18 years of age, held professionally recognised tennis coaching certificates/qualifications, were previously and/or currently involved in tennis coaching, and could read and understand English.

2.1.3. Analysis

Data obtained through the online questionnaire were exported to Microsoft Excel (V. 2112, Microsoft 365, MSO, Redmond, WA, USA) and formatted for statistical and descriptive analysis. A cluster analysis (R Package Version 1.0.7; [23]) categorised participants into 'less' and 'more' experienced coaches. Within this analysis, coaching and educational qualifications, and the total number of years and hours per week of coaching was used to determine the level of experience. The cluster analysis revealed that on average, less experienced coaches had lower levels of formal coaching education (Level 1 or 2 coaching accreditation) and eight years of coaching experience ranging between 11 and 20 h per week, whereas more experienced coaches had higher levels of formal coaching education (Level 3 or 4 coaching accreditation) and twenty-eight years of coaching experience ranging between 21 and 30 h per week. For questions where participants were able to select multiple responses, answers were grouped into 'single' or 'multiple' responses for analysis. For example, when coaches were asked what specific forehand grip positions they taught in their lessons, only selecting the 'Eastern forehand' was considered a single response, whereas selecting both 'Eastern forehand' and 'Semi-Western' was considered a multiple response.

2.1.4. Coach Demographics

Two hundred and twenty-six accredited tennis coaches (less experience: n = 140; more experience: n = 86; Male 86.7%, female 12.4%, prefer not to disclose 0.9%; age: 41.1 ± 13.9 years; experience coaching: 15.8 ± 11.8 years) across 40 countries took part in this study, with 65% of respondents from United States, Austria, Slovenia, Australia, and the United Kingdom (Table 1). Most participants were male, the age and number of years coaching was lower for less experienced coaches, and more experienced coaches coached a greater percentage of athletes between the ages of 11 and 17 (Table 1).

Table 1. Demographics of coaches across experience levels.

	Coaching Experience	
	Less (n = 140)	**More (n = 86)**
Gender (%)		
Male	85.0	89.5
Female	14.3	9.3
Not disclosed	0.7	1.2
Age (years, mean ± SD)	34.4 ± 11.3	52.0 ± 10.6
Coaching time (years, mean ± SD)	8.1 ± 4.6	28.4 ± 9.0
Coached age group (years, %)		
3 to 6	21.4	22.1
7 to 10	61.4	44.2
11 to 14	63.6	79.1
15 to 17	41.4	55.8
18+	42.1	48.8

Statistical analysis was performed in Jamovi (V 2.3.12.0, Jamovi Project, 2022). Data normality was checked via visual inspection of Quantile–Quantile plots, and based on this inspection, data were analysed using non-parametric statistics. For categorical variables (as expressed in the example above), the Chi-Squared test (χ^2) was used to assess the statistical association between groups, and Cramer's V to calculate effect sizes (0.10 small; 0.30 medium; 0.50 large), as previously used within a cohort of tennis coaches [24]. Where appropriate, the Kruskal–Wallis test was used to assess the statistical significance specifically for the likelihood of using PCTs during the coach's training sessions. All analyses were compared between less and more experienced coaches, with the alpha level set at 0.05.

3. Results

3.1. Coach Perceptions of Foundational Development

When asked to rank foundational athlete development concepts (training grip positions; physical conditioning; technique development; court movement; transferring concepts from training to match-play) on a scale of 1 (most important) to 5 (least important), there were no statistical associations between those ranked 1–4 among less and more experienced coaches ($p > 0.050$). There was a significant association at ranking level five ($\chi^2 = 13.7$, $p = 0.008$, $V = 0.246$), where less experienced coaches indicated that for foundational development, transferring concepts from training to match-play was the least important (56.5%) compared with more experienced coaches, who stated that physical conditioning was least important (41.7%). Technique development was either the first or second most important aspect of foundational development, irrespective of experience level (Table 2). Of these concepts, there was a significant association for how challenging these aspects are during foundational development ($\chi^2 = 3.9$, $p = 0.047$, $V = 0.132$). Compared with more experienced coaches, less experienced coaches responded with a lower percentage of singular responses (less experienced: 52.9%; more experienced: 66.3%) and a higher percentage of multiple responses (less experienced: 47.1%; more experienced: 33.7%). Approximately half of the coaches selected that transferring concepts from training into match-play was difficult, whereas physical conditioning was chosen the least (Table 3).

Table 2. Contingency table of accredited tennis coaches' responses to what aspects are most important during foundational tennis player development.

	Less Experienced					More Experienced					
Level of Importance (1 Most; 5 Least)	**TGP**	**PC**	**TD**	**CM**	**MP**	**TGP**	**PC**	**TD**	**CM**	**MP**	***p***
Percentage (%)											
1	37.2	8.6	40.7	8.6	4.9	29.1	5.8	46.5	11.5	7.1	0.584
2	21.5	12.1	42.8	19.2	4.4	19.7	5.9	34.9	30.3	9.2	0.092
3	21.4	15.7	10.8	44.3	7.8	17.5	13.0	11.5	41.7	16.3	0.371
4	9.3	35	5.1	24.2	26.4	14.0	33.6	5.8	10.6	36.0	0.087
* 5	10.6	28.6	0.6	3.7	56.5	19.7	41.7	1.3	5.9	31.4	0.008 *

TGP = training grip positions; PC = physical conditioning; TD = technique development; CM = court movement; MP = transferring concepts from training to match-play. Asterisk (*) refers to a significant association $p < 0.050$.

Table 3. Frequency count (expressed as percentages) of accredited tennis coaches' perceptions of what aspects are most challenging during foundational tennis player development.

	Experience Level	
Developmental Concepts	**Less**	**More**
Percentage (%)		
TGP	30.7	23.3
PC	22.9	15.1
TD	45.0	39.5
CM	30.0	31.4
MP	46.4	54.7

TGP = training grip positions; PC = physical conditioning; TD = technique development; CM = court movement; MP = transferring concepts from training to match-play. The presented test of association result ($\chi^2 = 3.9$, $p = 0.047$) represents answers that were grouped into 'single' or 'multiple' responses for each developmental concept.

3.1.1. Grip Position Practices by Coaches and Associated Perceptions

Irrespective of experience level, coaches indicated that grip positions should be adhered to between the ages of 7 and 10 years old (less experienced = 66.7%; more experienced = 68.4%); however, there was no significant association. For coaching grip positions in the serve, forehand, and double-handed backhand, there were no significant associations between experience levels for singular (e.g., Continental) or multiple (e.g., Continental and Eastern forehand) taught grips, or the age at which they were implemented by coaches ($p > 0.050$). A trend was observed that the Continental, Eastern forehand, and Semi-western forehand grip positions are mainly taught by coaches. In the serve and dominant hand for double-handed backhands, the Continental was the taught grip position, whereas in the forehand and non-dominant hand for double-handed backhands, the Eastern forehand and Semi-western grip position were the most taught by coaches. When asked at what age they (the coach) would implement the specific grip position for an athlete, the serve grip was predominantly taught between 7 and 10 years of age (less experienced coaches) or between 11 and 14 years old (more experienced coaches), and between 7 and 10 years for the forehand and backhand, irrespective of coach experience level (Tables 4 and 5). Less experienced coaches (61.4%) indicated that their athletes use their own grip positions rather than the coach's suggested grip compared with more experienced coaches (55.8%); however, there was no significant association. There was a significant association for the perceived reasons why athletes 'revert' from their coach-instructed grip positions ($\chi^2 = 6.4$, $p = 0.011$, $V = 0.219$). More experienced coaches responded with singular causes more (less experience: 33.6%; more experience: 56.1%; e.g., discomfort from suggested grip use) compared with less experienced coaches who responded with multiple responses more (less experienced: 66.4%; more experienced: 43.9%; e.g., discomfort from suggested grip use and not confident). The most frequent perceived causes (by the coach) for 'reverting' grip positions by athletes are hand discomfort (less experienced: 58.1%; more experienced: 50%) and out of habit (Table 4; less experienced: 61.6%; more experienced: 56.3%).

Table 4. Frequency count (expressed as percentages) of accredited tennis coaches' practices for grip positions across strokes, and the perceptions of reasons why athletes revert to their preferred grip positions.

Strokes and Grip Position Variables	Experience Level		*p*
	Less	More	
Percentage (%)			
Serve			0.852
Continental	93.6	93.9	
Forehand			0.936
Eastern forehand	48.6	48.8	
Western	5.7	8.1	
Semi-western	67.9	65.1	
Continental	4.3	2.3	
Other	5.0	9.3	
Double-handed backhand			0.394
Continental/Eastern forehand	59.3	47.7	
Continental/Semi-western	25.7	31.4	
Eastern backhand/Semi-western	12.9	14.0	
Eastern backhand/Continental	8.6	9.3	
Eastern backhand/Eastern forehand	7.1	10.5	
Continental/Continental	6.4	3.5	
Other	5.7	7.0	
Perceived causes of reverting grip			0.011 *
Discomfort from suggested grip use	58.1	50.0	
Hand grip not strong enough	20.9	22.9	
They refuse to	3.5	6.3	
Out of habit	61.6	56.3	
Not confident	44.2	20.8	
Other	10.5	18.8	

Presented test of association (χ^2) results represent answers that were grouped into 'single' or 'multiple' responses for each variable of the serve, forehand, double-handed backhand, and perceived causes of reverting grip. Asterisk (*) refers to a significant association $p < 0.050$.

Table 5. Frequency count (expressed as percentages) of accredited tennis coaches' practices for what age they implement grip positions across strokes.

Age Range	Experience Level					
	Serve		Forehand		Backhand	
	Less	More	Less	More	Less	More
Percentage (%)						
3 to 6	17.9	0.0	32.1	36.0	31.4	26.7
7 to 10	67.9	15.3	55.0	57.0	55.7	66.3
11 to 14	12.1	68.2	10.0	4.7	10.0	4.7
15 to 17	0.7	15.3	0.7	1.2	0.7	1.2
18+	1.4	1.2	2.1	1.2	2.1	1.2
p	0.946		0.936		0.446	

Presented test of association (χ^2) results represent answers that were grouped into 'single' or 'multiple' responses for each variable of the serve, forehand, and backhand strokes.

3.1.2. Coach Perceptions from Using a Physically Constraining Tool

There was no statistical association ($p > 0.050$) between less and more experienced coaches for any question regarding the use of PCTs. Approximately half of the coaches indicated that using a grip position tool would facilitate improved learning of tennis strokes. Of the coaches that responded with either 'yes' or 'unsure' for the previous question, slightly less (less experienced: 43.0%; more experienced: 49.3%) indicated that using a PCT would facilitate skill transfer from training into match-play environments, with 'unsure' responses increasing irrespective of coach experience (Table 6). Of the same participants, 65% of coaches indicated that they would use a PCT during their training if readily available.

Table 6. Frequency count (expressed as percentages) of accredited tennis coaches' perceptions on using a physically constraining tool to facilitate learning and transfer from training into match-play, and the likelihood of coaches implementing a physically constraining tool into their training.

	Experience Level						p
	Less			More			
Training Tool Scenario	Yes	Unsure	No	Yes	Unsure	No	
Percentage (%)							
Learn	51.5	35.1	13.6	44.1	36.0	19.7	0.392
Transfer	43.0	43.8	13.2	49.3	39.1	11.6	0.703
Mean ± SD							
Likelihood of use		64.2 ± 23.5			66.3 ± 24.2		0.532

Likelihood of use variable represents the test of association results (Kruskal–Wallis one-way ANOVA, $p = 0.532$).

4. Discussion

The purpose of this study was to explore the current perceptions of accredited tennis coaches regarding foundational development, including grip positions in youth athletes, and opinions on using a PCT for developing grip positions. Our hypotheses were supported as coaches, irrespective of experience level, and the priorities during foundational tennis development were similar from levels 1 to 3; however, more experience indicated that physical conditioning is the least important component during foundational development, whereas less experienced coaches stated that transferring concepts from training to match-play is the least important. In relation to grip positions, the coaches' main perceived reasons for why their athletes 'revert' their grip positions were hand discomfort and habit, with 65% of coaches would use a PCT device to develop grip positions if readily available.

4.1. Foundational Tennis Development

Tennis is a complex sport that requires the cohesive development of technical, physical, mental, and tactical characteristics from an early age. Conventionally, a coach takes on the role of an instructor to help develop these characteristics through purposeful and deliberate practice [25]. The results of this study showed that irrespective of the experience level, coaches emphasised the importance of technical training, as technique development and training grip positions were indicated as the most important areas during foundational tennis development. This implies that many coaches may initially focus on stroke execution with new athletes, which is a fundamental aspect in tennis to create efficient and effective shot mechanics [1]. Well-developed shot mechanics are crucial for shot performance so that favourable outcomes (e.g., winners and forced errors) can be achieved, as well as to reduce the risk of overuse and acute injuries [4,26,27]. To develop shot mechanics, coaches use purposeful methods that are likely constrained by their own experiences and knowledge. For example, common tennis coaching practices include instructing athletes to 'arabesque' or perform ball throwing, actions that are designed to develop serve technique [28,29]. These studies, using task and instructional constraints of technique instruction and representative actions, demonstrate the complex nature of developing a tennis serve, which may extend into other areas of foundational tennis development including the use of certain grip positions.

Coaches indicated that transferring concepts from training into match-play is the most challenging area of foundational tennis development. This may suggest that coaches struggle with certain practices in relation to skilful transfer during foundational tennis training for match-play performance. The ability to perform well in tennis can be dependent on (but not limited to) physical development [30], effective shot mechanics [1], and game (tactical) understanding [31]. Developing game understanding, which is arguably a difficult developmental process, can be achieved through early exposure to 'game sense' activities. The game sense approach is associated with a modal for 'Teaching Games for Understanding' [32], with an integration/addition of contextual information for learning within games or game-like scenarios [31]. Game sense differentiates from the traditional pedagogical framing of sports teaching as a technical-to-tactical progression [32], and rather involves 'game-context' skill development which integrates technical and tactical development synchronously [31]. Game-context, commonly used in contemporary skill development methods, involves training the ability to cope with pressure, decision making, timing for technique, the use of space, and managing risk [33]. Irrespective of coach experience level, this may reflect the persistence of traditional and linear pedagogical practices to skill development for the current cohort of coaches. This possibly alludes to a lack of 'game sense' practices being used by the current cohort of coaches; however, without assessing the direct perceptions of coaches about their understanding of game sense and practices for skill transfer from training into match-play, this cannot be confirmed.

4.2. Grip Positions

Grip positions are a fundamental contribution to effective techniques that are developed during the initial stages of learning tennis [1]. The serve may be considered the most complex of strokes performed in tennis. Classed as a serial skill, the serve relies on the interplay between shot selection, ball-toss positioning, temporal organisation of key kinematic events, and coordinated shot mechanics [12,34,35]. This complexity may explain why more experienced coaches may not enforce adherence to the continental grip position for the serve until later in development, compared with less experienced coaches. Despite the fundamental nature of grip positions for effective serve performance, more experienced coaches may rather focus on the temporal and kinematic attributes for effective serves, which include (but are not limited to) 'leg drive' coordination with shoulder mechanics [36], and dominant-arm long-axis internal rotation [37]. These results may also reflect the ages of athletes taught by the coaches as demographic backgrounds have previously been shown to affect survey responses [38]. Less experienced coaches predominantly taught athletes between 7 and 10 years old compared with more experienced coaches who taught athletes between 11 and 17 years old. Given coaches indicated that they teach grip positions for the serve in different age groups, this presents a possible response bias.

Adapting to a new grip position or stroke technique in tennis is important to continue developing with evolving physical and tactical match-play characteristics. Over half of coaches indicated that students 'revert' their grip positions from what they were instructed to use, with the primary perceived causes being discomfort and out of habit. In more experienced coaches, the frequency of used grip positions across the forehand and double-handed backhand is greater compared with less experienced coaches, who are still in favour of the Eastern and Semi-Western grips. This is consistent with the previous literature as the majority of the top 100 professional players (male and female) use the Eastern and Semi-Western grips as the top hand in the double-handed backhand [15]. Also evident in sub-elite tennis, athletes reported using the Eastern (24.9%) and Semi-Western (60.5%) grips for the forehand stroke [5]. It is important to note that grip influences the kinematics of the swing and subsequently post-impact ball characteristics [1,27]. The Eastern is considered to be a "traditional" forehand grip, featured with greater horizontal racket head velocity contribution to ball speed, compared with the Semi-Western, which features increased vertical racket head velocity [3], possibly imparting greater ball spin compared with the Eastern grip. Both are considered versatile to use across playing surfaces as they allow athletes to adapt their swing technique with varying incoming ball speeds and heights. It would be most appropriate to conceptualise the athlete in a nonlinear nature, and that their movement behaviour emerges as an adaptive pattern. Athletes are constantly interacting with affordances, resulting in self-organised movement responses in a complex and dynamic performance environment [10,11]. In relation to grip positions in tennis, every stroke exchange between opponents (e.g., serve and return, forehand to backhand on the baseline) provide critical sources of information that athletes engage with to prepare and perform effective task outcomes (e.g., returning the serve), commonly requiring an adaptive grip position. Naturally emerging a grip, an approach that involves using multiple grip positions during a stroke, could benefit athletes, allowing them to naturally build grip positions across different scenarios with associated techniques through discovery and movement exploration.

Interestingly, a lower number of coaches (up to 8% for the forehand) expressed that they use/allow the Western grip in their methods for tennis development. These results are consistent with anecdotal coaching practices as there is a negative connotation associated with the Western grip; it is deemed detrimental to tennis performance as no professionals at the time used the Western grip for the double-handed backhand, as evidenced in [15]. This may align with traditional tennis development, where coaches may subconsciously express 'an ideal model' for their athletes [39], which possibly extends to the use of the Eastern forehand or Semi-Western grips. This is supported by the larger percentage of coaches that use the Eastern or Semi-Western grip positions in their practice across all strokes. The current data may imply that the knowledge of stroke execution, both benefits and restrictions when using a Western grip position, is limited. Should coaches not restrict stroke development to only Eastern forehand and Semi-Western grips in groundstrokes and permit the Western grip within their acceptable grip range, then this may provide the opportunity for their athletes to develop a grip naturally. Coaching requires a mixture of instinctive and intuitive processes to inform decision making for effective development [40], possibly requiring an interplay between traditional and contemporary coaching methods.

4.3. Physically Constraining Tools for Grip Positions

The use of PCTs for stroke development is a common practice in sports coaching that has previously been assessed during the golf drive [13]; however, to date, there is no empirical evidence on the efficacy of PCTs in relation to grip-specific skill development [14]. Almost half of coaches (less experienced: 51.5%; more experienced: 44.1%) believed that using a grip position training device would improve the learning and performance of grip positions, with a smaller number unsure about the learning effects of the tool (less experienced: 35.1%; more experienced: 36.0%). Coaches welcome the use of PCTs in their practice as 65% of coaches indicated that they would use such device if readily available. Only up to 20% of coaches also indicated that the tool would not facilitate the ability to learn or transfer a new grip position from training and into a match-play. This might suggest that coaches have reservations about the effectiveness of PCTs for skill development in regard to grip positions.

A PCT could be used to blend traditional and contemporary based coaching methods. Haptic (vibration or tactile information) and kinaesthetic (instantaneous information about the "feeling" of movement) feedback are fundamentally incorporated into PCTs. Physically constraining tools encourage athletes to maintain a consistent grip position during training under different task or environmental constraints, facilitating an adaptation towards the preferred grip position. It is currently unknown how effective these devices are in creating biomechanical or performance changes in either acute or longitudinal settings. If PCTs deliver constructive, permanent changes in grip position, they would enable coaches to focus their attention on other aspects of tennis performance.

4.4. Limitations and Future Directions and Practical Applications

A limitation of this study was that participants possibly did not have English as their first language, which may have led to possible misinterpretations of questions. However, the authors made their best attempt to minimise interpretations through the piloting process. In addition, being able to read and understand English was a requirement for participation and was expected when the questionnaire was completed. In future, the context for responses from coaches in the form of semi-structured interviews will be important for gaining a better understanding of the thought processes underpinning coaching decisions. This research demonstrated that coaches welcome the idea of using PCTs in practice, with approximately 65% indicating that they would use a PCT in training if readily available. However, there are possible reservations about the ability of PCTs to facilitate skilful learning and transfer. Therefore, it is important to assess the efficacy (biomechanics and skill acquisition) of PCTs for sport-specific skill development.

From a practical application perspective, these findings contribute to a greater understanding of the perceptions of and methods for grip position development within tennis. It also provides an initial perspective regarding the use and implementation of PCTs for skill development. It has previously been expressed that the experiential knowledge of coaches is a highly valuable resource which provides complementary information to support the empirical understanding of performance in sports and to guide future research questions [16,17]. Collectively, these findings provide valuable insights for tennis practitioners by detailing the perspectives of accredited tennis coaches' on grip positions and various aspects of foundational tennis development. This study explored the best practices for grip positions tailored to specific strokes, as well as coaches' opinions on using a PCT. These findings serve as a compass for future investigations, emphasising the importance of aligning research with current coaching practices. Furthermore, the inclusion of coach-led questioning contributes to the ongoing evolution of best practices in developmental-level tennis coaching.

5. Conclusions

This study investigated the perspectives and considerations of accredited tennis coaches on grip positions and foundational development. Irrespective of the experience level, this study showed that coaches rated the importance of technique development as coaches indicated that the Continental, Semi-western, and Eastern forehand grip positions were the most predominantly taught grips and that grip positions are the second-most important contributor to foundational development. There was a significant association between less and more experienced coaches for the reasons why their students revert grip positions, with more experienced coaches only having singular causes compared with less experienced coaches, who responded more often with multiple responses. The most frequent reasons given for reverting grip positions were hand discomfort and out of habit, a common barrier for foundational tennis development. Approximately 65% of coaches would use a PCT to assist in coaching their preferred grip positions to athletes; however, there are possibly reservations about skilful learning and transfer when using a PCT for grip positions. The perceptions and considerations of more experienced coaches may offer practical guidance for less experienced coaches aiming to develop grip positions effectively, similarly for other racket- and club-based sports that require effective grip positions for shot performance. Future research should aim to determine further context behind coaching decisions with regard to grip positions during foundational development, and to assess the efficacy and both the acute and longitudinal effects of PCTs for sport-specific skill development in tennis.

Author Contributions: Conceptualization, N.A.B. and A.H.R.; methodology, N.A.B.; validation, N.A.B.; data curation, N.A.B. and M.H.; writing—original draft preparation, N.A.B.; writing—review and editing, N.A.B., A.H.R., M.D., M.H. and K.J.M.; supervision, A.H.R., M.D. and K.J.M.; project administration, N.A.B. All authors have read and agreed to the published version of the manuscript.

Funding: This research was supported by the Australian Government Research Training Program (RTP) Scholarship, administered by La Trobe University.

Institutional Review Board Statement: The study was conducted according to the guidelines of the Declaration of Helsinki, and approved by the Institutional Human Ethics Committee of La Trobe University (HEC20336; date of approval: 3 November 2020).

Informed Consent Statement: Informed consent was obtained from all participants involved in the study.

Data Availability Statement: The original contributions presented in the study are included in the article, and further inquiries can be directed to the corresponding author.

Conflicts of Interest: The authors declare no conflicts of interest.

References

1. Elliott, B. Biomechanics and tennis. *Br. J. Sports Med.* **2006**, *40*, 392–396. [CrossRef]
2. Carson, H.J.; Richards, J.; Mazuquin, B. Examining the influence of grip type on wrist and club head kinematics during the golf swing: Benefits of a local co-ordinate system. *Eur. J. Sport Sci.* **2019**, *19*, 327–335. [CrossRef]
3. Elliott, B.; Takahashi, K.; Noffal, G. The Influence of Grip Position on Upper Limb Contributions to Racket Head Velocity in a Tennis Forehand. *J. Appl. Biomech.* **1997**, *12*, 182–196. [CrossRef]
4. Genevois, C.; Reid, M.; Rogowski, I.; Crespo, M. Performance Factors Related to the Different Tennis Backhand Groundstrokes A review. *J. Sports Sci. Med.* **2015**, *14*, 194–202.
5. Tagliafico, A.S.; Ameri, P.; Michaud, J.; Derchi, L.E.; Sormani, M.P.; Martinoli, C. Wrist Injuries in Nonprofessional Tennis Players: Relationships with Different Grips. *Am. J. Sports Med.* **2009**, *37*, 760–767. [CrossRef]
6. Busuttil, N.A.; Reid, M.; Connolly, M.; Dascombe, B.; Middleton, K.J. A kinematic analysis of the upper limb during the topspin double-handed backhand stroke in tennis. *Sports Biomech.* **2020**, *21*, 1046–1064. [CrossRef]
7. Busuttil, N.A.; Connolly, M.; Roberts, A.H.; Reid, M.; Dascombe, B.J.; Middleton, K.J. Grip position affects upper limb kinematic chain during tennis double-handed backhand topspin strokes: Considerations for transitioning tennis grip position technique. *Sports Biomech.* **2022**, 1–20. [CrossRef]
8. D'Arcy, M.; Heisler, S.; Quilling, E.; Struder, H.K.; Chevalier, A. The effect of grip position on golf driving accuracy and distance. *J. Sport. Sci.* **2021**, *39*, 1287–1294. [CrossRef]
9. Tennis Australia (Tennis Australia, Melbourne, Victoria, Australia). *Junior Development Course Workbook*; Tennis Australia: Melbourne, Australia, 2012.
10. Chow, J.Y.; Davids, K.; Button, C.; Renshaw, I. *Nonlinear Pedagogy in Skill Acquisition: An Introduction*, 1st ed.; Routledge: London, UK, 2015.
11. Moy, B.; Renshaw, I.; Davids, K. Variations in acculturation and Australian physical education teacher education students' receptiveness to an alternative pedagogical approach to games teaching. *Phys. Educ. Sport Pedagog.* **2013**, *19*, 349–369. [CrossRef]
12. Reid, M.; Whiteside, D.; Elliott, B. Effect of skill decomposition on racket and ball kinematics of the elite junior tennis serve. *Sports Biomech.* **2010**, *9*, 296–303. [CrossRef] [PubMed]
13. Yost, M.; Strauss, R.; Davis, R. The Effectiveness of the "Golfer's Groove" in Improving Golfers' Scores. *Res. Q. Exerc. Sport.* **1976**, *47*, 569–573. [CrossRef]
14. Busuttil, N.A.; Roberts, A.H.; Dunn, M.; Connolly, M.; Middleton, K.J. The use of physically constraining tools for grip-specific skill development in racket, stick and club sports: A scoping review. *J. Sport. Sci.* **2023**, *41*, 788–795. [CrossRef] [PubMed]
15. Eng, D.; Hagler, D. A novel analysis of grip variations on the two-handed backhand. *ITF Coach. Sport. Sci. Rev.* **2014**, *62*, 14–15.
16. Greenwood, D.; Davids, K.; Renshaw, I. How elite coaches' experiential knowledge might enhance research on sport performance. *Int. J. Sports Sci. Coach.* **2012**, *7*, 411–422. [CrossRef]
17. Greenwood, D.; Davids, K.; Renshaw, I. Experiential knowledge of expert coaches can help identify informational constraints on performance of dynamic interceptive actions. *J. Sport. Sci.* **2014**, *32*, 328–335. [CrossRef]
18. Drennan, J. Cognitive interviewing: Verbal data in the design and pretesting of questionnaires. *J. Adv. Nurs.* **2003**, *42*, 57–63. [CrossRef]
19. Willis, G.B. *Cognitive Interviewing: A Tool for Improving Questionnaire Design*, 1st ed.; Sage publishing Ltd.: Thousand Oaks, CA, USA, 2004.
20. Willis, G.B. *Questionnaire Pretesting*, 1st ed.; Sage publishing Ltd.: Thousand Oaks, CA, USA, 2016.
21. Harris, P.A.; Taylor, R.; Minor, B.L.; Elliott, V.; Fernandez, M.; O'Neal, L.; McLeod, L.; Delacqua, G.; Delacqua, F.; Kirby, F.; et al. The REDCap consortium: Building an international community of software platform partners. *J. Biomed. Inform.* **2019**, *95*, 103–208. [CrossRef]
22. Naderifar, M.; Goli, H.; Ghaljaie, F. Snowball sampling: A purposeful method of sampling in qualitative research. *Strides Dev. Med. Educ.* **2017**, *14*, e67670. [CrossRef]
23. Kassambara, A.; Mundt, F. Factoextra: Extract and Visualize the Results of Multivariate Data Analyses. R Package Version 1.0.7. Available online: https://CRAN.R-project.org/package=factoextra (accessed on 18 April 2022).
24. Crespo, M.; Martínez-Gallego, R.; Ramón-Llin, J. Tennis coaches' perceptions of COVID-19 impact on their health and professional activity: A multi-cultural approach. *Sustainability* **2021**, *13*, 5554. [CrossRef]
25. Ericsson, K.A.; Krampe, R.T.; Tesch-Romer, C. The Role of Deliberate Practice in the Acquisition of Expert Performance. *Psychol. Rev.* **1993**, *100*, 363–406. [CrossRef]
26. Elliott, B.; Reid, M.; Crespo, M. *Technique Development in Tennis Stroke Production*, 1st ed.; ITF Limited: London, UK, 2009.
27. Reid, M.; Elliott, B.; Crespo, M. Mechanics and learning practices associated with the tennis forehand: A review. *J. Sports Sci. Med.* **2013**, *12*, 225–231. [PubMed]

28. Reid, M.; Giblin, G. Another day, another tennis coaching intervention, but does this one do what coaches purport? *Sports Biomech.* **2015**, *14*, 180–189. [CrossRef]
29. Reid, M.; Giblin, G.; Whiteside, D. A kinematic comparison of the overhand throw and tennis serve in tennis players: How similar are they really? *J. Sport. Sci.* **2015**, *33*, 713–723. [CrossRef]
30. Kovacs, M. Applied physiology of tennis performance. *Br. J. Sports Med.* **2006**, *40*, 381–386. [CrossRef]
31. Pill, S.; Hewitt, M. Tennis coaching: Applying the game sense approach. *Strategies* **2017**, *30*, 10–16.
32. Bunker, D.; Thorpe, R. A model for the teaching of games in secondary schools. *Bull. Phys. Educ.* **1982**, *18*, 5–8.
33. den Duyn, N. *Game Sense: Developing Thinking Players Workbook;* Australian Sports Commission: Belconnen/Canberra Australia, 1997.
34. Reid, M.; Whiteside, D.; Elliott, B. Serving to different locations: Set-up, toss, and racket kinematics of the professional tennis serve. *Sports Biomech.* **2011**, *10*, 407–414. [CrossRef] [PubMed]
35. Whiteside, D.; Elliott, B.C.; Lay, B.; Reid, M. Coordination and variability in the elite female tennis serve. *J. Sport. Sci.* **2015**, *33* 675–686. [CrossRef]
36. Reid, M.; Elliott, B.; Alderson, J. Lower-limb coordination and shoulder joint mechanics in the tennis serve. *Med. Sci. Sports Exerc* **2008**, *40*, 308–315. [CrossRef]
37. Elliott, B.; Marshall, R.N.; Noffal, G.J. Contributions of upper limb segment rotations during the power serve in tennis. *J. Appl Biomech.* **1995**, *11*, 433–442. [CrossRef]
38. Gove, W.R.; Geerken, M.R. Response bias in surveys of mental health: An empirical investigation. *Am. J. Sociol.* **1977**, *82* 1289–1317. [CrossRef] [PubMed]
39. Fery, Y.; Morizot, P. Kinesthetic and visual image in modeling closed motor skills: The example of the tennis serve. *Percept. Mot Skills* **2000**, *90*, 707–722. [CrossRef] [PubMed]
40. Nash, C.; Collins, D. Tacit knowledge in expert coaching: Science or art? *Quest* **2006**, *58*, 465–477. [CrossRef]

applied sciences

MDPI

Article

Assessing the Probability of Winning a Point in Men's Padel: A Comprehensive Analysis

Iván Prieto-Lage [1,*], Xoana Reguera-López-de-la-Osa [2,*], Nicolás Durán-Rodríguez [1], Antonio José Silva-Pinto [1], Juan Carlos Argibay-González [1] and Alfonso Gutiérrez-Santiago [1]

[1] Observational Research Group, Faculty of Education and Sport, University of Vigo, 36005 Pontevedra, Spain; nicolasduranrodriguez.ndr@gmail.com (N.D.-R.); toze-pinto@hotmail.com (A.J.S.-P.); juan.carlos.argibay@uvigo.gal (J.C.A.-G.); ags@uvigo.es (A.G.-S.)

[2] Education, Physical Activity and Health Research Group (Gies10-DE3), Galicia Sur Health Research, Institute (IIS Galicia Sur), SERGAS-UVIGO, 36208 Vigo, Spain

* Correspondence: ivanprieto@uvigo.es (I.P.-L.); xreguera@uvigo.es (X.R.-L.-d.-l.-O.)

Abstract: Background—The number of studies on padel has grown significantly in recent years, reflecting the growing importance of the sport. However, more research is still needed on a comprehensive analysis of performance indicators. This study had a double objective: on the one hand, to analyze the probability of winning a point as a function of several variables and, on the other hand, to develop a match analysis. Methods—A total of 980 points from the Menorca 2020 World Padel Tour Master Final Men's category were examined using observational methodology. The participants were the eight pairs who competed in the final rounds of the tournament. To obtain the results, various analytical techniques were used, such as descriptive analysis and the chi-square test, with a significance level of $p < 0.05$. Results—The results indicated that most points were initiated on the first serve (88.5%) and were most often won by the serving pair (59.3%). Short rallies predominated (42.2%), with the serving pair most likely to win the point (71%). As the rally became longer, the probability of winning the point decreased, reaching 57% for medium rallies and 47% for long rallies. Almost half of the points were completed in less than 10 s, with an average point duration of 15 s. Most points were finished from the middle area and near the net (41.4% and 36%, respectively), mainly by smashes (25.9%) or volleys (28.9%), with the cross-court trajectory being the most effective. Conclusions—Short rallies (0–6 shots) were the most common, with an average point duration of approximately 15 s. Most points ended with a shot from the middle of the court, using a volley or a smash with a cross-court trajectory. There is a clear relationship between proximity to the net on the final shot and an increased probability of winning the point.

Keywords: notational analysis; performance; observational analysis; match statistics; padel coaching

1. Introduction

Padel, a racket sport that originated in Acapulco (Mexico) in 1969, has expanded significantly in recent years [1]. It currently has 50 national federations around the world [2]. Padel is played by individuals of various ages and competitive levels thanks to its straightforward rules and the sport's ability to adapt its physical demands to different skill levels [3]. In recent years, several professional circuits (A1 Padel, World Padel Tour, and Premier Padel) have coexisted. However, in 2024, the World Padel Tour and Premier Padel merged, with the latter becoming the most prestigious among professionals.

Despite its remarkable growth in the last decade, the sport has received limited attention from the scientific community [4]. It is therefore crucial to carry out a constant analysis of the factors influencing performance as the sport may be changing at a faster pace compared to other more established racket sports such as tennis, badminton or squash, which have also seen substantial variations in their performance indicators since the 2000s [5].

In the field of sport performance, research has been carried out that has focused on various aspects such as the validation of observational instruments [6–8], the time structure of the match [9–11], the anthropometric characteristics and physiological requirements of the athletes [12–14], and the analysis of the game at a technical–tactical level [15–21].

Knowledge of the structure of the game is essential to design tasks and training sessions aimed at optimizing players' performance. Unlike tennis [22,23], in padel, the serve (in reference to winning the point with this stroke) and the dominance from the back of the court are not determining factors for performance. Previous research has indicated that up to 80% of points are won from a position close to the net, using a variety of strokes, such as the volley (20–25%) and the tray and the smash (12–18%) [13,17,24]. From the start of the point, there is a constant battle for a position near the net as maintaining this position gives a tactical advantage over the opponent. Numerous studies have highlighted that the probability of winning the point increases when players maintain a position close to the net [11,25,26]. Although aces are rare in this sport, it has been shown that serving is more effective than returning as the serving pair wins approximately 62.5% of the points in the men's category [1].

As for the number of shots in each rally, an average of between nine and ten shots per point has been observed in both the men's and women's categories [26,27]. Research on time structure has revealed that padel is an intermittent sport, with an average duration in elite players of 9.30 ± 4.00 s per point and 9.38 ± 1.72 shots per point in matches of a 57.4 ± 11.6 min duration [11]. These studies have also shown that in the first few seconds of the rally, more points are lost due to unforced errors whereas as the rally progresses, unforced errors decrease and winners or forced errors increase [10]. As for the variety of strokes and their direction, volleys predominate (25.0–26.8%), as do ground strokes (15.5%), which tend to be mostly cross hits (62.5–65.5%) [17].

However, despite the information gathered in previous research, there has been a notable absence of studies that thoroughly address the probability of winning a point, taking into account different combinations of the most influential performance indicators in the sport. Therefore, the main purpose of this paper is to analyze the probability of winning a point in elite men's padel, considering factors such as the type of rally, the location of the players on the court where the last shot is played, the type of final shot, and the finishing area. This comprehensive approach will provide valuable information to deepen the understanding of padel performance and to improve match strategy in this sport.

2. Materials and Methods

2.1. Design

For the purpose of this research on high-level men's padel, we adopted an observational methodology [28]. The observational design [29] was characterized by being nomothetic as it covered all the points played in the final rounds of the World Padel Tour Master Final in Menorca in 2020. Moreover, it was a follow-up, as it analyzed a tournament from the quarter-finals onwards, and focused on a unidimensional dimension, with no concurrence of simultaneous behaviors.

2.2. Sample

Considering that the unit of analysis of this study comprised the points played in the World Padel Tour Master Final 2020 in the men's category, the final sample was made up of a total of 980 points. Participants included the 8 pairs competing in the quarter-final, semi-final, and final rounds. A total of seven matches were analyzed. Informed consent of the participants was not required because the data were not generated by experimentation and the video material was obtained secondarily [30]. The study was approved by the Ethics Committee of the Faculty of Education and Sport Sciences of the University of Vigo (application 07-280722).

2.3. Instruments

To carry out this study, we used the OBSPADEL-S20, an observation instrument designed to analyze the different actions present in the game of padel. The observation instrument was created ad hoc for this research and was based on criteria and categories previously used in padel studies (see Table 1 and Figure 1) [8,15,31].

Table 1. OBSPADEL observation instrument.

Criteria	Code	Description
Service	FS	The point is played with first serve
	SS	The point is played with second serve
	DF	Double fault
Rally lenght	SH	Short rally (0–6 shots).
	MD	Medium rally (7–12 shots).
	LN	Long rally (13+ shots).
Strike zone (see Figure 1)	SZ1	Zone between the end wall and the service line
	SZ2	Zone between the service line and three meters before the net
	SZ3	Zone between 3 meters in front of the net and the net
	SZ	Service zone
The finish zone (see Figure 1)	PST	Zone of the court parallel to the final stroke (player's parallel stroke)
	MST	The player hits the ball to the middle of the court
	CST	Zone of the court crossed to the final stroke (player's cross-court stroke)
	SNT	Final shot to the net
	SSC	Final shot to the opponent's side of the court directly
	SEC	Final shot to the end of the court directly
Winner	SW	The serving pair wins the point
	RW	The returning pair wins the point
Point Ending	SWW	The serving team wins with a winner
	SWFE	The serving team wins with a forced error by the opponent
	SWUE	The serving team wins with an unforced error by the opponent
	RWW	The returning team wins with a winner
	RWFE	The returning team wins with a forced error by the opponent
	RWUE	The returning team wins with an unforced error by the opponent
Final Stroke	ACE	Direct serve
	FHW	Forehand wall outlet
	BHW	Backhand wall outlet
	FHG	Forehand groundstroke
	BHG	Backhand groundstroke
	FHV	Forehand volley
	BHV	Backhand volley
	SM	Smash
	TR	Tray
	LB	Lob
	DS	Drop shot
	OT	Other (counter-wall, double wall, special stroke...)
Time	T	Duration of the point in seconds

Note: PST, MST, and CST (finish zone criterion) refer to the trajectory of the stroke in both winners and forced error points. (Acronyms in Table 1.)

The OBSPADEL-S20 consists of eight criteria that form a category system that meets the requirements of completeness and mutual exclusivity. Data recording was carried out using LINCE PLUS software version 2.1.0 [32].

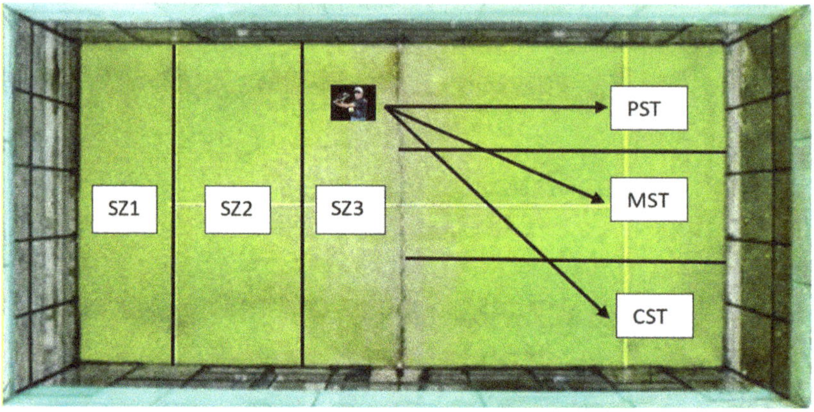

Figure 1. Court zone and direction of the final stroke. Note: SZ—strike zone, PST—parallel stroke, MST—middle zone stroke, and CST—cross stroke.

2.4. Procedure

The data collection was carried out by downloading the matches from the official World Padel Tour YouTube channel. Subsequently, all the files were combined into a single video of 12 h and 23 min. The editing of the matches was achieved using Wondershare Filmora software version X. These matches were downloaded in high definition (1080p, 1920 × 1080) and viewed on 27-inch monitors for analysis.

To ensure the quality and consistency of the data, a rigorous protocol was followed. Prior to the data quality check, carried out by two experts in padel and observation methodology, a comprehensive training program was conducted. One of the experts was a national paddle tennis coach with a degree in Physical Education and Sports Science while the other was a university professor specializing in racquet sports and observational methodology. This training consisted of nine two-hour sessions over a three-week period and used videos of men's padel matches from the 2020 season for the experts to become familiar with the observation tool.

In order to reinforce the integrity of the recording process [33], the quality of the recorded data was assessed by calculating intra-observer and inter-observer concordance using the Kappa coefficient [34]. The LINCE PLUS program facilitated this analysis. Both concordances were performed on points from padel matches that did not belong to the final sample (n = 300; 1/3 final sample). The intra-observer kappa was 0.96 for the first observer and 0.95 for the second observer while the inter-observer kappa was 0.94. Subsequently, observer 1 proceeded to analyze all items in the research sample.

Once the meticulous recording of all data was completed, an Excel file was generated documenting the sequence of actions at each of the points analyzed. The versatility of this Excel file allowed the data to be transferred to an SPSS file (Statistical Package for the Social Sciences), the software used to carry out various statistical analyses essential to the research.

2.5. Data Analysis

All statistical analyzes were carried out using SPSS version 25.0 (IBM-SPSS Inc., Chicago, IL, USA). Statistical significance was considered to be reached at $p < 0.05$.

First, a descriptive analysis of the study variables was carried out. To assess the differences between the categories of each criterion used (intra-criterion analysis), the chi-square test (χ^2) was used. The analysis of the probability of winning a point, as influenced by the combination of performance indicators selected by the research team, was carried out using the case selection and frequency analysis technique.

3. Results

3.1. Descriptive Analysis

Table 2 presents a descriptive analysis of the study, including the intra-criterion χ^2 test performed for the categories of each criterion.

Table 2. Distribution of points played in the World Padel Tour Menorca Master Final 2020 and χ^2 intra-criterion analysis.

Criterion	Cat.	n	%	χ^2	Criterion	Cat.	n	%	χ^2
Service *	FS	867	88.5	$\chi^2 = 582.252$	Winner	SW	581	59.3	$\chi^2 = 34.207$
	SS	112	11.4	$p < 0.001$		RW	399	40.7	$p < 0.001$
	DF	1	0.1		Final Stroke	FHW	117	11.9	$\chi^2 = 593.011$
Rally length	SH	414	42.2	$\chi^2 = 34.525$		BHW	54	5.5	$p < 0.001$
	MD	283	28.9	$p < 0.001$		FHG	55	5.6	
	LN	283	28.9			BHG	41	4.2	
Strike zone *	SZ1	220	22.4	$\chi^2 = 56.276$		FHV	151	15.4	
	SZ2	406	41.4	$p < 0.001$		BHV	132	13.5	
	SZ3	353	36.0			SM	254	25.9	
	SZ	1	0.1			TR	107	10.9	
The finish zone	PST	162	16.5	$\chi^2 = 182.236$		LB	46	4.7	
	MST	124	12.7	$p < 0.001$		OT	6	0.6	
	CST	262	26.7			DS	16	1.6	
	SNT	250	25.5						
	SSC	73	7.4		Point duration	1–10 s	439	44.8	$\chi^2 = 287.698$
	SEC	109	11.1			11–20 s	294	30.0	$p < 0.001$
Point ending	SWW	268	27.3	$\chi^2 = 230.113$		21–30 s	145	14.8	
	SWFE	75	7.7	$p < 0.001$		31+	102	10.4	
	SWUE	237	24.2						
	RWW	154	15.7						
	RWFE	52	5.3						
	RWUE	194	19.8						

* Note: The category with the lowest frequency value was eliminated for the χ^2 test. Acronyms are given in Table 1.

During the investigation, it was observed that most of the points were initiated with the first service, reaching 88.5%. In addition, short rallies were predominant, accounting for 42.2%. The middle area of the court was the location from where most of the final shots were executed, comprising 41.4% of the total number of cases. Almost 60% of the points were won by serving. In terms of how the points were completed, it is worth noting that points won on serve by winners (27.3% of the total) and unforced errors (24.2%) predominated. Points won by the receiving team through unforced errors constituted 19.8% of the total while winners accounted for 15.7%. The most commonly used finishing stroke was the smash (which included the smash ×3, smash ×4, fake smash, and smash over the back wall), with a percentage of 25.9%. Forehand and backhand volleys were also commonly observed, with percentages of 15.4% and 13.5%, respectively. In terms of the finishing area, it was evident that the predominant way of winning points was by cross-court shots (26.7%) while the majority of errors were made after hitting the net. Regarding the duration of the points, the most common time interval was 1 to 10 s, accounting for 44.8% of the cases, followed by 11 to 20 s, which made up 30%. The average point duration was 15.23 ± 11.6 s.

Statistically significant differences ($p < 0.05$) were observed between the categories of each of the criteria studied according to the results of the intra-criterion χ^2 test.

3.2. Analysis of the Probability of Winning a Point

The following is a detailed analysis of the probability of winning a point in padel, taking into account several variables of the game. This analysis has focused exclusively on points played on the first serve as they accounted for approximately 90% of the total in this study (see Table 3).

Table 3. Analysis of the probability of winning a point as a function of service, type of rally, and strike zone.

		Serving Team				Returning Team			
	Fr. (%)	Total	Won	Lost	Prob.	Total	Won	Lost	Prob.
First service	88.5	867	521	346	60	867	346	521	40
Second service	11.5	112	60	52	54	112	52	60	46
First Service–Short rally	42.9	372	264	108	71	372	108	264	29
First Service–Medium rally	28.1	244	139	105	57	244	105	139	43
First Service–Long rally	29.0	251	118	133	47	251	133	118	53
First Service–Short rally–Strike zone 1	12.6	30	12	18	40	79	4	75	5
First Service–Short rally–Strike zone 2	14.8	106	78	28	74	22	8	14	36
First Service–Short rally–Strike zone 3	15.6	89	73	16	82	46	34	12	74
First Service–Medium rally–Strike zone 1	5.3	15	3	12	20	31	4	27	13
First Service–Medium rally–Strike zone 2	13.0	62	35	27	56	51	20	31	39
First Service–Medium rally–Strike zone 3	9.8	47	33	14	70	38	28	10	74
First Service–Long rally–Strike zone 1	4.4	15	3	12	20	23	8	15	35
First Service–Long rally–Strike zone 2	13.8	53	32	21	60	67	41	26	61
First Service–Long rally–Strike zone 3	10.7	54	39	15	72	39	36	3	92

Note: Fr—frequency; Total—total points occurred in that match situation; Prob—probability (%).

Firstly, our findings indicate that the serving team wins 71% of the points in short rallies (0–6 shots). This percentage decreases to 57% in medium-length rallies (6–12 shots) and further drops to 47% in long rallies (13+ shots).

During a short rally, it is interesting to note that zone 3 is where you have the highest probability of winning a point, both on serve (82%) and on return (74%). In zone 2, the probabilities are somewhat lower in the service (74%) but considerably lower in the return (36%). Finally, in zone 1, the probabilities of winning the point are low in both pairs (4% for service and 0.5% for the return).

In medium-length rallies, we see a similar pattern although the odds of winning the point vary. The final hit from zone 3 gives the highest odds to both the serving team (70%) and the receiving team (74%), followed by zone 2 (56% to the serve and 39% to the return) and, finally, zone 1 (20% and 13%, respectively).

In the long rally, the same pattern is repeated. Zone 3 has the highest probability of success in both pairs (72% for service and 92% for the return), followed by zone 2 (60% and 61%) and finally zone 1 (20% and 35%).

3.3. Match Analysis

Table 4 presents a match analysis taking into account different performance indicators.

After analyzing all the matches, we observed that 11.1% of the points ended with a short rally and a final hit from zone 1. In these cases, the serving pair won 13.8% of those points through winners while the returning team (RT) won 18.2%. It is important to note that there was a high rate of points won on serve due to unforced errors (86.2% serving and 81.8% returning), with a predominance of hitting the net errors.

A total of 13.1% of the points culminated in a short rally and a final hit from zone 2. In this situation, the serving pair achieved 84.7% of the points by winners (22.2% RT) and there was a balance between those obtained with cross and parallel strokes in both pairs.

Table 4. Match analysis of points with first serve and according to rally length, strike zone, the finish zone, winner, and point ending.

Pattern	n = 980			Pattern	n = 980		
	Fr.	%			Fr.	%	
FS-SH-SW-SWFE	26	7.0		FS-SH-RW-RWFE	6	1.6	
FS-SH-SW-SWUE	101	27.2		FS-SH-RW-RWUE	62	16.7	
FS-SH-SW-SWW	137	36.8		FS-SH-RW-RWW	40	10.8	
FS-MD-SW-SWFE	25	10.2		FS-MD-RW-RWFE	14	5.7	
FS-MD-SW-SWUE	67	27.5		FS-MD-RW-RWUE	53	21.7	
FS-MD-SW-SWW	46	18.9		FS-MD-RW-RWW	39	16.0	
FS-LN-SW-SWFE	19	7.6		FS-LN-RW-RWFE	27	10.8	
FS-LN-SW-SWUE	44	17.5		FS-LN-RW-RWUE	48	19.1	
FS-LN-SW-SWW	55	21.9		FS-LN-RW-RWW	58	23.1	
FS-SH-ST1-SW	87 (109)	(11.1)	79.8	FS-SH-ST1-RW	22 (109)	(11.1)	20.2
FS-SH-ST1-SEC-SW	26	29.9		FS-SH-ST1-SEC-RW	4	18.2	
FS-SH-ST1-SSC-SW	7	8.0	75 (87) 86.2	FS-SH-ST1-SSC-RW	2	9.1	18 (22) 81.8
FS-SH-ST1-SNT-SW	42	48.3		FS-SH-ST1-SNT-RW	12	54.5	
FS-SH-ST1-PST-SW	3	3.4		FS-SH-ST1-PST-RW	1	4.5	
FS-SH-ST1-MST-SW	4	4.6	12 (87) 13.8	FS-SH-ST1-MST-RW	3	13.6	4 (22) 18.2
FS-SH-ST1-CST-SW	5	5.7		FS-SH-ST1-CST-RW	-	-	
FS-SH-ST2-SW	92 (128)	(13.1)	71.9	FS-SH-ST2-RW	36 (128)	(13.1)	28.1
FS-SH-ST2-SEC-SW	3	3.3		FS-SH-ST2-SEC-RW	4	11.1	
FS-SH-ST2-SSC-SW	3	3.3	14 (92) 15.3	FS-SH-ST2-SSC-RW	5	13.9	28 (36) 77.8
FS-SH-ST2-SNT-SW	8	8.7		FS-SH-ST2-SNT-RW	19	52.8	
FS-SH-ST2-PST-SW	27	29.3		FS-SH-ST2-PST-RW	4	11.1	
FS-SH-ST2-MST-SW	22	23.9	78 (92) 84.7	FS-SH-ST2-MST-RW	1	2.8	8 (36) 22.2
FS-SH-ST2-CST-SW	29	31.5		FS-SH-ST2-CST-RW	3	8.3	
FS-SH-ST3-SW	85 (135)	(13.8)	63.0	FS-SH-ST3-RW	50 (135)	(13.8)	37.0
FS-SH-ST3-SEC-SW	-	-		FS-SH-ST3-SEC-RW	4	8.0	
FS-SH-ST3-SSC-SW	3	3.5	12 (85) 14.1	FS-SH-ST3-SSC-RW	4	8.0	16 (50) 32.0
FS-SH-ST3-SNT-SW	9	10.6		FS-SH-ST3-SNT-RW	8	16.0	
FS-SH-ST3-PST-SW	24	28.2		FS-SH-ST3-PST-RW	12	24.0	
FS-SH-ST3-MST-SW	16	18.8	73 (85) 85.8	FS-SH-ST3-MST-RW	7	14.0	34 (50) 68.8
FS-SH-ST3-CST-SW	33	38.8		FS-SH-ST3-CST-RW	15	30.0	
FS-MD-ST1-SW	30 (46)	(4.7)	65.2	FS-MD-ST1-RW	16 (46)	(4.7)	34.8
FS-MD-ST1-SEC-SW	9	30.0		FS-MD-ST1-SEC-RW	4	25.0	
FS-MD-ST1-SSC-SW	4	13.3	27 (30) 90.0	FS-MD-ST1-SSC-RW	-	-	12 (16) 75.0
FS-MD-ST1-SNT-SW	14	46.7		FS-MD-ST1-SNT-RW	8	50.0	
FS-MD-ST1-PST-SW	1	3.3		FS-MD-ST1-PST-RW	1	6.3	
FS-MD-ST1-MST-SW	-	-	3 (30) 10.0	FS-MD-ST1-MST-RW	1	6.3	4 (16) 25.0
FS-MD-ST1-CST-SW	2	6.7		FS-MD-ST1-CST-RW	2	12.5	
FS-MD-ST2-SW	66 (113)	(11.5)	58.4	FS-MD-ST2-RW	47 (113)	(11.5)	41.6
FS-MD-ST2-SEC-SW	6	9.1		FS-MD-ST2-SEC-RW	7	14.9	
FS-MD-ST2-SSC-SW	6	9.1	31 (66) 47.0	FS-MD-ST2-SSC-RW	6	12.8	27 (47) 57.5
FS-MD-ST2-SNT-SW	19	28.8		FS-MD-ST2-SNT-RW	14	29.8	
FS-MD-ST2-PST-SW	8	12.1	35 (66)	FS-MD-ST2-PST-RW	3	6.4	
FS-MD-ST2-MST-SW	6	9.1	53.0	FS-MD-ST2-MST-RW	6	12.8	20 (47) 42.5
FS-MD-ST2-CST-SW	21	31.8		FS-MD-ST2-CST-RW	11	23.4	
FS-MD-ST3-SW	43 (85)	(8.7)	50.6	FS-MD-ST3-RW	42 (85)	(8.7)	49.4
FS-MD-ST3-SEC-SW	2	4.7		FS-MD-ST3-SEC-RW	3	7.1	
FS-MD-ST3-SSC-SW	2	4.7	10 (43) 23.4	FS-MD-ST3-SSC-RW	3	7.1	14 (42) 33.3
FS-MD-ST3-SNT-SW	6	14.0		FS-MD-ST3-SNT-RW	8	19.0	
FS-MD-ST3-PST-SW	8	18.6		FS-MD-ST3-PST-RW	10	23.8	
FS-MD-ST3-MST-SW	4	9.3	33 (43) 76.6	FS-MD-ST3-MST-RW	3	7.1	28 (42) 66.7
FS-MD-ST3-CST-SW	21	48.8		FS-MD-ST3-CST-RW	15	35.7	
FS-LN-ST1-SW	18 (38)	(3.9)	47.4	FS-LN-ST1-RW	20 (38)	(3.9)	52.6
FS-LN-ST1-SEC-SW	3	16.7		FS-LN-ST1-SEC-RW	3	15.0	
FS-LN-ST1-SSC-SW	1	5.6	15 (18) 83.3	FS-LN-ST1-SSC-RW	3	15.0	12 (20) 60.0
FS-LN-ST1-SNT-SW	11	61.1		FS-LN-ST1-SNT-RW	6	30.0	
FS-LN-ST1-PST-SW	2	11.1		FS-LN-ST1-PST-RW	2	10.0	
FS-LN-ST1-MST-SW	-	-	3 (18) 16.7	FS-LN-ST1-MST-RW	2	10.0	8 (20) 40.0
FS-LN-ST1-CST-SW	1	5.6		FS-LN-ST1-CST-RW	4	20.0	

Table 4. *Cont.*

Pattern	n = 980			Pattern	n = 980		
	Fr.	%			Fr.	%	
FS-LN-ST2-SW	58 (120)	(12.2)	48.3	FS-LN-ST2-RW	62 (120)	(12.2)	51.7
FS-LN-ST2-SEC-SW	8	13.8		FS-LN-ST2-SEC-RW	7	11.3	
FS-LN-ST2-SSC-SW	4	6.9	26 (58) 44.8	FS-LN-ST2-SSC-RW	6	9.7	21 (62) 33.9
FS-LN-ST2-SNT-SW	14	24.1		FS-LN-ST2-SNT-RW	8	12.9	
FS-LN-ST2-PST-SW	8	13.8		FS-LN-ST2-PST-RW	11	17.7	
FS-LN-ST2-MST-SW	8	13.8	32 (58) 55.2	FS-LN-ST2-MST-RW	8	12.9	41 (62) 66.1
FS-LN-ST2-CST-SW	16	27.6		FS-LN-ST2-CST-RW	22	35.5	
FS-LN-ST3-SW	42 (93)	(9.5)	45.2	FS-LN-ST3-RW	51 (93)	(9.5)	54.8
FS-LN-ST3-SEC-SW	-	-		FS-LN-ST3-SEC-RW	3	5.9	
FS-LN-ST3-SSC-SW	1	2.4	3 (42) 7.2	FS-LN-ST3-SSC-RW	3	5.9	15 (51) 29.4
FS-LN-ST3-SNT-SW	2	4.8		FS-LN-ST3-SNT-RW	9	17.6	
FS-LN-ST3-PST-SW	15	35.7		FS-LN-ST3-PST-RW	12	23.5	
FS-LN-ST3-MST-SW	6	14.3	39 (42) 92.8	FS-LN-ST3-MST-RW	10	19.6	36 (51) 70.6
FS-LN-ST3-CST-SW	18	42.9		FS-LN-ST3-CST-RW	14	27.5	

Note: Acronyms are given in Table 1.

A total of 13.8% of the points ended with a short rally and a final hit from zone 3. The values were very similar to those observed in zone 2 for the serving pair (85.8% won by winners) but different in the defending pair (68.8% winners). In both cases, winners with crossed trajectories predominated.

Although the situation where the point ended with a medium rally and a hit from zone 1 only occurred on 4.7% of occasions, it is interesting to note that the serving pair managed to win the point in 10% of the cases by a winner while the defending pair did so in 25% of the cases. Unforced errors were more common from hitting the net.

When the final shot was executed from zone 2 and ended in a medium rally, it was observed that the serving pair achieved 53% of points through winners (42.5% RT), with a predominance of cross-court shots as the final trajectory in both teams. This situation occurred 11.5% of the time. It is interesting to note that the percentage of service winners decreased significantly compared to the short rally in the same zone but increased for the defending pair.

A total of 8.7% of the points ended after a medium rally and a final hit from zone 3. In this situation, up to 76.6% of the points won on serve were won by a winner (66.7% RT), again with a predominance of crossed shots in both teams. A decrease in the percentage of points won by winners was observed for the serving pair compared to the points won from this area in the case of short rallies, but no such decrease was observed for the defending pair.

When the point ended after a long rally and a stroke executed from zone 1, although this only occurred in 4% of the cases, the same tendency observed in the case of a medium rally was repeated. In this situation, there were higher percentages of winners for the pair receiving the service (16.7% and 40%, respectively).

A total of 12.2% of the points ended after a long rally and a final shot executed from zone 2. In this case, the serving pair won 55.2% of the points through winners (66.1% RT), predominantly with cross-court shots in both cases. In both pairs, the points won by unforced errors were mostly due to shots directed to the net.

Finally, points ending after a long rally and a final hit from zone 3 accounted for 9.5% of the points analyzed. In this situation, winners clearly predominated as a way of finishing the point, with 92.8% in the serving pair and 70.6% in the defending pair. Again, there was a high proportion of winners with cross-court shots although there was also a considerable percentage of winners with parallel shots.

4. Discussion

The aim of the research was to assess the probability of winning a point by considering a number of variables that affect performance as well as by providing a comprehensive analysis of matches. The data showed that the probability of winning a point by serving was higher in short rallies and decreased in medium and long rallies. A position close to the net increases the probability of winning the point. The research revealed that the most common type of rally is the short rally and that the average duration of points is 15 s. In addition, the most common trajectory of the final shots is the cross-court shot, executed over the middle of the court. Smashes and volleys predominate as final shots.

In the match analysis in this research, it was observed that the first serve is used on 90% of occasions and that double faults are infrequent, a result that coincided with previous research [1]. The probability of winning the point by serving the first serve was somewhat higher than by returning (60%), with rates similar to those observed in this sport previously [35].

Although it is uncommon to obtain direct points (aces) or indirect points with the serve [1], probably due to the regulatory restrictions of padel compared to racket sports such as tennis [18,36], this technical action allows one to secure an offensive position near the net [9]. This, according to experts [18,25], provides a tactical advantage to win the point. Previous research supports that a position close to the net favors winners or increases the likelihood of errors being made by the opposing team [15,26,37], a finding that we also confirmed in our study. The results of this research indicate that proximity to the net, whether serving or returning, increases the chances of winning the point.

Short rallies (0–6 shots) were the most common type of rally detected. However, analysis of the duration of the points revealed an average of 15 s, in line with recent studies [27] but marking a change from older research that reported a duration of 7–12 s [9–11,38]. It is possible that the technical–tactical and physical improvement of padel pairs is making it difficult to finish points quickly, a relevant aspect to consider in the planning of training sessions, especially from a conditional approach.

The type of rally plays a crucial factor in the chances of winning the point. In short rallies, the service pair won 73% of the points; however, this value dropped to 57% in medium rallies and dropped even further to 47% in long rallies. This pattern supports the idea that the tactical advantage in serving fades after the first six shots [1,36]. Consequently, in order to optimize training, it is suggested that the serving pair should seek to conclude the point quickly, taking advantage of their initial position close to the net, while the defending pair should prolong the rally, as following these guidelines significantly increases the chances of winning the point. In another sense, it is essential that coaches consider the option of creating training routines that cover both the return of serves to the server and the execution of defensive shots such as deep lobs to the corners of the court [39]. Previous studies have demonstrated that the lob is the most frequently utilized technique for reaching the net, a position on the court that subsequently increases the likelihood of winning points [20,39,40].

Points ending with shots from the middle area of the court were the most frequent in this study, as had been shown previously [15,41], although they did not represent the area with the highest percentage of winners, as has been observed recently [18]. From the middle zone, except in short rallies, where there was a predominance of winners in the serving pair, similar numbers of points won by winners and unforced errors were recorded. In contrast, from the area furthest from the net, more unforced errors were observed in any type of rally. On the other hand, in shots close to the net, regardless of the type of rally, a higher proportion of winners was evident. Once again, it was confirmed that the probability of winning the point increases as the pair gets closer to the net as they have more chances to get a winner. On the other hand, hitting from the back of the court increases the likelihood of errors [15]. This is because when players play close to the net, they generally try to finish the point with a winner [42] whereas when they play from areas away from the net, they have less of an angle to play the ball to the fence [43]. Although previous research did not establish an explicit probability, it did highlight the tactical importance of getting close to the net or shortening–lengthening the length of the rally depending on whether the team was on serve or return. It is relevant to note that a higher percentage of winners was observed in long rallies compared to medium-length rallies. This discrepancy could have been due to accumulated fatigue during the prolongation of the point.

As for the final hit, in our research, smashes (25.9%) stood out as the main option. This phenomenon can be attributed to the effectiveness of this stroke in padel, which is characterized by a relatively low rate of unforced errors. This stroke, aggressive and confident when the technique is mastered, is presumed to be a fundamental skill in professional players [3,8]. It is clear that players are looking for opportunities throughout the point to execute a smash, but training this shot from less comfortable positions could be a valuable training strategy, given its high performance as a finishing stroke. The combination of forehand and backhand volleys (28.9%) outperformed the smash as the final shot, highlighting the importance of also optimizing this technical skill to close out points [44].

In relation to the direction of the final stroke, our study confirmed that the majority of points end with cross-court strokes, almost twice as often as parallel strokes and three times as often as strokes aimed at the center of the court. Although we did not carry out an analysis of all rally points, as was achieved in other research [8,17], we can affirm that there is a clear tendency for the cross-court shot to be more effective in finishing a point. This observation aligns with previous findings [15] and is related to the difficulty of returning shots that bounce off the metal fence, the side wall, or the corner between the back wall and the side wall. This creates greater uncertainty for the opponent and increases the likelihood of mistakes [17].

Limitations and Future Perspectives

Only matches from the WPT Master Final, which brings together the eight best pairings on the men's tour, were analyzed. It is important to note that if the analysis had been carried out for one or more complete tournaments on the World Padel Tour circuit, with more rounds and participating pairings, the results could have been different. Furthermore, it is relevant to note that this observational study did not take into account aspects such as the positioning of the players and the strokes used throughout the rally, but focused only on the final stroke. This choice was based on the specific objective of the study, but future research could approach the analysis from other perspectives. It would be equally interesting to replicate this study in the female category to compare performance indicators between men and women.

5. Conclusions

This research enriches the knowledge about men's professional padel and provides valuable information to improve strategy and coaching.

The analysis revealed that nearly all points were played on the first serve, with a slightly higher probability of winning the point compared to starting with a second serve. It was observed that the probability of winning a point by serving was highest in short rallies and decreased progressively in medium and long rallies.

Regarding finishing shots, the smash was identified as the most frequently used technique to close points, followed by forehand and backhand volleys. Cross-court shots were more commonly used to finish points, either through winners or forced errors. Additionally, nearly half of the points concluded with a short rally, lasting between 1 and 10 s. The average duration of a point was estimated to be 15.23 s.

The probability of winning a point is influenced by factors such as service possession, type of rally, and court positioning. Generally, it was observed that in short rallies, the serving pair had a higher chance of winning the point while the chances diminished as the rally lengthened. Furthermore, the pair dominating the net had a higher probability of securing the point. The combination of a first serve, short rally, and a shot from zone 3 was found to be the most advantageous for the serving pair, with an 82% success rate. Conversely, the combination of a first serve, long rally, and a final shot from zone 3 offered the defending pair the highest chances of winning the point, with a 92% success rate.

For the serving pair, the highest probability of winning the point is achieved when the point ends with a short rally and the pair positions themselves close to the net to execute a cross-court finishing shot. Therefore, it is beneficial for the serving partner to show intensity from the start of the point, looking for winners from the middle area or near the net while keeping the opposing partner away from the net.

For the returning pair, it is crucial to initially focus on keeping the serving pair away from the net. As the rally progresses, the chances of winning the point increase significantly. In short and medium rallies, points are more likely to be won by forcing an error rather than hitting a winner. However, as the rally lengthens, the likelihood of winning the point with a winner increases, especially when utilizing cross-court trajectories.

These results have significant potential for enhancing both training and match strategies, providing a data-driven approach to improving performance on the court.

Author Contributions: Conceptualization, I.P.-L., A.J.S.-P., N.D.-R., X.R.-L.-d.-l.-O. and A.G.-S.; methodology, I.P.-L., J.C.A.-G., X.R.-L.-d.-l.-O. and A.G.-S.; software, I.P.-L., N.D.-R. and A.G.-S.; validation, J.C.A.-G., N.D.-R. and X.R.-L.-d.-l.-O.; formal analysis, I.P.-L. and A.G.-S.; investigation, I.P.-L., J.C.A.-G., A.J.S.-P., N.D.-R., X.R.-L.-d.-l.-O. and A.G.-S.; resources, I.P.-L., A.J.S.-P., J.C.A.-G., N.D.-R. and X.R.-L.-d.-l.-O.; data curation, I.P.-L., A.J.S.-P., J.C.A.-G. and A.G.-S.; writing—original draft, I.P.-L., N.D.-R., A.J.S.-P. and A.G.-S.; writing—review and editing, I.P.-L., X.R.-L.-d.-l.-O. and A.G.-S.; visualization, A.J.S.-P., J.C.A.-G. and N.D.-R.; supervision, I.P.-L., A.J.S.-P. and A.G.-S.; project administration, I.P.-L., J.C.A.-G., X.R.-L.-d.-l.-O. and A.G.-S.; funding acquisition, I.P.-L. and A.G.-S. All authors have read and agreed to the published version of the manuscript.

Funding: This study was funded by the Ministerio de Cultura y Deporte (https://www.culturaydeporte.gob.es/portada.html), Consejo Superior de Deportes (https://www.csd.gob.es/es) and European Union (https://european-union.europa.eu/index_es) under Project "Integración entre datos observacionales y datos provenientes de sensores externos: Evolución del software LINCE PLUS y desarrollo de la aplicación móvil para la optimización del deporte y la actividad física beneficiosa para la salud (2023)" EXP_74847, provided to A.G.-S. and I.P.-L.

Institutional Review Board Statement: The study was approved by the ethics committee of the Faculty of Education and Sport Science (University of Vigo, application 07-280722).

Informed Consent Statement: Not applicable.

Data Availability Statement: The raw data supporting the conclusions of this article will be made available by the authors on request.

Acknowledgments: This publication was made possible thanks to the research stays during the years 2023 and 2024 at the Instituto Politécnico de Viana do Castelo [IPVC]—Escola Superior de Desporto e Lazer.

Conflicts of Interest: The authors declare no conflicts of interest.

References

1. Sánchez-Alcaraz, B.J.; Muñoz, D.; Pradas, F.; Ramón-Llin, J.; Cañas, J.; Sánchez-Pay, A. Analysis of serve and serve-return strategies in elite male and female padel. *Appl. Sci.* **2020**, *10*, 11. [CrossRef]
2. International Padel Federation Federaciones Mundiales de Padel. Available online: https://www.padelfip.com/es/federaciones/ (accessed on 10 November 2023).
3. de Ossó, A.F.; Pecci, J.; Sánchez-Trigo, H.; Muñoz, D.; Escudero-Tena, A.; León, J. Differences between genders and competitive levels on technical-tactical parameters in padel: Implications for training. *Int. J. Sports Sci. Coach* **2024**, *19*, 1349–1356. [CrossRef]
4. Denche-Zamorano, A.; Escudero-Tena, A.; Pereira-Payo, D.; Adsuar, J.C.; Muñoz, D. Scientific mapping of the state-of-the-art in padel. A bibliometric analysis. *Int. J. Sports Sci. Coach* **2023**, *19*, 1275–1285. [CrossRef]
5. Krizkova, S.; Tomaskova, H.; Tirkolaee, E.B. Sport performance analysis with a focus on racket sports: A review. *Appl. Sci.* **2021**, *11*, 9212. [CrossRef]
6. Díaz, J.; Muñoz, D.; Muñoz, J.; Ibáñez, S.J. Design and Validation of an Observational Instrument for Final Actions in Padel. *Rev. Int. Med. Ciencias Act. Física Deport.* **2021**, *21*, 197–210. [CrossRef]
7. Escudero-Tena, A.; Muñoz, D.; García-Rubio, J.; Ibáñez, S.J. Analysis of the Actions of Net Zone Approach in Padel: Validation of the NAPOA Instrument. *Int. J. Environ. Res. Public Health* **2022**, *19*, 14. [CrossRef] [PubMed]

8. Mellado-Arbelo, Ó.; Baiget Vidal, E.; Usón, M.V. Analysis of game actions in professional male padel. *Cultura_Ciencia_Deporte* **2019**, *14*, 191–201. [CrossRef]
9. Marín, D.M.; Fernández, A.G.; Pérez, F.J.G.; García, J.D.; Sánchez, I.B.; Jiménez, J.M. Influence of Set Duration on Time Variables in Paddle Tennis Matches. *Apunt. Educ. Fis. Deport.* **2016**, *123*, 69–75. [CrossRef]
10. Courel-Ibáñez, J.; Sánchez-Alcaraz Martínez, B.J.; Cañas, J. Game performance and length of rally in professional padel players *J. Hum. Kinet.* **2017**, *55*, 161–169. [CrossRef]
11. Torres-Luque, G.; Ramirez, A.; Cabello-Manrique, D.; Nikolaidis, T.P.; Alvero-Cruz, J.R. Match analysis of elite players during paddle tennis competition. *Int. J. Perform. Anal. Sport* **2015**, *15*, 1135–1144. [CrossRef]
12. Pradas de la Fuente, F.; Cachón Zagalaz, J.; Otín Benedí, D.; Quintas Hijós, A.; Arraco Castellar, S.I.; Castellar Otín, C. Anthropometric, physiological and temporal analysis in elite female paddle players. *Retos* **2015**, *1*, 107–112. [CrossRef]
13. Castillo-Rodríguez, A.; Alvero-Cruz, J.R.; Hernández-Mendo, A.; Fernández-García, J.C. Physical and physiological responses in Paddle Tennis competition. *Int. J. Perform. Anal. Sport* **2014**, *14*, 524–534. [CrossRef]
14. Armstrong, C.; Reid, M.; Beale, C.; Girard, O. A Comparison of Match Load Between Padel and Singles and Doubles Tennis. *Int. J. Sports Physiol. Perform.* **2023**, *18*, 512–522. [CrossRef] [PubMed]
15. Sánchez-Alcaraz, B.J.; Martínez-Gallego, R.; Ramón-Llin Mas, J.; Crespo, M.; Muñoz, D.; López Martínez, J.M.; Sánchez-Pay, A. Professional padel tennis: Characteristics and effectiveness of the shots played to the fence. *Int. J. Sports Sci. Coach.* **2022**, *19*, 1324–1331. [CrossRef]
16. Escudero-Tena, A.; Sánchez-Alcaraz, B.J.; García-Rubio, J.; Ibáñez, S.J. Analysis of game performance indicators during 2015–2019 world padel tour seasons and their influence on match outcome. *Int. J. Environ. Res. Public Health* **2021**, *18*, 8. [CrossRef] [PubMed]
17. Ramón-Llin, J.; Guzmán, J.; Martínez-Gallego, R.; Muñoz, D.; Sánchez-Pay, A.; Sánchez-Alcaraz, B.J. Stroke Analysis in Padel According to Match Outcome and Game Side on Court. *Int. J. Environ. Res. Public Health* **2020**, *17*, 7838. [CrossRef] [PubMed]
18. Ungureanu, A.N.; Lupo, C.; Contardo, M.; Brustio, P.R. Decoding the decade: Analyzing the evolution of technical and tactical performance in elite padel tennis (2011–2021). *Int. J. Sport. Sci. Coach.* **2024**, *19*, 1306–1313. [CrossRef]
19. Almonacid, B.; Martínez, J.; Escudero-Tena, A.; Sánchez-Alcaraz, B.J.; Muñoz, D. Influence of the play score on external load parameters in men's and women's professional padel. *Cult. Cienc. Deport.* **2023**, *18*, 119–125. [CrossRef]
20. Escudero-Tena, A.; Ibáñez, S.J.; Vaquer Castillo, A.; Sánchez-Alcaraz, B.J.; Ramón-Llin, J.; Muñoz, D. Analysis of the return in professional men's and women's padel. *Int. J. Sports Sci. Coach* **2024**, *19*, 1375–1383. [CrossRef]
21. Martín-Miguel, I.; Muñoz, D.; Escudero-Tena, A.; Sánchez-Alcaraz, B.J. Analysis of Off-The-Wall Smash Shots in Men's and Women's Professional Padel. *Percept. Mot. Skills* **2024**, *131*, 843–860. [CrossRef]
22. O'Donoghue, P.G.; Brown, E.J. The importance of service in Grand Slam singles tennis. *J. Perform. Anal. Sport* **2008**, *8*, 70–78 [CrossRef]
23. Fitzpatrick, A.; Stone, J.A.; Choppin, S.; Kelley, J. Important performance characteristics in elite clay and grass court tennis match-play. *Int. J. Perform. Anal. Sport* **2019**, *19*, 942–952. [CrossRef]
24. García-Benítez, S.; Pérez-Bilbao, T.; Echegaray, M.; Felipe, J.L. The influence of gender on temporal structure and match activity patterns of professional padel tournaments. *Cultura_Ciencia_Deporte* **2016**, *11*, 241–247. [CrossRef]
25. Courel-Ibáñez, J.; Sánchez-Alcaraz, B.J.; Cañas, J. Effectiveness at the net as a predictor of final match outcome in professional padel players. *Int. J. Perform. Anal. Sport* **2015**, *15*, 632–640. [CrossRef]
26. Ramón-Llin, J.; Guzmán, J.; Llana, S.; Vučković, G.; James, N. Comparison of distance covered in paddle in the serve team according to performance level. *J. Hum. Sport Exerc.* **2013**, *8*, 738–742. [CrossRef]
27. Sánchez-Alcaraz, B.J.; Jiménez, V.; Muñoz, D.; Ramón-Llin, J. External training load differences between male and female professional padel. *J. Sport Health Res.* **2021**, *13*, 445–454.
28. Anguera, M.T.; Blanco-Villaseñor, A.; Losada, J.L.; Portell, M. Guidelines for designing and conducting a study that applies observational methodology. *Anu. Psicol.* **2018**, *48*, 9–17. [CrossRef]
29. Anguera, M.T.; Blanco-Villaseñor, A.; Hernández-Mendo, A.; Losada-López, J.L. Observational designs: Their suitability and application in sports psychology. *Cuad. Psicol. Deport.* **2011**, *11*, 63–76.
30. American Psychological Association Ethical principles of psychologists and code of conduct. *Am. Psychol.* **2002**, *57*, 1060–1073. [CrossRef]
31. Fernández-de-Ossó-Fuentes, A.I.; León-Prados, J.A. Herramienta de evaluación técnico-táctica en pádel/Technical and Tactical Assessment Tool for Paddle. *Rev. Int. Med. Ciencias Act. Física Deport.* **2017**, *68*, 693–714. [CrossRef]
32. Soto, A.; Camerino, O.; Iglesias, X.; Anguera, M.T.; Castañer, M. LINCE PLUS: Research Software for Behavior Video Analysis *Apunt. Educ. Física Esports* **2019**, *137*, 149–153. [CrossRef]
33. Blanco-Villaseñor, A.; Anguera, M.T. Evaluación de la calidad en el registro del comportamiento: Aplicación a deportes de equipo. In *Métodos Numéricos en Ciencias Sociales*; Oñate, E., García-Sicilia, F., Ramallo, L., Eds.; Centro Internacional de Métodos Numéricos en Ingeniería: Barcelona, Spain, 2000; pp. 30–48.
34. Cohen, J. Weighted kappa: Nominal scale agreement with provision for scaled disagreement of partial credit. *Psychol. Bull.* **1968**, *70*, 213–220. [CrossRef] [PubMed]
35. Ramón-Llin, J.; Guzmán, J.; Martínez-Gallego, R.; Muñoz, D.; Sánchez-Pay, A.; Sánchez-Alcaraz, B.J. Análisis de la situación en la pista de los jugadores en el saque y su relación con la dirección, el lado de la pista y el resultado del punto en pádel de alto nivel (Analysis of the situation on the court of the players in the serve and its relationship. *Retos* **2021**, *41*, 399–405. [CrossRef]

36. Ramón-Llin, J.; Guzmán, J.F.; Llana, S.; Martínez-Gallego, R.; James, N.; Vučković, G. The Effect of the Return of Serve on the Server Pair's Movement Parameters and Rally Outcome in Padel Using Cluster Analysis. *Front. Psychol.* **2019**, *10*, 1194. [CrossRef] [PubMed]
37. Escudero-Tena, A.; Gómez-Ruano, M.Á.; Ibáñez, S.J.; Sánchez-Alcaraz, B.J.; Muñoz, D. Importance of Maintaining Net Position in Men's and Women's Professional Padel. *Percept. Mot. Skills* **2023**, *130*, 2210–2225. [CrossRef] [PubMed]
38. Sañudo Corrales, B.; Del Hoyo Lora, M.; Carrasco Páez, L. Demandas fisiológicas y características estructurales de la competición en pádel masculino. *Apunt. Educ. Física Deport.* **2008**, *4*, 23–28.
39. Escudero-tena, A.; Fernández-cortes, J.; García-rubio, J.; Ibáñez, S.J. Use and efficacy of the lob to achieve the offensive position in women's professional padel. Analysis of the 2018 wpt finals. *Int. J. Environ. Res. Public Health* **2020**, *17*, 4061. [CrossRef] [PubMed]
40. Sánchez-Alcaraz, B.J.; Courel-Ibáñez, J.; Muñoz, D.; Infantes-Córdoba, P.; Sáenz de Zumarán, F.; Sánchez-Pay, A. Análisis de las acciones de ataque en el pádel masculino profesional. *Apunt. Educ. Física Deport.* **2020**, *142*, 29–34. [CrossRef]
41. Demeco, A.; de Sire, A.; Marotta, N.; Spanò, R.; Lippi, L.; Palumbo, A.; Iona, T.; Gramigna, V.; Palermi, S.; Leigheb, M.; et al. Match Analysis, Physical Training, Risk of Injury and Rehabilitation in Padel: Overview of the Literature. *Int. J. Environ. Res. Public Health* **2022**, *19*, 4153. [CrossRef]
42. Martínez-Gallego, R.; Ramón-Llin, J.; Crespo, M. A Cluster Analysis Approach to Profile Men and Women's Volley Positions in Professional Tennis Matches (Doubles). *Sustainability* **2021**, *13*, 6370. [CrossRef]
43. Courel-Ibanez, J.; Sánchez-Alcaraz Martinez, B.J.; Muñoz Marín, D. Exploring Game Dynamics in Padel: Implications for Assessment and Training. *J. Strength Cond. Res.* **2019**, *33*, 1971–1977. [CrossRef]
44. Lupo, C.; Condello, G.; Courel-Ibáñez, J.; Gallo, C.; Conte, D.; Tessitore, A. Effect of gender and match outcome on professional padel competition. *RICYDE Rev. Int. Cienc. Deport.* **2018**, *14*, 29–41. [CrossRef]

applied sciences

MDPI

Article

Sport and Physical Activity Participation by Weight Groups in School-Aged Hungarian Children

Martina Uvacsek *, Bernadett Wágner and Georgina Simkó

Department of Health Sciences and Sport Medicine, Hungarian University of Sports Science, 1123 Budapest, Hungary
* Correspondence: uvacsek.martina@tf.hu

Abstract: The aim of this study was to compare physical activity and organized sport participation survey data between different weight classifications in children. In the cross-sectional online data collection, 677 parents (42.8 ± 6.4 years old) provided information about 677 children (10.9 ± 2.5 years old). On average, 77% of the children achieved 60 min of MVPA/day and 63% participated in a club or organized sport. Most of them (63%) were in the healthy weight category, 14% of the children were underweight, and 22% of the children were overweight or obese. The parental support for physical activity was 83%. Club or organized sport participation (OR = 0.56 CI: 0.34–0.91; $p < 0.02$) and a parent with a higher educational level (OR = 0.25 CI:0.14–0.43; $p < 0.01$) were found to be preventive for obesity. Football was the most popular and highly chosen sport activity. Regarding sport activities with parents, cycling, walking, and football were the most popular, independently of the weight classification of the child. The overweight and obese children had almost the same participation rate in sport activities than others. Increased physical activity might be explained by the daily physical education in schools and governmental support. Further studies and measures are needed to prevent overweight and obesity in children of parents with a lower educational level.

Keywords: physical activity; children; organized sport; obesity; healthy lifestyle

1. Introduction

The increased prevalence of obesity in children and youth in many developed and developing countries is a serious public health concern. The obesity problem is more dramatic in boys than in girls [1]. According to a Health Behaviour in School-aged Children (HBSC) study in Hungary, the prevalence of overweight children is higher than the international average [2]. While the cause of obesity is a multifactorial complex interaction between environmental, genetic, behavioural, and socioeconomic factors, it is often considered to be a result of increased energy intake and less energy expenditure. Interestingly, in some countries, energy intake has not increased significantly in recent decades, but there has been a worldwide decline in energy expenditure due to a reduction in physical activity [3–5]. An increase in physical inactivity associated with increased screen time is an important and likely contributing factor for obesity. Therefore, limiting screen time is an important general recommendation [6]. It is generally accepted that a healthy diet and increased physical activity are the main factors that can prevent overweight and obesity. Increased levels of physical activity has several beneficial effects on the health and well-being of children and adolescents [6,7].

Preventive programs and strategies are needed to reduce the prevalence of childhood obesity, including greater support for physical activity-based programs in government policies, families, and sport clubs and organizations [5,8]. The most popular tool for health promotion worldwide is participation in organized sports [9]. Sports club membership is associated with higher levels of moderate-to-vigorous physical activity (MVPA) and less daily physical inactivity. Sport club participation or organized sport activities can successfully increase physical activity and fitness and reduce adiposity [10,11]. Sports club membership during adolescence generally leads to high levels of leisure-time physical activity in adulthood [12,13]. Therefore, involving children and youth in an organized sport can increase the number of people living a healthy lifestyle. Changing building environments and school environments to support active transportation is also generally recommended, but this strategy requires high financial and governmental support [14,15].

Previous studies showed positive associations between parental and child overweight in all countries. Positive and negative correlations were found between parental education and the child's weight classification [16]. The parental factors associated with child overweight were reported in a 12-country study where in countries like Colombia or Kenya, the parental education was negatively associated with the weight status of the child. In Western countries such as the UK, Finland, Australia, or Canada, the odds ratios were lower than 1, but only in the USA and Brazil was parental education indicated as a significant preventive factor [3]. A cross-sectional study based on data from 123,487 6-to-9-year-old children from 24 countries in the WHO European Region has generally found an inverse relationship between the prevalence of childhood overweight/obesity and parental education in high-income countries [17]. The relationship between maternal and paternal education and the child's weight classification and physical activity appear to be related to the developmental stage of different countries [3]. Parental support for children's physical activity is essential. The parental role in promoting children's healthy behaviour and parental involvement in youth sports have been investigated in many countries [18–20].

There is a lack of information about children's physical activity or sport participation based on the weight classification of children. There is a discrepancy between the BMI and PA results reported by the HBSC research group. The overall PA in children is lower than expected despite the introduced daily PE in schools. The aim of this study was to collect survey data about the overall physical activity levels and participation in an organized sport and active transportation and compare the results between the different weight classifications of school-aged children. The second aim was to identify significant factors that could be used in obesity prevention programs targeted at Hungarian children to achieve healthier lifestyles.

2. Materials and Methods

Prior to any data collection, ethical approval was received from the Hungarian University of Sports Science (MTSE-OKE KEB/08/2023). This study was a cross-sectional survey study. The data were collected in spring 2023 using social media platforms and internet correspondence. The research project and survey were sent to 1247 principals of primary schools and were shared in parental online groups. The survey started with an introduction for parents in which the inclusion criteria were written. Inclusion was being a parent of a school-age child (6–15 years old). To avoid bias, an increased sample size and the diversity of residency were targeted. After data cleaning the online data collection, 677 parents (42.8 ± 6.4 years old) provided information about 677 children (10.9 ± 2.5 years old). The 677 results (345 boys and 332 girls) were achieved from 611 different IP addresses. The identical IP addresses might be explained by family membership, meaning a parent filled in the questionnaire for more than one child. Informed consent was the first part of the questionnaire that was obtained from all participants prior to answering the questionnaire.

Our questionnaire was completed with the Qualtrics program and contained 37 questions. Parents completed this self-report questionnaire that captured the parent's age, sex, education, and residency and their child's sex, age, body height, weight, and physical activity behaviour.

In this report, we analyse the demographic variables and nine questions connected to physical activity. The questionnaire was compiled using the global matrix (GM) 4.0 indicators, definitions, and benchmarks [12]. The GM methods and physical activity indicator benchmarks for children and adolescents were published by Aubert et al. (2022) [10]. The global matrix on PA for children is an initiative launched under the leadership of the

Active Healthy Kids Global Alliance (AHKGA) to achieve a comprehensive understanding of the global variation in child and adolescent PA, related indicators, and key sources of influence. As an overall physical activity indicator, we wanted to know what percentage of children and youth meet the global health-related physical activity recommendation. The question was "Do you think your child accumulates at least 60 min of moderate-vigorous physical activity per day on average?" "Yes/No". We used recommended questions for the organized sport, physical activity, active transportation, and family and peers indicators. The questions for club sport were "Does your child participate in club sport?", "Yes/No", "If yes, what kind of sport?"; "Does your child participate in organized sport but not in a sport club? (in school or afterschool)", "Yes/No", "If yes, what kind of organized sport?"; "Does your child use active transportation to get to and from places? (walk, cycling, scooter, or other)", "Yes/No"; "Do you do physical activity together with your child?", "Yes/No", "If yes, what kind of activity?"; "Do you facilitate physical activity and sport opportunities for your child? (driving, volunteering, cheering, paying membership fees)", "Yes/No".

The weight status categories (underweight, healthy, overweight, obese) were determined by the World Health Organization (WHO)'s age- and gender-specific reference using the calculated body mass index [21].

For the odds ratio calculation, we needed two categories in which Yes/No questions were obvious, but in parental education or residency, we had to separate the results into two main groups. Those who reported attaining some college degree or postgraduate degree became part of a higher-educated group, and those who reported completing high school, some high school, or less than a high school education, remained in the other group. Two categories were created from all residency locations based on type: The capital of Hungary, county seats, and towns comprised one group. The municipalities, villages, and farms comprised the second group.

Data were analysed using TIBCO 14.00.15. Statistics and IBM SPSS Statistics 29.0. Descriptive statistics and frequency tables were used to describe the demographic characteristics of the children and parents. Means and standard deviations were calculated for continuous variables and frequencies, and percentages were reported for categorical variables. Chi-square tests were used to compare different participation rates of groups. Crosstabs were used to analyse the associations between obesity and different factors affecting physical activity, the odds ratios (OR), and 95% confidence intervals (CI). A bivariate regression model was also used for the equation of associations and for the assessment of the significance level.

3. Results

The characteristics of the children who participated in the study and their parents are presented in Table 1. On average, the parents were 42.8 ± 6.4 years old. Most (84%) of the parent respondents were mothers, and more than half (54%) had a higher education degree. A majority (68%) of the families lived in large population centres (towns, county seats, or in the capital of Hungary). Half (51%) of the children were male with a mean age of 10.98 ± 2.53 years. According to the BMI percentile cut-offs published by the WHO, most (63%) of the children were in the healthy weight category, 14% of the children were underweight, and 22% of the children were overweight or obese.

The participation rates of the children in physical activity categorized by weight status are presented in Table 2. On average, more than two-thirds of all the children achieved 60 min MVPA/day. The highest rate of participation in physical activity was in the underweight children group, and the lowest rate of participation in physical activity was found in overweight children. The difference between the two groups was significant ($p < 0.01$). On average, more than half of all the children participated in a sport club or organized sport or activity. The highest rate of participation was found in the healthy weight group, and the lowest rate of participation was in obese children. The difference between the two groups was also significant ($p < 0.02$). Using active transportation was similar for every group. Interestingly, the overweight and obese children's rates of using active transportation were slightly higher than the other weight classifications. Performing physical activity with their parents was the most common in healthy weight children and the least common characteristic in obese children, but this difference was not statistically significant. The parental support of physical activity was also generally high with the highest rate in underweight children and the lowest in overweight children.

Table 1. Characteristics of participants.

Children	
Total sample	677
Males	345 (51%)
Females	332 (49%)
Mean Age (years)	10.9 ± 2.5
Body Height (cm)	152.5 ± 15.0
Body Mass (kg)	43.1 ± 15.2
BMI (kg/m^2)	18.1 ± 4.1
Underweight	93 (14%)
Healthy	424 (63%)
Overweight	81 (12%)
Obese	69 (10%)
Parents	
Mother	572 (84%)
Father	76 (11%)
Other (grandparent)	24 (4%)
Mean Age (years)	42.8 ± 6.4
Education	
Primary and secondary school education	283 (42%)
Higher education	363 (54%)
Residency	
Capital, county seat or town	464 (68%)
Municipality, village or farm	213 (32%)

Table 2. Participation rate of children in physical activity in total sample and different weight classifications.

	Achieving MVPA > 60 min/day	Sport Club or Organized Sport	Active Transport	Activity with Parents	Parental Support
Total	77%	63%	80%	70%	83%
Underweight	81%	61%	79%	67%	88%
Healthy	79%	67%	80%	73%	85%
Overweight	63% [a]	55%	81%	69%	78%
Obese	74%	51% [b]	81%	63%	83%
	a	**b**	**NS**	**NS**	**NS**

a = significantly ($p < 0.05$) less than the underweight group, b = significantly ($p < 0.05$) less than the healthy group.

In Table 3, we report the odds ratios for obesity in different factors affecting physical activity. Achieving a minimum of 60 min of moderate-to-vigorous-intensity physical activity per day is a general recommendation from the WHO. This and participation in clubs or organized sport are frequently investigated factors. A preventive factor may include the use of active transportation and the parental behaviour of supporting physical activity in some way or carrying out an activity together with the child. We also analysed two demographic factors: the parental level of education and the residency of the family. In the first column, all the odds ratios were less than 1 (OR < 1) and seemed to be preventive factors for obesity, but only two associations were significant. Only the club sport or organized sport participation ($p < 0.02$) and the higher educational level of the parent ($p < 0.01$) were real preventive factors for obesity.

Table 3. Odds ratios for obesity in different factors affecting physical activity.

	Odds Ratio for Obesity	CI (95%)	p
Achieving MVPA > 60 min/day	0.74	0.40–1.37	0.34
Club sport or organized sport	0.56	0.34–0.91	<0.02
Active transport	0.97	0.46–2.05	0.95
Activity with parents	0.67	0.37–1.20	0.18
Parental support	0.75	0.28–1.98	0.56
Higher education of parents	0.25	0.14–0.43	<0.01
Residency (capital, county seat, or town)	0.83	0.48–1.39	0.48

Significance was calculated with binary logistic regression.

The order of chosen or preferred sports and the physical activity types by weight status are shown in Table 4. We separated participation in club sport from participation in organized sport, and we also present the types of activity performed together with a parent. The first three most preferred forms of activity are presented in Table 4. In club sports, football is the most preferred sport activity, even in the obese children. Only the overweight group preferred a different type of activity, namely martial arts. Martial arts were also in the top three most preferred choices of activity for obese and healthy weight children. Handball, dance, kayaking, and canoeing were also popular club sport activities.

Table 4. Order of preferred sports and physical activities and ratios in different weight status.

	Underweight	Healthy	Overweight	Obese
Club sport	Football (36%)	Football (21%)	Martial arts (31%)	Football (31%)
	Kayaking & Canoeing (13%)	Dance (15%)	Handball (17%)	Martial arts (19%)
	Martial arts (13%)	Martial arts (13%)	Football (10%)	Handball (15%)
Organized sport	Football (26%)	Dancing (14%)	Swimming (15%)	Football (36%)
	Swimming (14%)	Football (10%)	Football (15%)	Working out in gym (14%)
	Basketball (14%)	Swimming (8%)	Basketball (15%)	Gymnastics (9%)
Activity with parents	Cycling (59%)	Cycling (52%)	Cycling (51%)	Cycling (50%)
	Walking (31%)	Walking (32%)	Walking (42%)	Walking (30%)
	Football (23%)	Football (8%)	Football (13%)	Football (18%)

Football was also the most preferred organized sport activity in two groups. Interestingly, football demonstrated the highest participation rate in the obese group. The preferred activities of the obese children were different from those of children in the other weight classifications. For example, working out in a gym and gymnastics were not mentioned by children in other weight classifications. Swimming was popular in three groups and basketball in two.

Regarding activities with parents, we found that the same three activities were popular in the same order in all weight classifications. These were, in order from the most popular to the third most popular, as follows: cycling with a parent, then walking together, and finally playing football together.

4. Discussion

The aims of this study were to collect data about school children's overall physical activity and their participation in organized sport and active transportation, and then compare the results between the different weight classifications. We also tried to identify significant factors that could be used in obesity prevention interventions for Hungarian children. To our knowledge, this is the first study that reports children's sport and physical activity participation rates and the joint activity of parents and children based on weight status in Hungary.

Hungary has the highest obesity rate in Europe and the fifth highest prevalence of obesity in the world. In Hungary, as in other countries with relatively high proportions of overweight and obese adults, the rates have increased by about 1% annually. According to the Organization for Economic Co-operation and Development [22], 33% of Hungarian adults are obese and 67% are obese or overweight. The prevalence (22%) of overweight and obese children and youth in our study was higher than previously published (20%) in the Health Behaviour in School-aged Children (HBSC) study but closer to another Hungarian study in which the prevalence was 23% [2,23].

The rate of children and adolescents who achieved the minimum 60 min of daily moderate-to-vigorous physical activity in our study was 77%, which is much higher than published in the HBSC global report earlier or in Polish adolescents (17%) [24]. In the Global Matrix 4.0 report, the average of 57 countries was lower (27–33%) [9]. Our results are in agreement with those of a study conducted in Slovakia where 66% of adolescents met the PA recommendation [25]. An explanation might be that in Hungary, a national physical education curriculum including five sessions of 45 min per week (1 per weekday) and recommendations for extracurricular PA as well as school sports programs were gradually introduced in 2012 in all Hungarian schools. A recent study found that after the introduction of daily physical education in Hungarian schools, leisure time spent in sports and exercise increased significantly, regardless of gender and age group [26]. Another explanation might be that in the HBSC data collection, children fill in the questionnaires in an online form, and they often underestimate their own physical activity. According to a previous study using objectively measured PA in 9–12-year-old children living in Budapest, more than 90% of them achieved the 60 min recommendation on weekdays [27].

We have found that 63% of children participate in a club sport or organized sport, which is higher than in countries with similar economic and social environments. In Hungary, participation in a club sport means a higher level of sport activity with highly educated coaches and better facilities. Organized sport might be any kind of sport or leisure time activity that generally takes place at schools and is led by a physical education teacher or a coach who is not necessarily a member of any sport federations. In an earlier report, the participation in organized sport was 40% lower [28], but in the HBSC study, it was published that two-thirds of the children reported vigorous physical activity twice a week that was related to organized sport participation [2]. Similar results were found in Slovakia with 41% overall participation and 54% overall participation in Poland [24,25].

Despite the health benefits of active traveling, active travel to school has declined or stabilized at a relatively low level. European active travel to school data were relatively higher than in USA or Australia [29]. In our study, using active travel was reported by 80% of the participants, which is higher than previously reported in Slovakia (49%) or Poland (45%). Interestingly, active traveling declined more than 10% in Poland and Slovakia compared to an earlier HBSC publication where the overall rate of active traveling in four European countries (Poland, Slovakia, Czechia, and Germany) was 59% [30]. The question that was used in our study was the same as that used in those reports [24,25].

Parent–child joint physical activity in our study was 70% in general, which is higher than in the Slovak report (46%) or in Poland where the average was 40%. The parental support in our study, which meant the facilitation of physical activity and sport opportunities, was 83% in general, which was higher than expected. We did not find comparable results from Hungary, Poland, or Slovakia.

Our findings indicate that the higher education of parents is beneficial, which concurs with results from high-income or Western countries [3,16]. There is a lack of information about lower-educated parental health behaviours and parental involvement or support in youth sports.

Gender differences in physical activity are often reported in this field. A cross-sectional study in Serbia involving 301 children reported that more boys than girls played sports and that sport choice depended on gender. Boys preferred team sports, while girls were oriented more towards individual sports. The most popular sports for boys were football (28.3%), basketball (24.4%), volleyball (16.1%), and water polo (16.1%). The girls preferred to participate in gymnastics (37.8%), volleyball (21.8%), swimming (19.3%), and water polo (17.6%) [31]. Hebert et al. investigated the organized sport participation in Danish primary school children with parental help. According to their results, football was the most popular (20.7%), then handball (11.2%), gymnastics (8.3%), basketball (1.1%), and volleyball (0.8%). They found that children participating in football were less sedentary, performed more MVPA, and were more likely to achieve the recommended level of physical activity than children not participating in organized sport [32]. Our findings that football is the most popular type of activity in clubs and in organized sport concur with previous studies. Interestingly, martial arts have not previously been mentioned among popular activities, so they may be unique to Hungary. Hungary has several Olympic medals in martial arts like boxing and wrestling.

According to the WHO, walking, cycling, and other forms of active non-motorized transport are accessible and safe for everyone [21]. There is also a lack of information about parent–child joint activities. In general, the physical activity of the Hungarian population is mainly based on their work and housework activities. Physical activity achieved by transport or leisure time is not common, but a cross-sectional study found that walking or cycling is common in Hungarians living in county seats or towns and villages [33].

In our opinion, these results report the striving for a healthier lifestyle based on parental support and motivation.

The present study has several limitations. First, this study was cross-sectional rather than longitudinal, and the data might report only a short period of physical activity behaviour in school children. Second, the data were collected online, which might have also limited the accuracy of the data. There are many factors that can increase or decrease a child's participation in physical activity and sport, which were not measured in this study. The frequency and duration of sport or organized physical activity were not analysed. Eating habits and sedentary behaviour were not investigated in our study.

5. Conclusions

Based on our results, the physical activity and club and organized sport participation of children increased in Hungary. The overweight and obese children had almost the same participation rates in sport activities as children in other weight classifications. Higher education of parents and club sport or organized sport participation were preventive in childhood obesity. Football was the most popular type of club or organized sport activity and the third among joint activities with parents. The increased physical activity might be explained by the daily PE in schools and the governmental support of sport. Our results suggest that besides the introduced daily PE, other lifestyle interventions are needed to maintain or decrease the prevalence of overweight and obesity. Further studies and measures are needed to prevent overweight and obesity in children of parents with a lower educational level.

Author Contributions: Conceptualization, M.U. and B.W.; methodology, M.U.; formal analysis, M.U.; investigation, B.W.; writing—original draft preparation, M.U. and G.S.; writing—review and editing, M.U.; visualization, M.U. All authors have read and agreed to the published version of the manuscript.

Funding: This research received no external funding.

Institutional Review Board Statement: This study was conducted according to the guidelines of the Declaration of Helsinki and approved by the Ethics Committee of Hungarian University of Sports Science (MTSE-OKE KEB/08/2023; protocol data: 30 January 2023).

Informed Consent Statement: Informed consent was obtained from all subjects involved in the study.

Data Availability Statement: Data is contained within the article.

Conflicts of Interest: The authors declare no conflicts of interest.

References

1. Spotlight on Adolescent Health and Well-Being. Findings from the 2017/2018 Health Behaviour in School-Aged Children (HBSC) Survey in Europe and Canada. 2020.
2. Németh, Á.; Várnai, D. *Kamaszéletmód Magyarországon: Az Iskoláskorú Gyermekek Egészségmagatartása Elnevezésű, az Egészségügyi Világszervezettel Együttműködésben Megvalósuló Nemzetközi Kutatás 2018. Évi Felméréséről Készült Nemzeti Jelentés*; Németh, Á., Várnai, D.E., Eds.; ELTE PPK-L'Harmattan: Budapest, Hungary, 2019.
3. Muthuri, S.K.; Onywera, V.O.; Tremblay, M.S.; Broyles, S.T.; Chaput, J.-P.; Fogelholm, M.; Hu, G.; Kuriyan, R.; Kurpad, A.; Lambert, E.V.; et al. Relationships between Parental Education and Overweight with Childhood Overweight and Physical Activity in 9–11 Year Old Children: Results from a 12-Country Study. *PLoS ONE* **2016**, *11*, e0147746. [CrossRef]
4. Reilly, J.J.; Barnes, J.; Gonzalez, S.; Huang, W.Y.; Manyanga, T.; Tanaka, C.; Tremblay, M.S. Recent Secular Trends in Child and Adolescent Physical Activity and Sedentary Behavior Internationally: Analyses of Active Healthy Kids Global Alliance Global Matrices 1.0 to 4.0. *J. Phys. Act. Health* **2022**, *19*, 729–736. [CrossRef]
5. Schwarzfischer, P.; Gruszfeld, D.; Stolarczyk, A.; Ferre, N.; Escribano, J.; Rousseaux, D.; Moretti, M.; Mariani, B.; Verduci, E.; Koletzko, B.; et al. Physical Activity and Sedentary Behavior From 6 to 11 Years. *Pediatrics* **2019**, *143*, e20180994. [CrossRef] [PubMed]
6. Pearson, N.; Braithwaite, R.E.; Biddle, S.J.H.; Van Sluijs, E.M.F.; Atkin, A.J. Associations between Sedentary Behaviour and Physical Activity in Children and Adolescents: A Meta-analysis. *Obes. Rev.* **2014**, *15*, 666–675. [CrossRef] [PubMed]
7. Meng, C.; Yucheng, T.; Shu, L.; Yu, Z. Effects of School-Based High-Intensity Interval Training on Body Composition, Cardiorespiratory Fitness and Cardiometabolic Markers in Adolescent Boys with Obesity: A Randomized Controlled Trial. *BMC Pediatr.* **2022**, *22*, 112. [CrossRef]
8. Vehrs, P.R.; Barker, H.; Nomiyama, M.; Vehrs, Z.; Tóth, M.; Uvacsek, M.; Mitchel, U.H.; Johnson, A.W. Sex Differences in Dysfunctional Movements and Asymmetries in Young Normal Weight, Overweight, and Obese Children. *Children* **2021**, *8*, 184. [CrossRef] [PubMed]
9. Vella, S.A.; Cliff, D.P. Organised Sports Participation and Adiposity among a Cohort of Adolescents over a Two Year Period. *PLoS ONE* **2018**, *13*, e0206500. [CrossRef]
10. Aubert, S.; Barnes, J.D.; Demchenko, I.; Hawthorne, M.; Abdeta, C.; Abi Nader, P.; Adsuar Sala, J.C.; Aguilar-Farias, N.; Aznar, S.; Bakalár, P.; et al. Global Matrix 4.0 Physical Activity Report Card Grades for Children and Adolescents: Results and Analyses From 57 Countries. *J. Phys. Act. Health* **2022**, *19*, 700–728. [CrossRef]
11. Telford, R.M.; Telford, R.D.; Cochrane, T.; Cunningham, R.B.; Olive, L.S.; Davey, R. The Influence of Sport Club Participation on Physical Activity, Fitness and Body Fat during Childhood and Adolescence: The LOOK Longitudinal Study. *J. Sci. Med. Sport* **2016**, *19*, 400–406. [CrossRef] [PubMed]
12. Tremblay, M.S.; Barnes, J.D.; Demchenko, I.; Gonzalez, S.A.; Brazo-Sayavera, J.; Kalinowski, J.; Katzmarzyk, P.T.; Manyanga, T.; Reilly, J.J.; Wong, S.H.S.; et al. Active Healthy Kids Global Alliance Global Matrix 4.0—A Resource for Physical Activity Researchers. *J. Phys. Act. Health* **2022**, *19*, 693–699. [CrossRef] [PubMed]
13. Aira, T.; Vasankari, T.; Heinonen, O.J.; Korpelainen, R.; Kotkajuuri, J.; Parkkari, J.; Savonen, K.; Uusitalo, A.; Valtonen, M.; Villberg, J.; et al. Physical Activity from Adolescence to Young Adulthood: Patterns of Change, and Their Associations with Activity Domains and Sedentary Time. *Int. J. Behav. Nutr. Phys. Act.* **2021**, *18*, 85. [CrossRef]
14. Benjamin-Neelon, S.E.; Platt, A.; Bacardi-Gascon, M.; Armstrong, S.; Neelon, B.; Jimenez-Cruz, A. Greenspace, Physical Activity, and BMI in Children from Two Cities in Northern Mexico. *Prev. Med. Rep.* **2019**, *14*, 100870. [CrossRef]
15. Jacobs, J.; Crooks, N.; Allender, S.; Strugnell, C.; Backholer, K.; Nichols, M. Is the Physical Activity Environment Surrounding Primary Schools Associated with Students' Weight Status, Physical Activity or Active Transport, in Regional Areas of Victoria, Australia? A Cross-Sectional Study. *BMJ Open* **2021**, *11*, e045785. [CrossRef]
16. Seum, T.; Meyrose, A.-K.; Rabel, M.; Schienkiewitz, A.; Ravens-Sieberer, U. Pathways of Parental Education on Children's and Adolescent's Body Mass Index: The Mediating Roles of Behavioral and Psychological Factors. *Front. Public Health* **2022**, *10*, 763789. [CrossRef]
17. Buoncristiano, M.; Williams, J.; Simmonds, P.; Nurk, E.; Ahrens, W.; Nardone, P.; Rito, A.I.; Rutter, H.; Bergh, I.H.; Starc, G.; et al. Socioeconomic Inequalities in Overweight and Obesity among 6- to 9-year-old Children in 24 Countries from the World Health Organization European Region. *Obes. Rev.* **2021**, *22* (Suppl. S6), e13213. [CrossRef]

18. Neshteruk, C.D.; Mazzucca, S.; Vaughn, A.E.; Jones, D.J.; Ward, D.S. Identifying Patterns of Physical Activity and Screen Time Parenting Practices and Associations with Preschool Children's Physical Activity and Adiposity. *Prev. Med. Rep.* **2020**, *18*, 101068 [CrossRef]
19. Norman, Å.; Zeebari, Z.; Nyberg, G.; Elinder, L.S. Parental Support in Promoting Children's Health Behaviours and Preventing Overweight and Obesity—A Long-Term Follow-up of the Cluster-Randomised Healthy School Start Study II Trial. *BMC Pediatr.* **2019**, *19*, 104. [CrossRef]
20. Bonavolontà, V.; Cataldi, S.; Latino, F.; Carvutto, R.; De Candia, M.; Mastrorilli, G.; Messina, G.; Patti, A.; Fischetti, F. The Role of Parental Involvement in Youth Sport Experience: Perceived and Desired Behavior by Male Soccer Players. *Int. J. Environ. Res. Public. Health* **2021**, *18*, 8698. [CrossRef]
21. WHO. *WHO European Regional Obesity: Report 2022*; World Health Organization, Regional Office for Europe: Copenhagen, Denmark, 2022.
22. OECD. *Health at a Glance 2023: OECD Indicators*; Health at a Glance; OECD: Paris, France, 2023. [CrossRef]
23. Jakab, A.E.; Hidvégi, E.V.; Illyés, M.; Cziráki, A.; Kalmár, T.; Maróti, Z.; Bereczki, C. A Magasvérnyomás-Betegség Prevalenciája Túlsúlyos És Elhízott Magyar Gyermek- És Serdülőkorú Populációban. *Orv. Hetil.* **2020**, *161*, 151–160. [CrossRef] [PubMed]
24. Zembura, P.; Korcz, A.; Nałęcz, H.; Cieśla, E. Results from Poland's 2022 Report Card on Physical Activity for Children and Youth *Int. J. Environ. Res. Public. Health* **2022**, *19*, 4276. [CrossRef]
25. Bakalár, P.; Hnidková, L.; Ružbarská, B.; Ružbarský, P.; Slančová, T.K.; Kopčáková, J.; Kostičová, M.; Gába, A. First Report Card on Physical Activity for Children and Adolescents in Slovakia: A Comprehensive Analysis, International Comparison, and Identification of Surveillance Gaps. *Arch. Public Health* **2024**, *82*, 16. [CrossRef]
26. Dizmatsek, I.B.; Ling, J.; Faculty of Health Sciences and Wellbeing, University of Sunderland, Sunderland, United Kingdom, Tóth, L.; Hamar, P.; Soós, I.; Hungarian University of Sport Science, Budapest, Hungary. The Effect of the Introduction of Daily Physical Education Classes on the Leisure Activities of Hungarian Students. *Cogn. Brain Behav. Interdiscip. J.* **2022**, *26*, 1–17 [CrossRef]
27. Uvacsek, M.; Tóth, M.; Ridgers, N. Examining Physical Activity and Inactivity in 9–12 Years Old Children. *Acta Physiol. Hung.* **2011**, *98*, 313–320. [CrossRef]
28. Szmodis, M.; Zsákai, A.; Bosnyák, E.; Protzner, A.; Trájer, E.; Farkas, A.; Szőts, G.; Tóth, M. Reference Data for Ultrasound Bone Characteristics in Hungarian Children Aged 7–19 Years. *Ann. Hum. Biol.* **2017**, *44*, 704–714. [CrossRef]
29. González, S.A.; Aubert, S.; Barnes, J.D.; Larouche, R.; Tremblay, M.S. Profiles of Active Transportation among Children and Adolescents in the Global Matrix 3.0 Initiative: A 49-Country Comparison. *Int. J. Environ. Res. Public. Health* **2020**, *17*, 5997 [CrossRef] [PubMed]
30. Brindley, C.; Hamrik, Z.; Kleszczewska, D.; Dzielska, A.; Mazur, J.; Haug, E.; Kopcakova, J.; Marques, A.; Altenburg, T.; Demetriou, Y.; et al. Gender-Specific Social and Environmental Correlates of Active Travel to School in Four European Countries The HBSC Study. *Front. Public Health* **2023**, *11*, 1190045. [CrossRef]
31. Arsenovic, D.; Djokic, B.; Kovacevic, Z.; Stevanovic, D.; Janicijevic, K.; Janicijevic Petrovic, M.A.; Radevic, S.; Radovanovic, S Quality of Life of Children Engaged in Regular Physical Activities. *Iran. J. Public Health* **2022**, *51*, 1629–1636. [CrossRef]
32. Hebert, J.J.; Møller, N.C.; Andersen, L.B.; Wedderkopp, N. Organized Sport Participation Is Associated with Higher Levels of Overall Health-Related Physical Activity in Children (CHAMPS Study-DK). *PLoS ONE* **2015**, *10*, e0134621. [CrossRef]
33. Bácsné Bába, É.; Ráthonyi, G.; Müller, A.; Ráthonyi-Odor, K.; Balogh, P.; Ádány, R.; Bács, Z. Physical Activity of the Population of the Most Obese Country in Europe, Hungary. *Front. Public Health* **2020**, *8*, 203. [CrossRef] [PubMed]

applied sciences

MDPI

Article

Effects of Rowing on Cardiac Function in Breast Cancer Survivors: Sliding Seat Rowing vs. Fixed Seat Rowing

Juan Gavala-González [1,2], Mateo Real-Pérez [2,*], Juan Gamboa-González [2] and José Carlos Fernández-García [2,3]

[1] Department of Physical Education and Sports, Universidad de Sevilla, 41013 Sevilla, Spain; jgavala@us.es
[2] Researching in Sport Science: Grupo de investigación (CTS-563) del Plan Andaluz de Investigación, Universidad de Sevilla, 41003 Sevilla, Spain; juan_95.g@hotmail.com (J.G.-G.); jcfg@uma.es (J.C.F.-G.)
[3] Department of Didactics of Languages, Arts and Sport, Universidad de Málaga, Andalucía-Tech, IBIMA, 29010 Málaga, Spain
* Correspondence: mateo.realperez@gmail.com

Abstract: This longitudinal study aimed to analyze the effects of a team rowing-based training program on physical fitness and anthropometric parameters in female breast cancer survivors (n = 40; 56.78 ± 6.38 years). Participants were divided into two groups: one rowed in fixed seat rowing (FSR) boats (n = 20; 56.35 ± 4.89 years) and the other in sliding seat rowing (SSR) boats (n = 20; 57.20 ± 7.7 years). Both groups engaged in two 75-min sessions per week for 24 weeks. Significant improvements were observed in both groups in resting heart rate (FSR: −10.65 bpm; SSR: −8.45 bpm), heart rate at the beginning of the 6-min walk test (6 MWT) (FSR: −10.7 bpm; SSR: −11.25 bpm), and heart rate at the end of the test (FSR: −13.85 bpm; SSR: −20.35 bpm). Blood pressure improved significantly in both diastolic blood pressure (FSR: −12.35 mmHg; SSR: −19.25 mmHg) and systolic blood pressure (FSR: −13 mmHg; SSR: −16.95 mmHg). Additionally, both groups increased the distance covered in the 6 MWT (FSR: +63.05 m; SSR: +93.65 m). These results suggest that a rowing training program is a viable and safe activity for female breast cancer survivors, improving cardiac function, blood pressure, and cardiorespiratory capacity, particularly in sliding seat boats.

Keywords: rowing; breast cancer; physical activity; cardiac function; exercise

1. Introduction

The evolution of scientific knowledge is changing the paradigm of cancer from diagnosis and subsequent pharmacological treatment to a holistic and multidisciplinary approach that treats the individual through comprehensive therapeutic programs. In this regard, physical exercise has been postulated to play an important role in protecting against cancer [1]. As an example, it has been noted that the risk of breast cancer-related mortality appears to be significantly lower among survivors who adopt a physically active routine, in contrast to those who lead a sedentary lifestyle [2].

Breast cancer represents the most prevalent type of cancer in women, with 2.3 million diagnoses in 2020, and is the leading cause of cancer-related deaths in the female population on a global scale [3]. Despite this, the survival rate is close to 90% in most countries, so there is a high number of women who survive the disease for at least 5 years after initial treatment [4,5]. However, despite this high survival rate, it is important to note that the side effects associated with the disease and its treatment, such as cancer-related fatigue [6], lymphedema [7], cardiovascular disease [8,9], loss of bone mass [10], or psychological problems such as anxiety or depression [11], can persist for long periods of time, ranging from months to years.

If we focus on the side effects produced or exacerbated by the treatment of oncological diseases, we find that cardiovascular diseases and breast cancer share numerous risk factors such as age, diet, family history, alcohol consumption, obesity and overweight, level of physical activity, and tobacco use [8]. Yet, they share an even more relevant common risk factor, since current breast cancer treatments, based on chemotherapy, radiotherapy, and endocrine therapies, have a potentially deleterious effect related to cancer-induced cardiotoxicity and, consequently, to the development of cardiovascular disease [8,9]. Therefore, there is a need to examine which types of complementary non-pharmacological interventions can help to reduce the risk of developing cardiovascular disease in female breast cancer survivors.

The diagnosis of cancer is often accompanied by drastic changes in a person's life. Taking into account that the lifestyle adopted can positively influence the chances of survival of the disease [12], as well as protect against the possible sequelae of treatment [13,14], scientific evidence has shown that engaging in physical exercise can reduce the onset of symptoms associated with cancer treatment and improve physical fitness and mental health [1,6,15,16]. This research has shown that a controlled training program can produce significant improvements in aerobic capacity, as well as an increase in muscle mass and strength, in addition to improving functionality of the upper limbs in women with breast cancer [17–20]. The majority of the studies consulted affirm that physical activity positively influences health status, mood, and body composition, positively affecting the quality of life of survivors [15,16,21–23].

Despite the proven benefits of exercise and its positive impact on the health of women with breast cancer [1,8,24,25], the level of physical activity is significantly reduced during cancer treatment [26], and remains even lower than it was before diagnosis [25]. Unfortunately, studies have shown that women who have been diagnosed with breast cancer decrease their physical activity by 11%, falling even further in those who are treated with chemotherapy (50%) and radiotherapy (24%), compared to untreated women [26]. Fatigue, low motivation, kinesiophobia, fear of lymphedema, and difficulties in accessing sports facilities are the main barriers to participation in physical activities in cancer patients [4].

Additionally, we must also consider that persistent chronic pain and sensory changes are common sequelae following breast cancer surgery. Studies report that between 20% and 60% of women experience persistent pain, primarily felt in the anterior chest, arms, and axillae after breast cancer surgery, significantly worsening their quality of life [27,28]. This pain has a neuropathic character and is often attributed to the sectioning of the intercostobrachial nerve (ICBN), which frequently occurs during treatments involving lymphatic axillary dissection. This results in numbness of the upper limb and thoracic wall, and restriction of upper limb movement [29,30]. In this context, physical activity and physiokinetotherapy techniques can serve as fundamental tools in preventing associated problems and preserving mobility and muscle strength, improving functionality, posture, and reducing the risk of lymphedema in the areas most affected by this disease [31,32]. Therefore, it is important to promote strategies and activities that encourage adherence to physical activity, even during the treatment of the disease [33].

Within this context, programs based on rowing have now emerged as a possible non-pharmacological therapy to ameliorate the side effects of cancer and to slow the decline associated with cancer and its treatment [4,7,34,35]. Rowing is a water sport in which a boat is propelled by the use of oars. In this discipline, rowers use the oars as second-degree levers, moving them in the opposite direction to the forward motion of the boat. Some of the benefits associated with this type of rowing-based exercise indicate an improvement in the physical condition of the participants [4,36], mental and psychological health [37–39], prevention of lymphedema [7,40], and ultimately, an improvement in the quality of life of women rowers [4,34,35].

It is important to note that there are two main types of rowing: sliding seat rowing (SSR), characterized by movement of the seats to facilitate leg thrust, and fixed seat rowing (FSR), in which the rowers remain in a static seat during the exercise [41]. There are clear biomechanical differences in the technical movements between the two modalities, particularly with regard to the upper limbs. In FSR, overhead shoulder flexion is required to execute the necessary movements. In contrast, in SSR, the movement of the arms is performed at shoulder height, which helps to reduce the strain on the upper extremities and trunk [35].

Rowing was chosen because it involves the muscles of both the upper and lower extremities, as well as virtually every muscle in the body. Nevertheless, the distinguishing feature that sets it apart from most other sports is the cyclic and alternating action of flexion and extension of the upper and lower extremities, as well as the involvement of the stabilizing muscles of the trunk and back during the different phases of rowing [42,43].

Currently, limited evidence is available on the impact of rowing on cardiac function and blood pressure in breast cancer survivors [44]. Therefore, the aim of the following study will be to examine the influence of a rowing-based training program on cardiac function and aerobic capacity in female breast cancer survivors, as well as to compare the influence of boat type on the possible cardiovascular adaptations.

2. Materials and Methods

2.1. Design and Participants

This research is part of concurrent clinical trials. To support this, a 24-week training regimen, conducted twice a week, was developed for use in both FSR and SSR boats (Figure 1). Various breast cancer support groups were approached and given the opportunity to participate in a free 24-week rowing program, which included physical evaluations at the beginning and conclusion of the program. The only criteria for participation were a history of breast cancer and approval from their oncologist to engage in moderate physical activity.

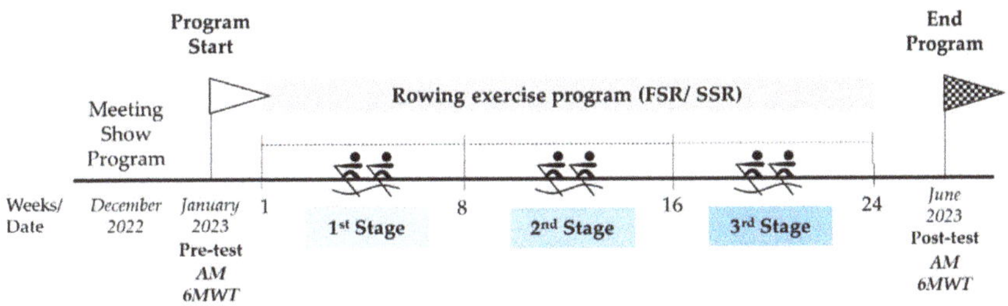

Figure 1. Timeline of the study. 6 MWT: 6-min walk test; AM: anthropometric measurements.

The participants (n = 40), aged 56.78 ± 6.38 years, were recruited on the condition that they had been diagnosed with breast cancer 6.58 ± 5.72 years previously, with varying degrees of involvement and with subsequent surgery, as shown in Table 1.

Table 1. Characteristics of the sample.

Breast (%)			
Right: 37.5	Left: 57.5	Both: 5.0	
Stage (%)			
I: 7.5	II: 37.5	III: 40.0	IV: 15.0
Surgery (%)			
Breast Conserving: 50.0	Total Mastectomy: 42.5	Double Mastectomy: 7.5	

After the initial selection, the nature of the study was explained to the participants, indicating that their anonymity would be maintained at all times, following the ethical considerations of Sport and Exercise Science Research [45] and with the principles included in the Declaration of Helsinki [46], which define the ethical guidelines for research in humans. The University of Malaga provided the identification number registered for the Ethics Committee: 65-2020-H, and the participants (Figure 2) provided written informed consent. Throughout the intervention and subsequently, we acted under the provisions of organic law 3/2018, of December 5, on the Protection of Personal Data and Guarantee of Digital Rights, regarding the protection of personal data under Spanish legislation.

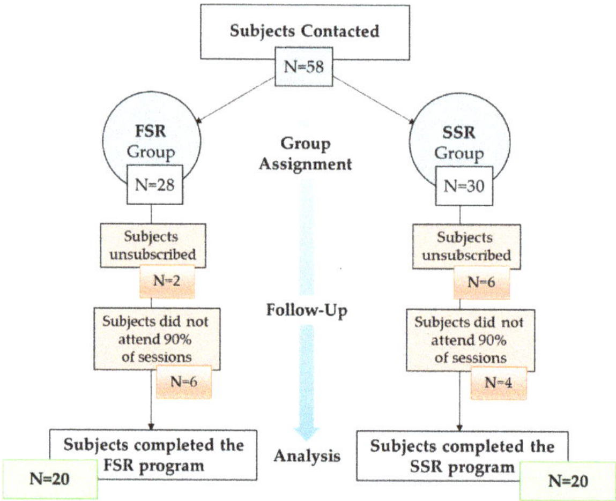

Figure 2. A flow diagram of the sample selected for this study.

2.2. Instruments

A Tanita model BC730 scale (Tanita Corporation, Tokyo, Japan), accuracy 0.1 kg, was used to weigh the subjects, and a SECA model 213 portable measuring rod (Seca GmbH & Co. KG, Hamburg, Germany), accuracy 0.1 cm, was used to measure height. The 6-min walk test was used to evaluate cardiac function, which is a valid and reliable test that assesses a person's cardiorespiratory capacity by measuring the maximum distance they can walk on a flat surface in 6 min. At the same time, heart rate per minute was monitored immediately before and after finishing the test using a Polar H10 chest strap (Polar Electro Oy, Kempele, Finland), which was fitted before the start of the test and transmitted the signal to the POLAR tablet application. For blood pressure measurement, the Omron M6 Comfort IT brachial blood pressure monitor (Omron Healthcare Co., Ltd., Kyoto, Japan) was used, which indicates systolic and diastolic blood pressure and pulse rate per minute.

2.3. Procedure

Among all the women who expressed interest, a series of physical fitness assessments were conducted. With equivalent anthropometric measurements (weight, height, BMI) and test results, a participant was assigned to one group (FSR or SSR). The participant with the most comparable results was assigned to the other group (SSR or FSR). Subjects participating in the study already engaged in moderate and regular physical activity. The participants were thus divided into two training groups with similar characteristics (Table 2):

Table 2. Descriptive analysis of study subjects according to training group.

	TOTAL (SSR + FSR)	Fixed Seat Rowing (FSR)	Sliding Seat Rowing (SSR)	Difference of Means (FSR-SSR)	*p*
Age (years) (SD)	56.78 (6.38)	56.35 (4.89)	57.2 (7.7)	−0.85 (2.04)	0.679
Height (cm) (SD)	162.05 (5.59)	161.9 (4.91)	162.2 (6.33)	−0.3 (1.79)	0.868
Weight (kg) (SD)	69.49 (9.8)	72.05 (8.11)	66.92 (10.85)	3.22 (3.11)	0.307
BMI (kg/m^2) (SD)	26.48 (3.58)	27.48 (2.73)	25.47 (4.09)	1.50 (1.18)	0.215
Rest HR (bpm) (SD)	94.33 (11.81)	96.1 (11.54)	92.55 (11.51)	3.55 (3.91)	0.241
Initial Test HR (bpm) (SD)	92.83 (12.76)	94.1 (14.21)	91.55 (10.58)	2.55 (4.05)	0.974
Final Test HR (bpm) (SD)	139.5 (18.44)	141,75 (18.67)	137.25 (17.44)	4.5 (6.32)	0.888
Diastolic BP (mmHg) (SD)	160.03 (13.37)	158.25 (12.8)	161.8 (13.35)	−3.55 (4.69)	0.405
Systolic BP (mmHg) (SD)	100.78 (10.19)	100.55 (10.51)	101 (9.59)	−0.45 (3.9)	0.856
6 MWT (m) (SD)	784.78 (103.64)	817.25 (51.1)	752.3 (127.37)	64.95 (44.43)	0.077

The 24-week rowing training program was divided into three 4-week stages. These stages progressively increased in intensity and were adjusted through the participants' subjective perception of effort using the Börg scale [47].

- Initial phase with mobility exercises, proprioceptive exercises, and postural control exercises. Main phase with rowing training. Final phase with stretching. Börg scale 5–6.
- Intermediate phase with mobility exercises, proprioceptive exercises, and postural control exercises. Main phase with rowing training. Final phase with stretching. Börg scale 6–7.
- Final phase with mobility exercises, proprioceptive exercises, and postural control exercises. Main phase with rowing training. Final phase with stretching. Börg scale 7–8.

Throughout the program, there were 2 days of training per week. Each session lasted 75 min. These sessions were supervised by a trainer who ensured attendance, correct execution of the tasks, and intensity of the sessions, in addition to excluding from the study those subjects who did not achieve at least 90% participation. Each training session had the same structure:

1. Initial part performed with warm-up, mobility, proprioceptive, and postural control exercises, all performed in a multipurpose room (5–10 min).
2. Cool down: Flexibility exercises to relax the muscles and bring the body back to its initial state after the effort (10–15 min).

2.4. Data Analysis

All analyses were performed with the IBM SPSS Statistics 25 statistical package. The significance level was set at $p < 0.05$. The adjustment of the different variables to the normal distribution was assessed by both graphic procedures and the Shapiro–Wilk test.

To determine whether there were differences as a result of the rowing training undertaken by the participants, the medians of each variable pre- and post-intervention were analyzed using the Wilcoxon test for related samples (paired data). In addition, the graphic analysis of the different variables was performed using boxplots or box and whisker plots. To analyze whether there were differences according to the rowing training performed by the participants, the data from the pre-test and post-test measurements were compared through the different tests. The estimated between-subject marginal means (Boat*Measurement) and the standard deviation were considered when quantifying the interaction between the variables and their longitudinal evolution through a repeated-measures ANOVA, applying the Bonferroni post hoc test.

3. Results

Table 3 shows the evolution of the results obtained after carrying out the rowing-based training protocol taking into account the measurements in both groups. There was a significant improvement in the mean values for cardiac variables, blood pressure and cardiorespiratory capacity after the intervention program.

Table 3. Within-subject analysis of the study variables after the intervention program.

	Pre-Test (SD)	Post-Test (SD)	$\Delta_{pre-post}$ (SD)	Student's t	Effect Size	p
Rest HR (bpm)	94.33 (11.81)	84.78 (11.27)	−9.55 (7.29)	8.275	1.154	0.000 **
Initial Test HR (bpm)	92.83 (12.76)	81.85/11.35)	−10.97 (7.59)	9.145	1.2	0.000 **
Final Test HR (bpm)	139.5 (18.44)	122.4 (19.17)	−17.1 (15.69)	6.891	2.481	0.000 **
Diastolic BP (mmHg)	160.03 (13.37)	144.23 (18.6)	−15.8 (16.36)	6.109	2.587	0.000 **
Systolic BP (mmHg)	100.78 (10.19)	85.8 (9.8)	−14.97 (10.86)	8.716	1.718	0.000 **
6 MWT (m)	784.78 (103.64)	863.13 (108.75)	+78.35 (62.57)	−7.92	9.893	0.000 **

Bpm = beats per minute; mmHg = millimetres of mercury; SD = standard deviation; MS = mean square. ** $p < 0.001$.

If we look at the differences obtained according to the type of vessel used in the training program (Table 4), we see that both the subjects who performed FSR and those who performed SSR significantly improved all the parameters related to cardiac function and cardiorespiratory capacity. Furthermore, in the SSR group, better results were obtained after the intervention protocol in all the variables of the study compared to the FSR group (Initial HR, Final HR, Diastolic BP, Systolic BP and the 6-min walk test [6 MWT]), except in Rest HR, which also shows a positive evolution.

Table 4. Within-subject analysis of the study variables according to boat type.

	Fixed Seat Rowing (FSR)			Sliding Seat Rowing (SSR)			Interaction Effect Boat Measurement		
	Pre-Test (SD)	Post-Test (SD)	$\Delta_{pre\text{-}post}$	Pre-Test (SD)	Post-Test (SD)	$\Delta_{pre\text{-}post}$	MS	F	p
Rest HR (bpm)	96.1 (11.54)	85.45 (11.28)	−10.65	92.55 (11.51)	84.1 (10.93)	−8.45	126.05	0.9	0.000 **
Initial test HR (bpm)	94.1 (14.21)	83.4 (12.86)	−10.7	91.55 (10.58)	80.3 (8.99)	−11.25	65.02	0.39	0.000 **
Final test HR (bpm)	141,75 (18.67)	127.9 (22.38)	−13.85	137.25 (17.44)	116.9 (12.47)	−20.35	202.5	0.59	0.000 **
Diastolic BP (mmHg)	158.25 (12.8)	145.9 (17.32)	−12.35	161.8 (13.35)	142.55 (19.2)	−19.25	126.05	0.7	0.000 **
Systolic BP (mmHg)	100.55 (10.51)	87.55 (8.11)	−13	101 (9.59)	84.05 (10.73)	−16.95	2.02	0.02	0.000 **
6 MWT (m)	817.25 (51.1)	880.3 (69.96)	+63.05	752.3 (127.37)	845.95 (132.58)	+93.65	42,185.02	4.25	0.000 **

Interaction Effect Boat Measurement refers to the influence of the type of boat used according to the training group on the variables. Bpm = beats per minute; mmHg = millimetres of mercury; 6 MWT = 6-min walk test; SD = standard deviation; MS = mean square. ** $p < 0.001$.

An in-depth analysis of the results is shown in Figure 3, considering the type of boat used in the training protocol and the evolution of the variables associated with cardiac function at rest, before starting the 6 MWT and at the end of the test. Both groups had significant improvements in resting heart rate (FSR: $\Delta_{pre\text{-}post}$ Rest HR = −10.65; $p = 0.000$; SSR: $\Delta_{pre\text{-}post}$ Rest HR = −8.45; $p = 0.000$), initial rate before the test (FSR: $\Delta_{pre\text{-}post}$ Initial HR = −10.7; $p = 0.000$; SSR: $\Delta_{pre\text{-}post}$ Initial HR = −11.25; $p = 0.000$) and final rate after the test (FSR: $\Delta_{pre\text{-}post}$ Final HR = −13.85; $p = 0.000$; SSR: $\Delta_{pre\text{-}post}$ Final HR = −20.35; $p = 0.000$).

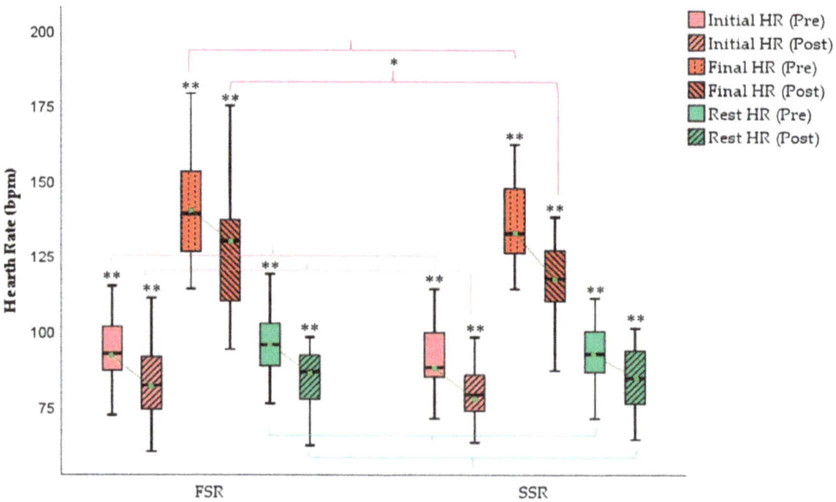

Figure 3. Comparison of cardiac variables before and after rowing training according to boat type. HR = heart rate; FSR = fixed seat rowing; SSR = sliding seat rowing. * $p < 0.05$; ** $p < 0.001$.

Figure 4 provides the blood pressure measurements obtained before and after the 6 MWT. Both the FSR and SSR groups showed significant improvements in systolic (FSR: $\Delta_{pre\text{-}post}$ Systolic BP = −13; $p = 0.000$; SSR: $\Delta_{pre\text{-}post}$ Systolic BP = −16.25; $p = 0.000$) and diastolic (FSR: $\Delta_{pre\text{-}post}$ Diastolic BP = −12.35; $p = 0.000$; SSR: $\Delta_{pre\text{-}post}$ Diastolic BP = −19.25;

$p = 0.000$) blood pressure, although these improvements were slightly greater in the women who rowed in the SSR group.

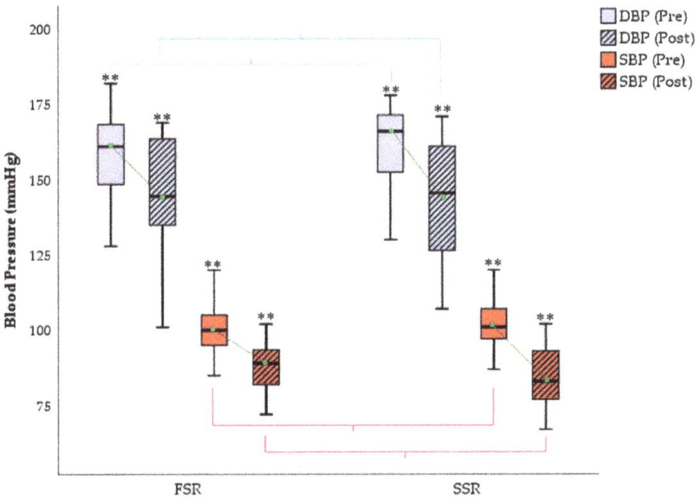

Figure 4. Comparison of blood pressure before and after rowing training according to boat type. BP = blood pressure; FSR= fixed seat rowing; SSR = sliding seat rowing. ** $p < 0.001$.

4. Discussion

In recent years, therapeutic programs based on rowing have been proposed as a type of non-pharmacological strategy that modulates adverse effects in female breast cancer survivors by involving moderate-intensity physical exercise that combines aerobic and muscle strength training [35]. The potential of this activity lies in a viable, sustainable, and safe model that can be tolerated by different age groups [7,35,44]. Consequently, recent studies have shown, after 4 years of follow-up, that women who participated in dragon boat training were able to maintain their cardiac parameters within normal ranges for their age (compared to healthy active individuals), despite chemotherapy treatment, in addition to not developing any type of cardiac condition during this period [44]. Other studies, conducted over 12 weeks in this type of vessel, have reported a 30% improvement in cardiorespiratory capacity, also measured through the 6 MWT [4]. Despite these improvements, there are no studies that verify which type of boat is more suitable when designing novel therapeutic programs based on rowing activity, since the muscle groups and exercise dynamics involved in fixed seat rowing differ from rowing on a sliding seat.

With this in mind, statistically significant improvements in cardiac function, systolic and diastolic blood pressure, and cardiorespiratory capacity can be observed when analyzing the results of our study. These improvements after implementation of the intervention protocol occur in both the FSR group and the rowers who participated in the SSR. When comparing the groups, a higher rate of improvement in resting heart rate can be seen in the FSR group, while the female breast cancer survivors who participated in the SSR group had greater improvements in the variables of heart rate before and after the 6 MWT, systolic and diastolic blood pressure, and distance traveled in the 6 MWT (directly correlated with the cardiorespiratory capacity and VO2max of the subjects). According to the data, although the rowing activity itself can promote cardiac adaptations that optimize the functioning of the cardiovascular system, with the SSR modality, greater adaptations occur comparatively considering the same time span (12 weeks).

Cardiac function adaptations were also found after a 12-week intervention when we compared the results, focusing on the variables of our study, with previous studies that used rowing training programs in breast cancer survivors [48]. The results showed a 10%

improvement in the systolic and diastolic blood pressure of the participating women. These results are consistent with other rowing studies, such as those by Stefani et al. [44], which showed significant improvements in diastolic function in women breast cancer survivors treated with chemotherapy after 4 years of dragon boat training [44], or by Serra et al. [49], who found that a 16-week resistance training program improved systolic and diastolic blood pressure by 5% in breast cancer survivors. These results indicate the positive impact that a professionally supervised intervention program based on rowing could have on myocardial function, even in women previously treated with chemotherapy [44].

This is important because one of the main problems associated with oncological treatments is chemotherapy-induced cardiotoxicity, which has direct and indirect adverse effects on the cardiovascular system [9,50,51]. As an example, it has been shown that the incidence of left ventricular dysfunction among patients treated with certain anticancer drugs, such as high-dose doxorubicin (700 mg/m^2), can reach 48%. The incidence of myocardial ischemia due to 5-fluorouracil (5-FU) can be as high as 10% [52,53]. Furthermore, between 26% and 93% of patients with arsenic trioxide show a prolonged QT interval, and many develop life-threatening ventricular tachyarrhythmias [54]. As a result, chemotherapy-induced cardiotoxicity has been associated with cardiovascular diseases such as myocardial dysfunction, heart failure, coronary artery disease, arrhythmias, arterial hypertension, thromboembolic disease, peripheral vascular disease, pulmonary hypertension, and pericardial complications [9,55].

In this context, clinical trials in breast cancer survivors based on pharmacological strategies (e.g., beta-blockers, angiotensin-converting enzyme inhibitors, etc.) have shown some benefits in the treatment of cardiovascular disease, but also adverse effects [8]. A rowing-based training program offers a non-pharmacological therapy that can safely contribute to achieving the goals proposed by the American College of Sports Medicine (ACSM), which recommends that cancer survivors perform at least 150 min of moderate physical activity or 75 min of vigorous exercise, as well as incorporating strength training, twice a week [56]. Reviews, such as that by Sturgeon et al. [10], suggest that aerobic exercise has a moderate effect on improving cardiac function in women with breast cancer, consistent with findings in disease-free populations. Furthermore, Gonzalo-Encabo et al. [8] after reviewing published studies, found that 16 weeks of aerobic and resistance training can reduce the risk of cardiovascular disease by 15% in Hispanic and Latina breast cancer survivors (at greater risk than the rest of the population of developing this type of disease).

Rowing is an activity that combines the benefits of aerobic exercise and strength training and can have a beneficial effect on cardiovascular health in female breast cancer survivors [48]. In this study, we can see a directly proportional relationship between cardiorespiratory capacity, heart rate, and blood pressure in female rowers who participated in both training groups. Better cardiorespiratory capacity improves the heart's ability to maintain function and pump blood with less effort [57]. Exercise can also improve the regulation of the autonomic nervous system, reducing the activity of the sympathetic nervous system (which increases blood pressure and heart rate) and increasing that of the parasympathetic nervous system (which decreases heart rate) [9,26]. Our study showed an overall improvement of 9–10 beats less at rest after 12 weeks of training. In addition, exercise-induced improvement of endothelial function [8] may lead to improved arterial health contributing to the prevention of diseases such as hypertension. As we can see, after 24 weeks of rowing training, diastolic blood pressure decreased overall by 10%, while systolic blood pressure decreased by 15%. Moreover, these results were more prominent in the SSR group rowing on a sliding seat boat than in the FSR group, which rowed on a fixed seat boat.

In our case, we have used rowing as a novel discipline since, prior to our studies, there was no literature on this activity, which, like dragon boating, is conducted on water. Despite being a minimally injurious social sport that exercises the entire body through symmetrical movement, rowing does not have the same tradition as dragon boating [40,58]. Furthermore, our country has a strong tradition of rowing, not only at the competitive

Olympic level (sculling) but also deeply rooted in coastal culture and tradition (fixed seat rowing). This is why we distinguished these two groups.

On the other hand, the risk of lymphedema following axillary surgery, such as axillary lymph node dissection, is a significant concern for breast cancer patients [59]. Engaging in physical activities, including rowing, poses potential risks and benefits. Rowing, which involves repetitive upper body movements and considerable exertion, can potentially exacerbate lymphedema due to increased fluid accumulation and stress on the lymphatic system. However, controlled and supervised physical activities have been shown to be beneficial in maintaining lymphatic function and reducing the risk of lymphedema, improving circulation and acting on the muscle as a pump during muscle contraction, which promotes venous and lymphatic drainage [7,60]. It is crucial for patients to consult with healthcare providers to develop personalized exercise programs that consider the type and extent of surgery, current physical condition, and risk factors for lymphedema. Proper technique, gradual progression, and the use of compression garments during physical activity can also help mitigate the risks associated with rowing and other upper body exercises [7,58].

Despite advances in research on the relationship between physical exercise and non-pharmacological oncological therapy, there is still insufficient scientific evidence to develop an exercise prescription for most people with this disease [10]. More research is therefore needed to understand how physical activity and sport interact with the disease, what the consequences are for the individual and what the best strategies are for oncological rehabilitation through exercise [21,24].

The strength of this pioneering study is the data it provides on physical activity and rowing, not only demonstrating that rowing is a viable and safe sport for breast cancer survivors, but also which type of boat produces the greatest positive changes in cardiac function in the participants. However, the study also has some limitations related to the sample power of the participants. Our findings are based on a relatively small sample, due to the very specific population encompassed by the study, the complexity in its recruitment and subsequent follow-up during the intervention protocol.

5. Conclusions

The present study shows that a rowing-based therapeutic program, combining aerobic and muscular strength exercises, can be a viable and safe strategy to improve cardiovascular health in female breast cancer survivors. It has been demonstrated that 24 weeks of rowing training can significantly improve cardiac function, blood pressure, and cardiorespiratory capacity, and may mitigate the adverse effects of cardiotoxicity induced by cancer treatments. These results are particularly noteworthy in the group using SSR boats, which showed greater cardiovascular adaptations compared to the group using FSR boats. This novel study highlights the importance of further exploring and validating the beneficial effects of physical exercise in cancer rehabilitation, opening the door to new non-pharmacological therapeutic strategies to improve the health and well-being of this vulnerable population.

Author Contributions: Conceptualization, J.G.-G. (Juan Gavala-González), M.R.-P. and J.C.F.-G.; methodology, J.G.-G. (Juan Gavala-González) and J.G.-G. (Juan Gamboa-González); software, M.R.-P.; validation, J.C.F.-G., J.G.-G. (Juan Gavala-González) and J.G.-G. (Juan Gamboa-González); formal analysis, M.R.-P.; investigation, M.R.-P. and J.G.-G. (Juan Gamboa-González); resources, J.G.-G. (Juan Gamboa-González) and M.R.-P.; data curation, J.G.-G. (Juan Gavala-González); writing—original draft preparation, M.R.-P. and J.G.-G. (Juan Gamboa-González); writing—review and editing, M.R.-P., J.G.-G. (Juan Gavala-González) and J.C.F.-G.; visualization, J.G.-G. (Juan Gavala-González); supervision, J.C.F.-G.; project administration, J.G.-G. (Juan Gavala-González). All authors have read and agreed to the published version of the manuscript.

Funding: This research received no external funding.

Institutional Review Board Statement: The study was conducted in accordance with the Declaration of Helsinki and approved by the Institutional Review Board (or Ethics Committee) of the University of Malaga with the number 65-2020-H.

Informed Consent Statement: Informed consent was obtained from all subjects involved in the study.

Data Availability Statement: The Ethical Committee of the University of Malaga, which authorized this study, precludes ceding, showing, or disclosing to third parties by any means the database of this research (personal data, medical history, interviews, physical condition tests, and others) because it is considered confidential and sensitive information.

Conflicts of Interest: The authors declare no conflicts of interest.

References

1. Spanoudaki, M.; Giaginis, C.; Karafyllaki, D.; Papadopoulos, K.; Solovos, E.; Antasouras, G.; Sfikas, G.; Papadopoulos, A.N.; Papadopoulou, S.K. Exercise as a Promising Agent against Cancer: Evaluating Its Anti-Cancer Molecular Mechanisms. *Cancers* **2023**, *15*, 5135. [CrossRef] [PubMed]
2. Kim, J.; Choi, W.J.; Jeong, S.H. The Effects of Physical Activity on Breast Cancer Survivors after Diagnosis. *J. Cancer Prev.* **2013**, *18*, 193–200. [CrossRef] [PubMed]
3. World Health Organization. Cancer. Available online: https://www.who.int/es/news-room/fact-sheets/detail/cancer (accessed on 26 August 2023).
4. Moro, T.; Casolo, A.; Bordignon, V.; Sampieri, A.; Schiavinotto, G.; Vigo, L.; Ghisi, M.; Paoli, A.; Cerea, S. Keep Calm and Keep Rowing: The Psychophysical Effects of Dragon Boat Program in Breast Cancer Survivors. *Support. Care Cancer* **2024**, *32*. [CrossRef] [PubMed]
5. Hidrobo-Coello, J.F. Actividad Física Para Pacientes Con Diagnóstico de Cáncer. Guía de Prescripción Deportiva Para Ecuador. *Rev. Iberoam. Ciencias Act. Física Deport.* **2020**, *9*, 18–41. [CrossRef]
6. Prieto-Gómez, V.; Yuste-Sánchez, M.J.; Bailón-Cerezo, J.; Romay-Barrero, H.; de la Rosa-Díaz, I.; Lirio-Romero, C.; Torres-Lacomba, M. Effectiveness of Therapeutic Exercise and Patient Education on Cancer-Related Fatigue in Breast Cancer Survivors : A Randomised, Single-Blind, Controlled Trial with a 6-Month. *J. Clin. Med.* **2022**, *11*, 269. [CrossRef] [PubMed]
7. Iacorossi, L.; Gambalunga, F.; Molinaro, S.; De Domenico, R.; Giannarelli, D.; Fabi, A. The Effectiveness of the Sport "Dragon Boat Racing" in Reducing the Risk of Lymphedema Incidence: An Observational Study. *Cancer Nurs.* **2019**, *42*, 323–331. [CrossRef] [PubMed]
8. Gonzalo-Encabo, P.; Sami, N.; Wilson, R.L.; Kang, D.-W.; Ficarra, S.; Dieli-Conwright, C.M. Exercise as Medicine in Cardio-Oncology: Reducing Health Disparities in Hispanic and Latina Breast Cancer Survivors. *Curr. Oncol. Rep.* **2023**, *25*, 1237–1245. [CrossRef]
9. Amin, A.M.; Khlidj, Y.; Abuelazm, M.; Ibrahim, A.A.; Tanashat, M.; Imran, M.; Nazir, A.; Shaikhkhalil, H.; Abdelazeem, B. The Efficacy and Safety of Exercise Regimens to Mitigate Chemotherapy Cardiotoxicity: A Systematic Review and Meta-Analysis of Randomized Controlled Trials. *Cardio-Oncology* **2024**, *10*, 10. [CrossRef] [PubMed]
10. Sturgeon, K.M.; Kok, D.E.; Kleckner, I.R.; Guertin, K.A.; McNeil, J.; Parry, T.L.; Ehlers, D.K.; Hamilton, A.; Schmitz, K.; Campbell, K.L.; et al. Updated Systematic Review of the Effects of Exercise on Understudied Health Outcomes in Cancer Survivors. *Cancer Med.* **2023**, *12*, 22278–22292. [CrossRef] [PubMed]
11. Todorov, N.; Sherman, K.A.; Kilby, C.J. Self-Compassion and Hope in the Context of Body Image Disturbance and Distress in Breast Cancer Survivors. *Psychooncology* **2019**, *28*, 2025–2032. [CrossRef]
12. Harvie, M.; Howell, A.; Evans, D.G. Can Diet and Lifestyle Prevent Breast Cancer: What Is the Evidence? *Am. Soc. Clin. Oncol. Educ. B.* **2015**, *35*, e66–e73. [CrossRef] [PubMed]
13. Courneya, K.S.; Mackey, J.R.; Jones, L.W. Coping with Cancer: Can Exercise Help? *Phys. Sportsmed.* **2000**, *28*, 49–73. [CrossRef] [PubMed]
14. Roscoe, C.M.P.; Pringle, A.; Chandler, C.; Faghy, M.A.; Barratt, B. The Role of Physical Activity in Cancer Recovery: An Exercise Practitioner's Perspective. *Int. J. Environ. Res. Public Health* **2022**, *19*, 3600. [CrossRef] [PubMed]
15. Murri, A.; Vitucci, D.; Tranchita, E.; Grazioli, E.; Gori, S.; Modena, A.; Turazza, M.; Filippini, R.; Galeazzi, S.; Verzè, M.; et al. "OPERATION PHALCO"—Adapted Physical Activity for Breast Cancer Survivors: Is It Time for a Multidisciplinary Approach? *Cancers* **2023**, *15*, 34. [CrossRef] [PubMed]
16. Patsou, E.D.; Alexias, G.D.; Anagnostopoulos, F.G.; Karamouzis, M.V. Effects of Physical Activity on Depressive Symptoms during Breast Cancer Survivorship: A Meta-Analysis of Randomised Control Trials. *ESMO Open* **2017**, *2*, e000271. [CrossRef] [PubMed]
17. Mascherini, G.; Tosi, B.; Giannelli, C.; Grifoni, E.; Degl'innocenti, S.; Galanti, G. Breast Cancer: Effectiveness of a One-Year Unsupervised Exercise Program. *J. Sport. Med. Phys. Fit.* **2019**, *59*, 283–289. [CrossRef] [PubMed]
18. Sousa, B.L.S.C.; dos Santos Rosa, T.; Silvino, V.O.; Barros, E.M.L.; de Luca Corrêa, H.; do Prado, D.M.L.; Veras-Silva, A.S.; de Souza, M.D.; de Lima, C.E.B.; de Oliveira, L.F.L.; et al. Physical and Autonomic Functionality in Women with Breast Cancer Pre and Post Chemotherapy: A Case Control Study. *BMC Sports Sci. Med. Rehabil.* **2024**, *16*, 5. [CrossRef] [PubMed]

19. Rogers, L.Q.; Courneya, K.S.; Oster, R.A.; Anton, P.M.; Phillips, S.; Ehlers, D.K.; McAuley, E. Physical Activity Intervention Benefits Persist Months Post-Intervention: Randomized Trial in Breast Cancer Survivors. *J. Cancer Surviv.* **2023**, *17*, 1834–1846. [CrossRef] [PubMed]
20. Parkinson, J.; Bandera, A.; Crichton, M.; Shannon, C.; Woodward, N.; Hodgkinson, A.; Millar, L.; Teleni, L.; van der Meij, B.S. Poor Muscle Status, Dietary Protein Intake, Exercise Levels, Quality of Life and Physical Function in Women with Metastatic Breast Cancer at Chemotherapy Commencement and during Follow-Up. *Curr. Oncol.* **2023**, *30*, 688–703. [CrossRef] [PubMed]
21. Campbell, K.L.; Winters-Stone, K.M.; Wiskemann, J.; May, A.M.; Schwartz, A.L.; Courneya, K.S.; Zucker, D.S.; Matthews, C.E.; Ligibel, J.A.; Gerber, L.H.; et al. Exercise Guidelines for Cancer Survivors: Consensus Statement from International Multidisciplinary Roundtable. *Med. Sci. Sports Exerc.* **2019**, *51*, 2375–2390. [CrossRef]
22. Shachar, S.S.; Heiling, H.; Muss, H.B.; Meghan, D.; Wagoner, C.W.; Deal, A.M.; Nyrop, K.A. Physical Activity Intervention in Patients with Metastatic Breast Cancer During Active Treatment: Quality of Life and Function. *Oncologist* **2022**, *28*, 84-e70. [CrossRef] [PubMed]
23. Schleicher, E.; Mcauley, E.; Anton, P.; Ehlers, D.K.; Phillips, S.M.; Rogers, L.Q. Moderators of Physical Activity and Quality of Life Response to a Physical Activity Intervention for Breast Cancer Survivors Trial. *Res. Sq.* **2022**, *31*, 53. [CrossRef]
24. Schmitz, K.H.; Campbell, A.M.; Stuiver, M.M.; Pinto, B.M.; Schwartz, A.L.; Morris, G.S.; Ligibel, J.A.; Cheville, A.; Galvão, D.A.; Alfano, C.M.; et al. Exercise Is Medicine in Oncology: Engaging Clinicians to Help Patients Move through Cancer. *CA Cancer J. Clin.* **2019**, *69*, 468–484. [CrossRef] [PubMed]
25. Goldschmidt, S.; Schmidt, M.E.; Steindorf, K. Long-Term Effects of Exercise Interventions on Physical Activity in Breast Cancer Patients: A Systematic Review and Meta-Analysis of Randomized Controlled Trials. *Support. Care Cancer* **2023**, *31*, 17–21. [CrossRef] [PubMed]
26. García-Chico, C.; López-Ortiz, S.; Peñín-Grandes, S.; Pinto-Fraga, J.; Valenzuela, P.L.; Emanuele, E.; Ceci, C.; Graziani, G.; Fiuza-Luces, C.; Lista, S.; et al. Physical Exercise and the Hallmarks of Breast Cancer: A Narrative Review. *Cancers* **2023**, *15*, 324. [CrossRef]
27. Kaur, N.; Kumar, R.; Jain, A.; Saxena, A.K. Sensory Changes and Postmastectomy Pain Following Preservation of Intercostobrachial Nerve in Breast Cancer Surgery: A Prospective Randomized Study. *Indian J. Surg. Oncol.* **2021**, *12*, 108–113. [CrossRef] [PubMed]
28. Cirocchi, R.; Matteucci, M.; Randolph, J.; Duro, F.; Properzi, L.; Avenia, S.; Amato, B.; Iandoli, R.; Tebala, G.; Boselli, C.; et al. Anatomical Variants of the Intercostobrachial Nerve and Its Preservation during Surgery, a Systematic Review and Meta-Analysis. *World J. Surg. Oncol.* **2024**, *22*, 92. [CrossRef] [PubMed]
29. Heidinger, M.; Weber, W.P. Axillary Surgery for Breast Cancer in 2024. *Cancers* **2024**, *16*, 1623. [CrossRef] [PubMed]
30. Slavu, I.M.; Tulin, A.; Filipoiu, F.; Dogaru, A.; Munteanu, O.; Anca Monica, O.M.; Tulin, R.; Ursut, B. Axillary Lymphadenectomy: Safe Dissection Through a Correct Technique. *Cureus* **2024**, *16*, e52434. [CrossRef] [PubMed]
31. Marco Continente, C.; Luesma Bartolomé, M.J.; Santander Ballestín, S. Influence of Physical Activity on the Prevention, Antineoplastic Treatment and Survival of Patients with Breast Cancer. *Rev. Senol. Patol. Mamar.* **2021**, *34*, 220–235. [CrossRef]
32. Fernández, D.; Mielgo, J.; Caballero, A.; Córdova, A.; Lázaro, M.; Fernández, C. Actividad Física En Pacientes Oncológicos de Cáncer de Mama: ¿Terapia Médica Deportiva No Farmacológica? Revisión Sistemática. *Arch. Med. Deport.* **2020**, *37*, 266–274.
33. Courneya, K.S.; Segal, R.J.; Gelmon, K.; Mackey, J.R.; Friedenreich, C.M.; Yasui, Y.; Reid, R.D.; Proulx, C.; Trinh, L.; Dolan, L.B.; et al. Predictors of Adherence to Different Types and Doses of Supervised Exercise during Breast Cancer Chemotherapy. *Int. J. Behav. Nutr. Phys. Act.* **2014**, *11*, 85. [CrossRef] [PubMed]
34. Gavala-González, J.; Torres-Pérez, A.; Fernández-García, J.C. Impact of Rowing Training on Quality of Life and Physical Activity Levels in Female Breast Cancer Survivors. *Int. J. Environ. Res. Public Health* **2021**, *18*, 7188. [CrossRef] [PubMed]
35. Asensio-García, M.D.R.; Tomás-Rodríguez, M.I.; Palazón-Bru, A.; Hernández-Sánchez, S.; Nouni-García, R.; Romero-Aledo, A.L.; Gil-Guillén, V.F. Effect of Rowing on Mobility, Functionality, and Quality of Life in Women with and without Breast Cancer: A 4-Month Intervention. *Support. Care Cancer* **2021**, *29*, 2639–2644. [CrossRef] [PubMed]
36. Gavala-González, J.; Gálvez-Fernández, I.; Mercadé-Melé, P.; Fernández-García, J.C. Rowing Training in Breast Cancer Survivors: A Longitudinal Study of Physical Fitness. *Int. J. Environ. Res. Public Health* **2020**, *17*, 4938. [CrossRef] [PubMed]
37. Blanzola, C.; O'Sullivan, P.; Smith, K.; Nelson, R. The Benefits of Dragon Boat Participation for Breast Cancer Survivors. *Ther. Recreation J.* **2016**, *50*, 242–246. [CrossRef]
38. McDonough, M.H.; Patterson, M.C.; Weisenbach, B.B.; Ullrich-French, S.; Sabiston, C.M. The Difference Is More than Floating: Factors Affecting Breast Cancer Survivors' Decisions to Join and Maintain Participation in Dragon Boat Teams and Support Groups. *Disabil. Rehabil.* **2019**, *41*, 1788–1796. [CrossRef] [PubMed]
39. Parry, D.C. The Contribution of Dragon Boat Racing to Women's Health and Breast Cancer Survivorship. *Qual. Health Res.* **2008**, *18*, 222–233. [CrossRef] [PubMed]
40. Unruh, A.M.; Elvin, N. In the Eye of the Dragon: Women's Experience of Breast Cancer and the Occupation of Dragon Boat Racing. *Can. J. Occup. Ther.* **2004**, *71*, 138–149. [CrossRef] [PubMed]
41. Gavala-González, J. *Las Modalidades Del Remo: El Remo En Banco Fijo*; Universidad de Sevilla: Sevilla, Spain, 2019.
42. Yoshiga, C.C.; Higuchi, M. Rowing Performance of Female and Male Rowers. *Scand. J. Med. Sci. Sports* **2003**, *13*, 317–321. [CrossRef] [PubMed]

43. Volianitis, S.; Yoshiga, C.C.; Secher, N.H. The Physiology of Rowing with Perspective on Training and Health. *Eur. J. Appl. Physiol.* **2020**, *120*, 1943–1963. [CrossRef] [PubMed]
44. Stefani, L.; Galanti, G.; Di Tante, V.; Klika, R.J.; Maffulli, N. Dragon Boat Training Exerts a Positive Effect on Myocardial Function in Breast Cancer Survivors. *Phys. Sportsmed.* **2015**, *43*, 307–311. [CrossRef] [PubMed]
45. Harriss, D.; Macsween, A.; Atkinson, G. Standards for Ethics in Sport and Exercise Science Research. *Int. J. Sports Med.* **2017**, *38*, 1126–1131. [PubMed]
46. Ebihara, A. World Medical Association Declaration of Helsinki. *Jpn. Pharmacol. Ther.* **2000**, *28*, 983–986. [CrossRef]
47. Börg, G. Psychophysical Bases of Perceived Exertion. *Med. Sci. Sports Exerc.* **1982**, *14*, 377–381. [CrossRef] [PubMed]
48. Gavala-González, J.; Gálvez-Fernández, I.; Mercadé-Melé, P.; Fernández-García, J.C. Cardiac Effects of a Rowing Training Program in Breast Cancer Survivors. *Sustainability* **2021**, *13*, 6805. [CrossRef]
49. Serra, M.C.; Ryan, A.S.; Ortmeyer, H.K.; Addison, O.; Goldberg, A.P. Resistance Training Reduces Inflammation and Fatigue and Improves Physical Function in Older Breast Cancer Survivors. *Menopause* **2018**, *25*, 211–216. [CrossRef] [PubMed]
50. Howden, E.; Foulkes, S.; Dillon, H.; Bigaran, A.; Wright, L.; Janssens, K.; Comie, P.; Costello, B.; La Gerche, A. Traditional Markers of Cardiac Toxicity Fail to Detect Marked Reductions in Cardiorespiratory Fitness among Cancer Patients Undergoing Anti-Cancer Treatment. *Eur. Heart J. Cardiovasc. Imaging* **2021**, *22*, 451–458. [CrossRef] [PubMed]
51. Ginzac, A.; Bernadach, M.; Molnar, I.; Duclos, M. Adapted Physical Activity for Breast Cancer Patients Treated with Neoadjuvant Chemotherapy and Trastuzumab Against HER2 (APACAN2): A Protocol for a Feasibility Study. *Front. Oncol.* **2021**, *11*, 744609. [CrossRef] [PubMed]
52. Zamorano, J.L.; Lancellotti, P.; Muñoz, D.R.; Aboyans, V.; Asteggiano, R.; Galderisi, M.; Habib, G.; Lenihan, D.J.; Lip, G.Y.H.; Lyon, A.R.; et al. 2016 ESC Position Paper on Cancer Treatments and Cardiovascular Toxicity Developed under the Auspices of the ESC Committee for Practice Guidelines: The Task Force for Cancer Treatments and Cardiovascular Toxicity of the European Society of Cardiology (ESC). *Eur. Heart J.* **2016**, *37*, 2768–2801. [CrossRef] [PubMed]
53. Frickhofen, N.; Beck, F.J.; Jung, B.; Fuhr, H.G.; Andrasch, H.; Sigmund, M. Capecitabine Can Induce Acute Coronary Syndrome Similar to 5-Fluorouracil. *Ann. Oncol.* **2002**, *13*, 797–801. [CrossRef] [PubMed]
54. Lenihan, D.J.; Kowey, P.R. Overview and Management of Cardiac Adverse Events Associated with Tyrosine Kinase Inhibitors. *Oncologist* **2013**, *18*, 900–908. [CrossRef] [PubMed]
55. Odynets, T.; Briskin, Y.; Ikkert, O.; Todorova, V.; Yefremova, A. Cardiopulmonary Function in Breast Cancer Patients versus Healthy Control Women. *Physiother. Q.* **2020**, *28*, 6–10. [CrossRef]
56. Rock, C.L.; Thomson, C.A.; Sullivan, K.R.; Howe, C.L.; Kushi, L.H.; Caan, B.J.; Neuhouser, M.L.; Bandera, E.V.; Wang, Y.; Robien, K.; et al. American Cancer Society Nutrition and Physical Activity Guideline for Cancer Survivors. CA. *Cancer J. Clin.* **2022**, *72*, 230–262. [CrossRef] [PubMed]
57. Ross, R.; Blair, S.; Arena, R.; Church, T.; Després, J.; Franklin, B.; Haskell, W.; Kaminsky, L.; Levine, B.; Lavie, C.; et al. Importance of Assessing Cardiorespiratory Fitness in Clinical Practice: A Case for Fitness as a Clinical Vital Sign. *Circulation* **2016**, *134*, 653–699. [CrossRef] [PubMed]
58. Harris, S.R.; Niesen-Vertommen, S.L. Challenging the Myth of Exercise-Induced Lymphedema Following Breast Cancer: A Series of Case Reports. *J. Surg. Oncol.* **2000**, *74*, 95–98. [CrossRef] [PubMed]
59. Hara, Y.; Otsubo, R.; Shinohara, S.; Morita, M.; Kuba, S.; Matsumoto, M.; Yamanouchi, K.; Yano, H.; Eguchi, S.; Nagayasu, T. Lymphedema After Axillary Lymph Node Dissection in Breast Cancer: Prevalence and Risk Factors—A Single-Center Retrospective Study. *Lymphat. Res. Biol.* **2022**, *20*, 600–606. [CrossRef] [PubMed]
60. Fukushima, T.; Tsuji, T.; Sano, Y.; Miyata, C.; Kamisako, M.; Hohri, H.; Yoshimura, C.; Asakura, M.; Okitsu, T.; Muraoka, K.; et al. Immediate Effects of Active Exercise with Compression Therapy on Lower-Limb Lymphedema. *Support. Care Cancer* **2017**, *25*, 2603–2610. [CrossRef] [PubMed]

applied sciences

MDPI

Article

Anthropometric Parameters and Body Composition in Elite Lead Climbers and Boulderers—A Retrospective Study

Agata Ginszt [1], Grzegorz Zieliński [2], Aleksandra Dolina [2], Estera Stachyra [3], Monika Zaborek-Łyczba [1], Jakub Łyczba [1], Piotr Gawda [2] and Michał Ginszt [3,*]

[1] Interdisciplinary Scientific Group of Sports Medicine, Department of Sports Medicine, Medical University of Lublin, 20-093 Lublin, Poland; agata.zysko97@gmail.com (A.G.); zaborelli00@gmail.com (M.Z.-Ł.); jakublyczba7@gmail.com (J.Ł.)

[2] Department of Sports Medicine, Medical University of Lublin, 20-093 Lublin, Poland; grzegorz.zielinski@umlub.pl (G.Z.); aleksandrabys@umlub.pl (A.D.); piotr.gawda@umlub.pl (P.G.)

[3] Department of Rehabilitation and Physiotherapy, Medical University of Lublin, 20-059 Lublin, Poland; estera.zieba.umlub@gmail.com

* Correspondence: michal.ginszt@umlub.pl

Abstract: Based on previous research studies and systematic reviews, success in sport climbing seems to be determined by variables such as strength, power, or endurance. However, besides strength-endurance parameters, several other factors may influence the performance of sports climbing. Moreover, there is a lack of research assessing differences in body composition and anthropometric parameters between lead climbing and bouldering—the two most common sport climbing subdisciplines. The presented research analyzed the connection between body mass, body height, body mass index, and the best result in sport climbing among male lead climbers and boulderers. Additionally, we investigated differences in starting climbing age and climbing experience in both climbing subdisciplines. We analyzed 422 male sport climbers' profiles in two categories: "Route Ranking: Top-10 climbs last 12 months" for lead climbers and "Boulder Ranking: Top-10 climbs last 12 months" for boulderers based on the 8a.nu world ranking website. The results showed that the "Elite" and "Higher Elite" lead climbers had lower body mass and lower body height. These differences were also observed between "Elite" and "Higher Elite" lead climbers. The "Higher Elite" group started climbing at a younger age and had a more extended period to achieve the most challenging route than "Elite" climbers in both subdisciplines. Our results suggest that lower body mass and lower body height can be key factors in lead climbing performance.

Keywords: sport climbing; lead climbing; bouldering; body composition; anthropometry

1. Introduction

Over the last few decades, a significant increase in interest in sports climbing has been observed [1]. It is a relatively young sport discipline included in the Tokyo 2020 Olympic Games program [2]. The subdisciplines of sports climbing presented in Tokyo were lead climbing, bouldering, and speed climbing. The first two subdisciplines are the most frequently trained sport climbing styles [2–4]. There are many differences between bouldering and lead climbing regarding the length of the climbing route, belaying methods, and the nature of physical effort. In bouldering, the climber ascends short technical boulder routes up to 4–5 m on low walls using crash mats instead of ropes [4,5]. The climbing routes in lead climbing are much longer (10 to 40 m) and, thus, contain more movements than in bouldering. In lead climbing, the climber is attached to a rope clipped into permanent bolts using "quickdraws", spaced intermittently from the bottom up [3–5]. Different forms of sport climbing require different sets of skills and physiological conditions [2]. Nevertheless, only a few previous research studies have compared the physical characteristics of sport climbers between lead climbing and bouldering subdisciplines. Lead climbing is characterized by more static, slow, and controlled movements than bouldering [6]. Moreover, lead climbers are more capable of longer routes than boulderers, with a shorter climbing duration (30 s for bouldering vs. 2–7 min for lead climbing). On the other hand, bouldering routes are shorter, but the movements are performed with maximum effort [4,5]. This suggests that bouldering can be classified as a strength subdiscipline, while lead climbing is characterized by endurance effort [5]. Several studies showed that boulderers are characterized by higher explosive strength of the forearm muscles compared to lead climbers [6–8]. The differences between lead climbers and boulderers were also observed at the genetic level and concern the functional polymorphism of the ACTN3 gene, which, depending on the genotype, is associated with the strength or endurance of skeletal muscles [9].

According to the systematic review by Saul et al. [10], the anthropometric data connected with success in sports climbing are large bone-to-tip pulp associated with generating a higher lifting force, and great forearm volume is an indirect parameter of muscle mass. Moreover, in several research studies, body mass values differ significantly between sport climbers and controls [11,12]. However, differences in body mass and height can vary within the groups because the researchers tried to recruit subjects of similar age and body size to compare physiological parameters like strength and endurance. Therefore, this generates difficulty in interpreting this data type in studies analyzing other main motor and physiological parameters. Several studies showed differences in anthropometrical, physiological, and strength-endurance parameters between elite sport climbers, less advanced athletes, and controls [13]. However, so far, there are no studies comparing body composition, anthropometric parameters, or the age of peak performance between lead climbers and boulderers.

Thus, the present study investigated the relationship between age, climbing experience, and anthropometric data (body mass, body height) and the best result achieved by male sport climbers in bouldering and lead climbing in natural rock formations.

2. Materials and Methods

2.1. Participants

The analysis was carried out with the consent of the Bioethics Committee of the Medical University of Lublin (KE-0254/93/2020). For the study, the competitors' profiles from "www.8a.nu (accessed on 30 August 2020)" were analyzed in two categories: "Route Ranking: Top-10 climbs last 12 months" and "Boulder Ranking: Top-10 climbs last 12 months". The www.8a.nu website consists of volitional self-reporting data that serve as experimental variables. The first 500 profiles were analyzed in each category. The data are made public voluntarily and free of charge. The values of the ascent difficulty level have been adopted according to the recommendation of the International Rock Climbing Research Association (IRCRA) [14]. The rock-climbing ascent difficulty level values have been converted from the French scale for lead climbing and from the Font scale for bouldering to the IRCRA level [14].

The following exclusion criteria were applied: profile incompleteness (lack of at least one record in the athlete's profile), sports classification below the "Elite" level, and female sex due to the small number of female athletes in the "Elite" and "Higher Elite" categories included in the www.8a.nu ranking.

Based on the above criteria, 422 male profiles were qualified for the study. The "Route Ranking: Top-10 lead climbs last 12 months" category included 164 lead climbers (average age = 28 $\pm$ 8 years), 86 lead climbers in the "Elite" group (IRCRA = 26 $\pm$ 1), and 78 lead climbers in the "Higher Elite" group (IRCRA = 29 $\pm$ 1). In comparison, 258 boulderers (average age 27 $\pm$ 6) were qualified for the "Boulder Ranking: Top-10 climbs last 12 months" category, including 114 boulderers in the "Elite" group (IRCRA = 26 $\pm$ 1) and 144 boulderers in the "Higher Elite" group (IRCRA = 29 $\pm$ 1).

2.2. Procedure and Data Preparation

Four independent researchers conducted the data collection from the www.8a.nu ranking website. Two of them assessed athletes' profiles in lead climbing. The others assessed sport climbers' profiles in bouldering. After analysis of the athletes' profiles and initial qualification for the present research, the authors analyzed the qualified profiles among themselves. After double-checking the examination, the qualified athletes' profiles did not differ between the two independent studies. The extracted and examined parameters from the www.8a.nu ranking website included the hardest lead climbing route or boulder ascent in Red Point (RP) style, age when climbing the hardest route or boulder, years of climbing experience, body mass, and body height. After obtaining and checking the above-mentioned data, additional parameters were calculated. Body mass index (BMI) was calculated based on body height and body mass. The time to achieve the best climbing ascent was calculated based on the year of climbing the hardest route or boulder and the year of starting climbing based on the formula:

$$\text{The time to achieve} = \text{the year of the hardest climb} - \text{the year of starting climbing} \quad (1)$$

Based on the hardest route or hardest boulder ascent, the sport climbers were qualified for the "Elite" and "Higher Elite" groups according to IRCRA standards. The qualification of the athletes to one of the groups was carried out using the IRCRA scale, which is used to classify climbing routes for statistical calculations [14]. The "Elite" level for lead climbers was determined between 24 and 27 IRCRA points (between 8a+ and 8c on the French scale). The "Higher Elite" level for lead climbers was determined between 28 and 32 IRCRA points (between 8c+ and 9b+ on the French scale). The "Elite" level for boulderers was marked between 24 and 27 IRCRA points (between 7C and 8A+ on the Font scale). The "Higher Elite" level for boulderers was determined between 28 and 32 IRCRA points (between 8B and 8C+ on the Font scale).

2.3. Statistical Analyses

The analysis of the obtained results was performed as described below:

1. Comparison of the age of starting climbing, age when climbing the hardest route, time to achieve the hardest route, body mass, body height, and BMI between the "Elite" and "Higher Elite" groups in the lead climbing.
2. Comparison of the age of starting climbing, age when climbing the hardest route, time to achieve the hardest route, body mass, body height, and BMI between the "Elite" and "Higher Elite" groups in bouldering.
3. Comparison of the age of starting climbing, age when climbing the hardest route, time to achieve the hardest route, body mass, body height, and BMI between the "Elite" and "Higher Elite" groups between lead climbers and boulderers.
4. Comparison of the age of starting climbing, age when climbing the hardest route, time to achieve the hardest route, body mass, body height, and BMI collectively in the "Elite" and "Higher Elite" groups between lead climbers and boulderers.

Statistical analyses were performed using the IBM SPSS STATISTICS 21 program (IBM Corp., Armonk, NY, USA). The Shapiro–Wilk test and the Kolmogorov–Smirnov test (with the Lilliefors correction) were applied first to verify the normality of the distribution. When the distribution was close to normal, the ANOVA parametric test was used, and when it was non-normal, the non-parametric Kruskal–Wallis test was used. The level of significance was determined at $p < 0.05$.

3. Results

The results of the Shapiro–Wilk normality test in "the age of starting climbing" and "age when climbing the hardest route" in "Elite" and "Higher Elite" lead climbers were close to normal. Thus, the ANOVA parametric test was used. In other cases, the distribution deviated from normality. Therefore, the non-parametric Kruskal–Wallis test ($\times 2$) was used.

3.1. Lead Climbing vs. Boulderers

The comparison of the climbers in the "Elite" groups between the lead climbers and boulderers showed that the lead climbers started to climb at a younger age (14.3 ± 4.7 years vs. 16.3 ± 5.3 years; $p = 0.001$) and had a longer time to achieve the hardest route than boulderers (11.1 ± 4.8 years vs. 8.6 ± 5.1 years; $p = 0.001$) (Tables 1 and 2). The remaining parameters were not statistically significantly different ($p > 0.05$).

Table 1. Characteristics of sport climbers (mean values ± standard deviation).

Group	N	Age (Years)	Age of Starting Climbing (Years)	Body Mass (kg)	Body Height (cm)	BMI (kg/m^2)	IRCRA Scale Result	Time to Achieve the Hardest Route (Years)	Age When Climbing the Hardest Route (Years)
ELC	86	27.5 ± 7.2	14.3 ± 4.7	65.7 ± 9.1	175.5 ± 8.6	21.3 ± 2.3	26.6 ± 0.6	11.1 ± 4.8	25.4 ± 6.4
HELC	78	28.8 ± 8.2	12.5 ± 5.1	63.3 ± 8.4	173.3 ± 6.3	21.0 ± 1.9	29.1 ± 1.0	13.3 ± 5.3	25.8 ± 6.8
EB	114	26.4 ± 6.7	16.3 ± 5.3	66.5 ± 7.5	176.3 ± 7.3	21.3 ± 1.5	26.6 ± 0.6	8.6 ± 5.1	24.9 ± 6.3
HEB	144	27.0 ± 6.2	13.0 ± 4.7	66.8 ± 8.8	176.1 ± 7.6	21.5 ± 2.2	29.4 ± 1.0	12.2 ± 5.4	25.3 ± 5.8
AEC	200	26.9 ± 6.9	15.5 ± 5.1	66.1 ± 8.2	175.9 ± 7.9	21.3 ± 1.9	26.6 ± 0.6	9.7 ± 5.1	25 ± 6
AHEC	222	27.7 ± 7.0	12.8 ± 4.9	65.6 ± 8.8	175.1 ± 7.3	21.3 ± 2.1	29.3 ± 1.0	12.6 ± 5.4	25.4 ± 6.2
ALC	164	28.1 ± 7.7	13.5 ± 5.0	64.5 ± 8.8	174.4 ± 7.6	21.2 ± 2.1	27.8 ± 1.4	12.1 ± 5.2	25.6 ± 6.6
AB	258	26.8 ± 6.4	14.5 ± 5.3	66.7 ± 8.2	176.2 ± 7.5	21.4 ± 1.9	28.1 ± 1.6	10.6 ± 5.5	25.1 ± 6.0

ELC—elite lead climbers; HELC—higher elite lead climbers; EB—elite boulderers; HEB—higher elite boulderers; AEC—all elite climbers; AHEC—all higher elite climbers; ALC—all lead climbers; AB—all boulderers.

Table 2. Comparison between sport climbers' groups.

Subdiscipline	Sport Level	Age of Starting Climbing (p)	Body Mass (p)	Body Height (p)	BMI (p)	Time to Achieve the Hardest Route (p)	Age When Climbing the Hardest Route (p)
LC	E / HE	0.016 * $x^2 = 5.911$	0.013 * $x^2 = 6.127$	0.008 * $x^2 = 7.111$	0.334 $x^2 = 0.934$	0.008 * $x^2 = 7.051$	0.735 $x^2 = 0.115$
B	E / HE	0.001 * $x^2 = 22.752$	0.929 $x^2 = 0.008$	0.722 $x^2 = 0.126$	0.821 $x^2 = 0.051$	0.001 * $x^2 = 33.550$	0.495 $x^2 = 0.466$
LC / B	E	0.001 * $x^2 = 23.074$	0.797 $x^2 = 0.453$	0.877 $x^2 = 0.262$	0.581 $x^2 = 1.082$	0.001 * $x^2 = 35.503$	0.648 $x^2 = 0.869$
LC / B	HE	0.081 $x^2 = 5.026$	0.008 * $x^2 = 7.065$	0.019 * $x^2 = 5.512$	0.170 $x^2 = 3.547$	0.002 * $x^2 = 9.597$	0.532 $x^2 = 0.532$
LC / B	All	0.024 * $x^2 = 5.130$	0.008 * $x^2 = 7.065$	0.019 * $x^2 = 5.512$	0.054 $x^2 = 3.709$	0.002 * $x^2 = 9.597$	0.532 $x^2 = 0.532$

LC—lead climbers; B—boulderers; E—elite climbers; HE—higher elite climbers; *—statistically significant difference.

The comparison of the "Higher Elite" climbers between lead climbers and boulderers showed that the lead climbers had lower body mass (63.3 ± 8.4 kg vs. 66.8 ± 8.8 kg; $p = 0.008$), lower body height (173.3 ± 6.3 cm vs. 176.1 ± 7.6 cm; $p = 0.019$), and a longer time to achieve the hardest route (13.3 ± 5.3 years vs. 12.2 ± 5.4 years; $p = 0.002$) in comparison with boulderers (Tables 1 and 2). The remaining parameters were not significantly different ($p > 0.05$).

The comparison of the collective groups "All Lead Climbers" and "All Boulderers" showed that the lead climbers started climbing at a younger age (13.5 ± 5.0 years vs. 14.5 ± 5.3; $p = 0.024$), had a lower mass (64.5 ± 8.8 kg vs. 66.7 ± 8.2; $p = 0.008$), lower height (174.4 ± 7.6 cm vs. 176.2 ± 7.5 cm; $p = 0.019$), and a longer time to achieve the hardest route (12.1 ± 5.2 years vs. 10.6 ± 5.5 years; $p = 0.002$) in comparison with the boulderers (Tables 1 and 2). BMIs and age at the time of climbing the most difficult route were not significantly different within all groups ($p > 0.05$) (Table 2).

3.2. Elite vs. Higher Elite Sport Climbers

When comparing the "Higher Elite" and "Elite" groups in lead climbing, the "Higher Elite" group started climbing at a younger age (12.5 ± 5.1 years vs. 14.3 ± 4.7 years; $p = 0.016$), had lower mass (63.3 ± 8.4 kg vs. 65.7 ± 9.1 kg; $p = 0.013$), lower height (173.3 ± 6.3 cm vs. 175.5 ± 8.6 cm; $p = 0.008$), and a longer climbing time to achieve the hardest route (13.3 ± 5.3 years vs. 11.1 ± 4.8 years; $p = 0.008$) (Tables 1 and 2).

When comparing the "Higher Elite" and "Elite" groups in bouldering, the "Higher Elite" group started climbing at a younger age (13.0 ± 4.7 years vs. 16.3 ± 5.3 years; $p = 0.001$) and had a longer climbing time to achieve the hardest route (12.2 ± 5.4 years vs. 8.6 ± 5.1 years; $p = 0.001$) (Tables 1 and 2). BMI and age at the time of climbing the most difficult route were not significantly different within all groups ($p > 0.05$) (Table 2).

4. Discussion

Due to the great interest in sports climbing, an increasing number of investigations are trying to prove which physiological and psychological parameters or training factors influence success in sports climbing subdisciplines. Training-modified parameters seem to be most important in shaping the climber's physical form [15]. However, anthropometric data can also influence sports climbing performance [10]. Therefore, the presented study aimed to analyze the relationship between age, climbing experience, anthropometric data, and the best result in sport climbing achieved by male sport climbers in bouldering and lead climbing.

In the presented study, a higher level of climbing performance was associated with starting training at an earlier age in lead climbing and bouldering. According to Myer et al. [16], initiating integrative neuromuscular training early in youth may help increase training abilities in the future and set the stage for even more significant gains in physical fitness during their post-pubertal years. However, the current literature lacks reports on the optimal age to initiate sport climbing training. Despite earlier reports suggesting that the level of sport climbing is mainly made up of variables that can be learned [15], the presented study showed that the lead climbers at the "Higher Elite" level had a lower body mass and lower height than the "Elite" lead climbers. Therefore, height and body mass may be important factors concerning the sport level among lead climbers. The possible mechanism of the influence of body mass on the climbing level in lead climbing may be associated with a longer period of effort during sports climbing. Since gravity is an important factor in climbing activity, lower body mass puts less gravitational force on the climber's body and enables them to exert prolonged efforts on the climbing wall. Thus, lower body mass during a longer time on the climbing wall can affect the slower fatigue of the athlete and result in better sports performance. Moreover, shorter climbers can be at a bit of an advantage in dynamic moves because they are forced to adapt to this issue earlier in their climbing progression. On the other hand, lower body mass may be less important than strength capabilities in the bouldering subdiscipline. Boulderers are often associated with greater muscle mass and, thus, with greater overall body mass. Moreover, boulderers are characterized by higher explosive strength than lead climbers, which also involves muscle and body mass [6–8]. Hence, lower body mass seems to be a more important factor in the lead climbing subdiscipline than in the bouldering subdiscipline, which is also confirmed by the results of this study. Moreover, lower body mass can relate to a lower body fat percentage, which has also been demonstrated in several research studies [13]. Body fat reduction may contribute to muscular and cardio-respiratory endurance as well as to the development of speed and agility, which can be essential for climbing performance [17].

The participants' BMI and age in none of the analyzed combinations reached statistical significance. The age at which the most difficult route was climbed was similar in all groups and was about 25 years. Thus, the age of peak performance in sports climbing is similar to that in other sports disciplines. The studies conducted by Ganse et al. note that the peak performance age is between 25 and 27 years in athletic disciplines [18]. Similar conclusions were reached by Haugen et al. on world-class track-and-field athletes [19]. However, the age of elite competition climbers is lower since they enter world-level competitions at the age of 16. It can be because young elite sport climbers tend to climb in natural rock formations less nowadays and leave that type of climbing for a later age, after a competitive career. In addition, frequent training camps and a large number of climbing competitions, both national and international, do not allow for frequent rock climbing.

Moreover, the average BMI of sport climbers in the presented study was 21.00. This is consistent with the literature review carried out by Saul et al., in which the average BMI was 21.66 (n = 1610). Although Saul et al. indicate that low fat and large forearm volume were important features in successful sports climbing, there was no association between BMI and sports climbing achievements during lead climbing and bouldering [10]. On the other hand, a lower BMI may be a prophylactic factor for climbing injuries. According to Lion et al., a BMI above 21 will predispose to injuries of the flexor tendon pulleys in the fingers [20].

The presented results confirm the assumptions of the studies by Laffaye et al., postulating that success in sport climbing is influenced by both training factors and anthropometric variables [21]. However, the authors emphasize that the training component explained 46% of the total variance, while anthropometric variables explained only 4%. Moreover, the previously indicated studies do not answer the question of which anthropometric features differentiate sport climbers at different levels of advancement. Thus, it suggests the need for long-term observation of sports climbers from an early age to their senior career.

The lead climbers had a longer time to achieve the most challenging route than the boulderers in both "Elite" and "Higher Elite" groups. This may be because lead climbing is a less force-dependent subdiscipline than bouldering. Moreover, the effort in lead climbing is based more on the endurance parameters of the sport climber. Peak endurance performance is maintained until 35 years of age, followed by modest decreases until 50–60 years of age [22]. On the other hand, skeletal muscle power starts declining after the age of 30, which can affect bouldering performance in older athletes [23].

The presented research has several practical applications. Our results provide an innovative insight into the performance analysis of world-class sport-climbing athletes. Previously, no study had analyzed anthropometric and body composition parameters on such a large group of the best sports climbers in the world. It may be helpful for athletes, coaches, and sports clubs to set realistic goals and evaluate their success strategies in sports climbing subdisciplines, especially within lead climbing and bouldering. The comparison between the lead climbers and boulderers showed that the lead climbers started to climb at a younger age and had a longer time to achieve the most challenging route than the boulderers. This may indicate the need for the early specialization of sport climbers in the lead climbing subdiscipline. The observations also provide a starting point for future research to explore the mechanisms underlying maximum climbing performance development, considering anthropometric parameters in sport climbers. Hence, future research observing the development of young sport climbers in terms of specialization in particular subdisciplines should be conducted, considering anthropometric, physiological, and psychological data.

The presented study has several limitations. Firstly, the results obtained are based on data from the www.8a.nu rank website, which consists of self-reported data. The research parameters are limited to the athletes' age, body mass, body height, and sports experience due to the lack of other parameters in the 8a.nu database. More parameters, such as somatotype, total skeletal muscle mass, subcutaneous fat mass, bone mass, cardiopulmonary capacity, and limb size, should also be included in future research. Moreover, the age of starting to climb and the age when climbing the hardest route parameters are difficult to correlate with the actual sports duration of the climbers over the years. Therefore, other methods should be adopted in future studies to measure the actual sports activity duration of athletes. Secondly, the study sample consists only of male athletes. Thus, future research should include the female population. Thirdly, generalizing the findings is limited by a need for more information about performance at sport climbing competitions among the included sport climbers. Therefore, future research should consider rock climbing ascents and competition performance.

5. Conclusions

The lead climbers had a lower body mass, a lower body height, and la onger time to achieve the most challenging route than the boulderers. Body height and body mass are essential to the sports level of "Elite" and "Higher Elite" lead climbers. Therefore, our study suggests that lower body mass and height are more crucial for lead climbing performance than for bouldering. A younger starting age and more extended sporting experience are the critical points in the "Higher Elite" level in both subdisciplines.

Author Contributions: Conceptualization, A.G., G.Z. and M.G.; methodology, A.G., G.Z. and M.G.; formal analysis, G.Z. and M.G.; investigation, A.D., E.S., M.Z.-Ł. and J.Ł.; data curation, A.G., G.Z. and M.G.; writing—original draft preparation, A.G., G.Z. and M.G.; supervision, M.G.; project administration, G.Z., P.G. and M.G.; funding acquisition, M.G. All authors have read and agreed to the published version of the manuscript.

Funding: This research received no external funding.

Institutional Review Board Statement: The analysis was carried out with the consent of the Bioethics Committee of the Medical University of Lublin (approval code KE-0254/93/2020 and approval date 30 April 2020).

Informed Consent Statement: Not applicable.

Data Availability Statement: The data presented in this study are available on request from the corresponding author. The data are not publicly available due to privacy.

Conflicts of Interest: The authors declare no conflicts of interest.

References

1. Woollings, K.Y.; McKay, C.D.; Kang, J.; Meeuwisse, W.H.; Emery, C.A. Incidence, Mechanism and Risk Factors for Injury in Youth Rock Climbers. *Br. J. Sports Med.* **2015**, *49*, 44–50. [CrossRef] [PubMed]
2. Lutter, C.; El-Sheikh, Y.; Schöffl, I.; Schöffl, V. Sport Climbing: Medical Considerations for This New Olympic Discipline. *Br. J. Sports Med.* **2017**, *51*, 2–3. [CrossRef] [PubMed]
3. Fanchini, M.; Violette, F.; Impellizzeri, F.M.; Maffiuletti, N.A. Differences in Climbing-Specific Strength between Boulder and Lead Rock Climbers. *J. Strength Cond. Res.* **2013**, *27*, 310–314. [CrossRef] [PubMed]
4. Zieliński, G.; Pająk-Zielińska, B. Bouldering & Chronic Traumatic Encephalopathy—That Is Repeated Mild Traumatic Brain Injury from Climbing. *Med. Hypotheses* **2024**, *185*, 111317. [CrossRef]
5. Stien, N.; Saeterbakken, A.H.; Hermans, E.; Vereide, V.A.; Olsen, E.; Andersen, V. Comparison of Climbing-Specific Strength and Endurance between Lead and Boulder Climbers. *PLoS ONE* **2019**, *14*, e0222529. [CrossRef] [PubMed]
6. White, D.J.; Olsen, P.D. A Time Motion Analysis of Bouldering Style Competitive Rock Climbing. *J. Strength Cond. Res.* **2010**, *24*, 1356–1360. [CrossRef] [PubMed]
7. Levernier, G.; Laffaye, G. Four Weeks of Finger Grip Training Increases the Rate of Force Development and the Maximal Force in Elite and Top World-Ranking Climbers. *J. Strength Cond. Res.* **2019**, *33*, 2471–2480. [CrossRef]
8. Fryer, S.; Stone, K.J.; Sveen, J.; Dickson, T.; España-Romero, V.; Giles, D.; Baláš, J.; Stoner, L.; Draper, N. Differences in Forearm Strength, Endurance, and Hemodynamic Kinetics between Male Boulderers and Lead Rock Climbers. *Eur. J. Sport. Sci.* **2017**, *17*, 1177–1183. [CrossRef]
9. Ginszt, M.; Michalak-Wojnowska, M.; Gawda, P.; Wojcierowska-Litwin, M.; Korszeń-Pilecka, I.; Kusztelak, M.; Muda, R.; Filip, A.A.; Majcher, P. ACTN3 Genotype in Professional Sport Climbers. *J. Strength Cond. Res.* **2018**, *32*, 1311–1315. [CrossRef]
10. Saul, D.; Steinmetz, G.; Lehmann, W.; Schilling, A.F. Determinants for Success in Climbing: A Systematic Review. *J. Exerc. Sci. Fit.* **2019**, *17*, 91–100. [CrossRef]
11. Fryer, S.; Stoner, L.; Scarrott, C.; Lucero, A.; Witter, T.; Love, R.; Dickson, T.; Draper, N. Forearm Oxygenation and Blood Flow Kinetics during a Sustained Contraction in Multiple Ability Groups of Rock Climbers. *J. Sports Sci.* **2015**, *33*, 518–526. [CrossRef] [PubMed]
12. Levernier, G.; Samozino, P.; Laffaye, G. Force-Velocity-Power Profile in High-Elite Boulder, Lead, and Speed Climber Competitors. *Int. J. Sports Physiol. Perform.* **2020**, *15*, 1012–1018. [CrossRef] [PubMed]
13. Ginszt, M.; Saito, M.; Zięba, E.; Majcher, P.; Kikuchi, N. Body Composition, Anthropometric Parameters, and Strength-Endurance Characteristics of Sport Climbers: A Systematic Review. *J. Strength Cond. Res.* **2023**, *37*, 1339–1348. [CrossRef] [PubMed]

14. Draper, N.; Giles, D.; Schöffl, V.; Konstantin Fuss, F.; Watts, P.; Wolf, P.; Baláš, J.; Espana-Romero, V.; Blunt Gonzalez, G.; Fryer, S.; et al. Comparative Grading Scales, Statistical Analyses, Climber Descriptors and Ability Grouping: International Rock Climbing Research Association Position Statement. *Sports Technol.* **2015**, *8*, 88–94. [CrossRef]
15. Mermier, C.M.; Janot, J.M.; Parker, D.L.; Swan, J.G. Physiological and Anthropometric Determinants of Sport Climbing Performance. *Br. J. Sports Med.* **2000**, *34*, 359–365, discussion 366. [CrossRef] [PubMed]
16. Myer, G.D.; Lloyd, R.S.; Brent, J.L.; Faigenbaum, A.D. How Young Is "Too Young" to Start Training? *ACSMs Health Fit. J.* **2013**, *17*, 14–23. [CrossRef]
17. Espada, M.C.; Ferreira, C.C.; Gamonales, J.M.; Hernández-Beltrán, V.; Massini, D.A.; Macedo, A.G.; Almeida, T.A.F.; Castro, E.A.; Pessôa Filho, D.M. Body Composition Relationship to Performance, Cardiorespiratory Profile, and Tether Force in Youth Trained Swimmers. *Life* **2023**, *13*, 1806. [CrossRef] [PubMed]
18. Ganse, B.; Ganse, U.; Dahl, J.; Degens, H. Linear Decrease in Athletic Performance During the Human Life Span. *Front. Physiol.* **2018**, *9*, 1100. [CrossRef] [PubMed]
19. Haugen, T.A.; Solberg, P.A.; Foster, C.; Morán-Navarro, R.; Breitschädel, F.; Hopkins, W.G. Peak Age and Performance Progression in World-Class Track-and-Field Athletes. *Int. J. Sports Physiol. Perform.* **2018**, *13*, 1122–1129. [CrossRef]
20. Lion, A.; van der Zwaard, B.C.; Remillieux, S.; Perrin, P.P.; Buatois, S. Risk Factors of Hand Climbing-Related Injuries. *Scand. J. Med. Sci. Sports* **2016**, *26*, 739–744. [CrossRef]
21. Laffaye, G.; Levernier, G.; Collin, J.-M. Determinant Factors in Climbing Ability: Influence of Strength, Anthropometry, and Neuromuscular Fatigue. *Scand. J. Med. Sci. Sports* **2016**, *26*, 1151–1159. [CrossRef] [PubMed]
22. Tanaka, H.; Seals, D.R. Endurance Exercise Performance in Masters Athletes: Age-Associated Changes and Underlying Physiological Mechanisms. *J. Physiol.* **2008**, *586*, 55–63. [CrossRef] [PubMed]
23. Gava, P.; Kern, H.; Carraro, U. Age-Associated Power Decline from Running, Jumping, and Throwing Male Masters World Records. *Exp. Aging Res.* **2015**, *41*, 115–135. [CrossRef] [PubMed]

applied sciences

MDPI

Article

The Impact of Cardiorespiratory and Metabolic Parameters on Match Running Performance (MRP) in National-Level Football Players: A Multiple Regression Analysis

Radivoje Radaković [1,2], Borko Katanić [3,*], Mima Stanković [4], Bojan Masanovic [5] and Suzana Žilić Fišer [6]

1 Institute of Information Technologies, University of Kragujevac, 34000 Kragujevac, Serbia; dididisport1@gmail.com
2 Bioengineering Research and Development Center, 34000 Kragujevac, Serbia
3 Montenegrin Sports Academy, 81110 Podgorica, Montenegro
4 Faculty of Sport and Physical Education, University of Niš, 18000 Niš, Serbia; mima.stankovic974@gmail.com
5 Faculty of Sport and Physical Education, University of Montenegro, 81400 Nikšić, Montenegro; bojanma@ucg.ac.me
6 Faculty of Electrical Engineering and Computer Science, Institute of Media Communications, University of Maribor, 2000 Maribor, Slovenia; suzana.zilicfiser@gmail.com
* Correspondence: borkokatanic@gmail.com

Abstract: The aim of the study was to examine the association between cardiorespiratory and metabolic parameters and match running performance (MRP) in highly trained football players. The sample of participants consisted of 41 national-level football players (aged 23.20 ± 3.40 years, body height 182.00 ± 5.15 cm, and body mass 76.86 ± 6.06 kg) from the Serbian Super league. For the purposes of this research, the following measurements were applied. A maximal multistage progressive treadmill test, with a direct measurement of maximal oxygen consumption (VO_2max) (using Fitmate MED, Cosmed, Rome, Italy) was conducted, alongside continuous heart rate monitoring. Capillary blood samples were taken from the hyperemic area using specific test strips, and, after sample collection, lactate concentration was immediately determined using a lactate analyzer. MRP variables were analyzed according to the BioIRC model of motion structure analysis, based on existing standards for profiling movement intensity. The results of multiple regression analysis indicated an association between cardiac parameters and total distance (R2 = 54.3%, p = 0.000), high-speed running (R2 = 46.4%, p = 0.000), and jogging (R2 = 33.6%, p = 0.004). Regression analysis revealed an association between cardiorespiratory parameters and total distance (R2 = 24.8%, p = 0.014), and high-speed running (R2 = 20%, p = 0.039). Meanwhile, no association was found between lactate concentration and running performance. The explanation for these regression analysis results is based on the observation that functional abilities represent significant potential for expressing movement performance, a crucial condition for success in football.

Keywords: physical performance; cardiovascular endurance; lactate concentration; maximal heart rate; professional soccer players; running performance analysis; VO_2max

1. Introduction

In recent years, the demands of modern football have changed, increasing significantly, and this trend certainly continues day after day [1]. Football, as a characteristic intermittent sport, requires players to execute multiple activities that require agility, strength, speed, balance, stability, flexibility, and endurance, implying that the physical conditioning of players is an extremely complex procedure [2]. In terms of training application, modern football and growing demands impose the need for the highest quality professional and scientific approach [3]. In competitive conditions of top-level football play, it is necessary to have high levels of functional abilities to adequately respond to the physical and technical/tactical demands of the game, including the ability to perform a large number of high-intensity movements, delay the onset of fatigue, and mitigate its impact on efficiency in the game [4,5].

Measurements in football show that both the aerobic and anaerobic pathways of metabolism make significant contributions to match performance [6]. During a football game, the aerobic energy system provides approximately 90% of the energy. In this regard, elite football players must have high aerobic endurance fitness to play for 90 min and recover between high-intensity sprints [7]. One of the best measures of cardiorespiratory fitness and endurance capacity performance is the maximal aerobic power, denoted by VO_2max [8]. Generally speaking, maximal oxygen consumption (VO_2max) represents the maximum work rate at which the body can absorb and use oxygen when engaging in maximal exercise. Given the demands of team sports, such as the ability to change direction during high-intensity running, the primary focus for players should be on endurance and metabolic conditioning [9].

Working muscle oxygen deficiency is thought to be a controlling factor in the metabolic alterations that lead to the depletion of muscle glycogen stores and the suppression of glycolytic enzyme activity. This is thought to be one of the main causes of the decline in efficiency and, consequently, the emergence of indicators of muscular tiredness [10]. The VO_2max of elite soccer players is typically between 50 and 75 mL/kg/min, but different values higher than 70 mL/kg/min have been identified [11].

During competitive matches, professional players typically operate at approximately 80–90% of their maximum heart rate, which corresponds to approximately 75–80% of the VO_2max [12]. Increasing VO_2max is believed to enhance players' tactical and technical performance by 7%. Additionally, this implies more efficient ball contacts and a greater number of longer sprints during a game, which increases the likelihood of scoring a goal [13]. It has been confirmed that leading football teams in the league have higher VO_2max values compared to weaker teams [14]. Therefore, the efficiency of the cardiorespiratory system is considered one of the most crucial components of the physical readiness of football players [5].

The match running performance (MRP) of football players has been the focus of researchers in recent years [15,16]. It has been established that, in professional football, players can cover total distances ranging from 9 to 14 km during matches, of which 5–15% are covered by high-intensity running [17]. Two important energy components determine energy expenditure in the game: the way players move and the way they control the ball. The energy expenditure of forward running is lower than that of backward and lateral running [18,19]. A football match's progression is typically associated with a gradual decline in the speed of runs, a fall in the number of sprints, and a shortening of the distance covered at maximum speed, especially in the later part of the game [20]. The culprit of this decrease in speed and in the frequency of sprints has been identified as a sharp decrease in glycogen in the working muscles of the players as the match moves forward. This viewpoint is supported by an increase in the blood lactate of players in the latter stages of matches [21]. More rapid elimination of lactate from the blood as the game progresses is a significant concern because it determines, at least in part, how quickly an athlete will become fatigued [22]. Working muscle oxygen deficiency is thought to be a regulatory factor in the metabolic changes that cause the depletion of muscle glycogen resources and the inhibition of glycolytic enzyme activity. A greater lactate threshold indicates that a player can maintain greater average intensity in a task without lactate accumulation [21].

Anaerobic threshold (AT) and VO_2max measurements are frequently used to assess aerobic fitness. It is important to note that players with higher values of VO_2max during high-intensity activities achieve lower blood lactate concentrations compared to players with lower VO_2max values [23]. The majority of the published studies on the relationship between lactate threshold and endurance have shown a strong correlation, indicating that training-induced improvements in cardiorespiratory endurance are significantly associated with improvements in lactate threshold [24,25]. While outdoor tests can be used to indirectly evaluate both VO_2max and AT, laboratory treadmill testing provides the most reliable measurement [26]. A previous study [26] has analyzed the correlation of cardiorespiratory fitness and team performance, player position, and physical characteristics. The mentioned study shows that cardiorespiratory fitness does not differentiate between age, weight, height, team performance, and player position, but VO_2max varies with age, weight, height, and BMI [26]. The study also found a strong correlation between the physical requirements of player positions throughout a match and the aerobic capacity of players playing those positions, which should be considered in soccer training [13]. In addition, Doncaster et al. [27] reported that measures of ventilatory equivalent, a determinant of running economy, at all sub-maximal exercise intensities were inversely related to the volume and percentage of very-high-intensity activities.

Today, it is known that coaches and sports scientists can tailor training plans based on well-defined physiological parameters such as VO_2max, maximum heart rate, and blood lactate concentration [28]. Although recent studies have revealed an association between cardiorespiratory parameters and running performances, such as high-intensity running [29,30] and total distance covered [31], it should be emphasized that conflicting results have been obtained in the study by Metaxas et al. [32], where no association between VO_2max and MRP was found. Therefore, these findings need to be verified. Regarding the association between lactate and MRP, only one study has shown an association between lactate levels and the total distance covered [33]. However, it is important to note that this study focused on young footballers. Additionally, a commonality among all mentioned studies is the limited number of observed parameters. Furthermore, there is a lack of studies that comprehensively assess the physiological parameters of players in a single sample. Therefore, there is a need for a study that will more thoroughly investigate this area. To the authors' knowledge, this is the first study to report the effect of a wide set of variables, cardiorespiratory and metabolic parameters, on match running performance. More importantly, this study is the only one with a national-level sample of football players in the territory of Serbia. Hence, the purpose of this study was to determine the association between cardiorespiratory and metabolic parameters and running performance in highly trained football players. In this regard, hypotheses have been formulated indicating that (i) there is an association between cardiovascular and running performance; (ii) there is an association between cardiorespiratory parameters and running performance; and (iii) there is an association between metabolic parameters and running performance. This study will contribute to understanding the relationship between cardiorespiratory and metabolic parameters and running performance among highly trained football players in Serbia, and will determine which cardiovascular and metabolic parameters are associated with specific running speeds.

2. Materials and Methods

2.1. Participants

The sample of participants in this cross-sectional study consisted of 41 elite football players (aged 23.20 $\pm$ 3.40 years, with a body height of 182.00 $\pm$ 5.15 cm, and a body mass of 76.86 $\pm$ 6.06 kg; Table 1). All players were members of the Serbian Super League, which is the top-tier national football competition. That is, according to categorization, they are highly trained/national level athletes [34]. The criteria for inclusion in the study were players aged $\geq$ 18 to $\leq$35 years, with a training age of $\geq$6 years, without a recent injury (>12 months) or any illness at that moment. Randomly, 4 teams out of 16 were selected from the league. Then, every other player was chosen through randomization. In the end, we selected 44 players to participate. Out of those, we gathered all the data for 41 players. All participants voluntarily participated and were informed about the purpose, benefits, and risks of the study, and they all provided written consent to participate in the study. Additionally, all data have been anonymized to ensure the confidentiality of the players and teams. Therefore, all procedures conducted in the study involving human participants were in accordance with the Helsinki Declaration and were approved by the

Ethics Committee of the Faculty of Medical Sciences, University of Kragujevac (decision number: 01-15731; date 29 December 2021).

Table 1. Sample description.

	Mean	SD	Min	Max
Age	23.20	3.40	18.00	32.00
Body height (cm)	182.00	5.15	172.00	192.00
Body mass (kg)	76.86	6.06	63.00	88.00

2.2. Procedures

The testing of football players was conducted in March 2022. Laboratory tests were performed in a room where the temperature was 20–23 °C and the air humidity was 55–60% so that the microclimatic conditions corresponded to the recommended ones. All measurements were performed in the morning, at approximately the same time (11 a.m.). On the day of testing, participants did not train in the morning as they needed to be rested, and, afterwards, they resumed their daily obligations. A multistage progressive treadmill test was conducted. After warming up, they performed 3 min of running on a treadmill at a speed of 5 km/h; the speed and incline were determined to increase at precise time intervals. The criteria for stopping the test were the fulfillment of 2 out of 4 conditions: VO_2max plateau reached (2 mL/kg/min); HR max reached; respiratory exchange coefficient (RER) > 1.2; the appearance of subjective complaints. The performance data of players' running performance were collected using performance analysis software during official football matches. It should be emphasized that during the research, the participants did not have a break in training but rather continued with their daily routines.

2.3. Anthropometric Characteristics

Anthropometric assessments were conducted following the guidelines of the International Biological Program [35]. A Tefal 6010 scale (Rumilly, Haute-Savoie, France) was used to measure body mass, and the result was read from the scale's display with an accuracy of 0.1 kg. Body height was measured using an anthropometer (GPM, Zurich, Switzerland), and the measurement result was read with an accuracy of 0.1 cm.

2.4. Cardiorespiratory Parameters

For the purposes of this research, a maximum multistage progressive treadmill test was applied (Technogym Run Exciting 9000, Fairfield, NJ, USA). After positioning the subjects, a mask (Hans Rudolph, Kansas City, MO, USA) was secured with elastic straps to prevent air leakage, and the VO_2max value was directly measured (Cosmed's FitMate Med, Rome, Italy). After securing the mask, a heart rate monitor (Polar Pro Team System, Kempele, Finland) was placed with the strap positioned around the chest, just below the nipples, and fastened. The heart rate monitor was placed directly on bare skin to enable successful measurement with constant heart rate monitoring. Cardiovascular and respiratory parameter values were automatically recorded every 15 s. The subject walked and ran during the test at different intensities and on varying inclines. A standardized stepwise continuous test protocol was employed [36,37].

2.5. Lactate Concentration

To define lactate thresholds, capillary blood lactate levels (measured in mmol/L) were used at the end of each phase of the step-continuing test. Capillary blood samples were obtained from a hyperemic lobe using special test strips. After acquiring a sample, the lactate concentration was determined immediately using a lactate analyzer (Lactate Scout, EKF SensLab, Leipzig, Germany). The sensitivity and accuracy of lactate concentration measurement using the Lactate Scout analyzer (EKF SensLab, Leipzig, Germany) were scientifically validated [38]. Based on the obtained results, the metabolic efficiency index was calculated, which represents the ratio of blood lactate concentration at the 4th and 10th minutes of recovery.

2.6. Match Running Performance (MRP)

For recording matches using the BioIRC Tracking Motion system (BioIRC, Kragujevac, Serbia), two identical Sony NEX-VG10 video cameras (Sony, Tokyo, Japan) were used, both in full-HD resolution, along with one high-speed control camera. The algorithmic part of the video-processing software for tracking the running performance (RP) of players was based on determining the similarity measure of the statistical color distribution of objects [39]. The software for analysis tracked player RP across the entire field, alternately analyzing video footage of each half of the field, depending on the current player's activities. The analysis speed on the computer (with Intel(R) Core2Duo E6750@2.66 GHz, 2 GB RAM, Win7 32-bit; Intel, Santa Clara, CA, USA) was approximately 4 frames per second. Match videos were processed in multiple stages. For video file analysis purposes, the videos were compressed using the XVID codec in MOV format, with a frame rate of 30 frames per second.

2.7. Cardiovascular and Metabolic Variables

The independent variables in this study can be categorized into three groups: cardiac parameters, parameters related to cardiovascular system efficiency, and lactate-related parameters. A total of eight cardiovascular variables were divided into two groups of four each. The first group included heart parameters such as maximum heart rate (HRmax), heart rate at the anaerobic threshold (HR AT), heart rate at the first minute of recovery (HR 1′), and heart rate at the second minute of recovery (HR 2′). The second group consisted of parameters associated with cardiovascular system efficiency, including maximum oxygen uptake (VO_2max), running efficiency (VO_2max/v), and cardiorespiratory efficiency (VO_2max/HR). Lactate metabolism variables comprised lactate at 4 min (LA 4′), lactate at 10 min (LA 10′), metabolic recovery index (Index LA), and metabolic efficiency index (Index ME); Table 2.

Table 2. Cardiovascular and metabolic variables.

No.	Variable	Abbreviation
1.	Maximum heart rate	HRmax
2.	Heart rate at the anaerobic threshold	HR AT
3.	Heart rate at the first minute of recovery	HR 1′
4.	Heart rate at the second minute of recovery	HR 2′
5.	Maximum oxygen uptake	VO_2max
6.	Running efficiency	VO_2max/v
7.	Cardiorespiratory efficiency	VO_2max/HR
8.	Lactate at 4 min	LA 4′
9.	Lactate at 10 min	LA 10′
10.	Metabolic recovery index	Index LA
11.	Metabolic efficiency index	Index ME

2.8. MRP Variables

The determination of MRP variables was conducted according to the BioIRC motion structure analysis model, based on existing standards for profiling movement intensities with respect to basic physical (movement speed) and physiological (physiological and biochemical changes at given speeds) parameters. Based on this model, five categories of movement intensity for players during the match were defined, and a sixth variable representing total player movement was calculated based on the measured variables [40–42].

The dependent variables were MRP variables including sums of movement (in meters) within specific speed ranges: walking (<8 km/h), jogging (8–15 km/h), running (15.1–19 km/h), high-speed running (19.1–23 km/h), sprinting (>23 km/h), and the total distance (total; Table 3).

Table 3. MRP variables.

No.	Variable	Abbreviation
1.	Walking (from 0 to 8 km/h)	<8 km/h
2.	Jogging (from 8 to 15 km/h)	8–15 km/h
3.	Running (from 15.1 to 19 km/h)	15.1–19 km/h
4.	High-speed running (from 19.1 to 23 km/h)	19.1–23 km/h
5.	Sprinting (over 23 km/h)	>23 km/h
6.	Total distance	Total

2.9. *Statistics*

For all data obtained through testing, basic central and distributional parameters were calculated, including the mean, standard deviation, minimum, maximum, and range. To assess the normality of the distribution of results, skewness and kurtosis were used. Pearson's correlation analysis was employed to explore the univariate association between physiological parameters and MRP. The classification of correlation coefficients followed the suggested guidelines: an r value of ≤0.35 denoted a low or weak correlation, an r value ranging from 0.36 to 0.67 indicated a modest or moderate correlation, an r value from 0.68 to 1.0 represented a strong or high correlation, and an r value greater than 0.90 signified a very high correlation [43]. The residual statistics diagram was used to assess the independence of residuals. Multivariate relationships among the predictors and criteria were evaluated using multiple regression analysis. Based on the formula n = 20 + 5k (where k represents the number of predictors), which was proposed by the authors [44] as optimal, considering the principle based on the rate of change in reliability criteria relative to the number of participants, this study calculated that it is optimal to use 4 predictor variables. The coefficients R, R^2, and p were calculated for linear multiple regression. Evaluation of the model was assessed through R2, which indicates the proportion of variance in the dependent variable explained by the model. Meanwhile, the statistical significance of the model was evaluated in the ANOVA test section. The assessment of each independent variable in the model was calculated based on standardized coefficients (Beta) to determine the contribution of each variable to the final equation [45]. Statistical significance was set at $p < 0.05$. Data analysis was performed using IBM SPSS Statistics software, version 26 (Statistical Package for Social Sciences, v26.0, SPSS Inc., Chicago, IL, USA).

3. Results

3.1. *Descriptive Cardio-Respiratory, Metabolic, and Running Performance Parameters*

The results in Table 4 for 41 national-level football players showed that the values of skewness within the normal distribution range from −1 to 1, with kurtosis ranging from −2.75 to 2.75 for all variables, except for the variable Index La.

Table 2 presents descriptive parameters for the top football players, and it was noticeable that the average value of HRmax was 192.90 ± 7.95 bpm, with a significant range, where the minimum value of Hrmax was 174.00, and the maximum was 207.00 bpm. The average value of VO_2max was 61.15 ± 3.89 mL/kg/min, with a noticeable range between the minimum and maximum values (ranging from 53.40 to 69.20 mL/kg/min). Lactate value at 4 min of rest averaged 9.42 ± 1.73 mmol/L. Concerning the total distances covered by the players, they averaged 10,799.79 ± 1143.70 m, with the smallest recorded total distance during the game being 8429.52 m, and the largest reached being 12,602.25 m. The participants covered an average distance of 4522.56 m by walking, as well as 4193.87 m while jogging. When they ran (15.1–19 km/h), they covered a distance of 983.55 m. Then, at higher speeds (high-speed running and sprinting), they covered 611.45 m and 488.38 m, respectively.

Table 4. Cardio-respiratory, metabolic, and match running performance parameters of national-level football players.

	Mean	SD	Min	Max	Range	Skew	Kurt
HRmax (bpm)	192.90	7.95	174.00	207.00	33.00	−0.30	−0.68
HR AT (bpm)	167.20	8.02	152.00	180.00	28.00	−0.07	−0.92
HR 1′ (bpm)	170.05	12.67	140.00	193.00	53.00	−0.48	−0.06
HR 2′ (bpm)	129.44	17.52	103.00	174.00	71.00	0.70	−0.01
VO_2max (ml/kg/min)	61.15	3.89	53.40	69.20	15.80	0.16	−0.27
VO_2max/v ($mL{\cdot}kg{\cdot}min^1/km/h$)	2.93	0.21	2.59	3.38	0.79	0.48	−0.32
VO_2max/HR	0.32	0.02	0.27	0.36	0.09	0.15	−0.60
La 4′ (mmol/L)	9.42	1.73	6.50	14.10	7.60	0.36	−0.25
La 10′ (mmol/L)	6.94	1.37	3.80	11.70	7.90	0.67	2.74
Index LA	39.01	31.77	−2.35	165.79	168.14	1.79	5.01
Index ME	2.29	0.45	1.56	3.33	1.77	0.52	−0.43
<8 km/h (m)	4522.56	450.43	3301.36	5243.99	1942.63	−0.58	0.34
8.1–15 km/h (m)	4193.87	831.19	2580.46	5850.53	3270.07	0.08	−0.57
15.1–19 km/h (m)	983.55	247.63	502.00	1393.53	891.53	−0.22	−1.27
19.1–23 km/h (m)	611.45	154.36	319.33	885.60	566.27	0.22	−0.75
>23 km/h (m)	488.38	144.99	261.26	893.85	632.59	0.76	0.36
Total (m)	10,799.79	1143.70	8429.52	12,602.25	4172.73	−0.11	−0.71

Legend: Mean—arithmetic mean; SD—standard deviation; Min—minimal value; Max—maximal value; Skew—skewness, measure of asymmetry; Kurt—kurtosis, measure of flattening.

3.2. Correlation Analysis

Based on Table 5, it is noticeable that cardiorespiratory parameters moderately correlate with speeds of movement at 8.1–15 km/h, 19.1–23 km/h, and total distance (−0.28–−0.045). Additionally, heart rate correlates with total distance (0.29–0.50) and heart rate at 2 min with speeds of movement of 8.1–15 km/h and 19.1–23 km/h, and the total distance. On the other hand, lactate does not significantly correlate with maximal running speeds in general.

Table 5. Pearson's correlation coefficients between MRP and predictor variables.

	<8 km/h	8.1–15 km/h	15.1–19 km/h	19.1–23 km/h	>23 km/h	Total
HR max	0.27 *	0.18	0.10	0.26	0.01	0.30 *
HR AT	0.09	−0.21	−0.20	−0.16	−0.14	−020
HR 1′	0.25	0.18	0.07	0.23	0.11	0.29 *
HR 2′	−0.16	−0.42 **	−0.22	−0.50 **	−0.10	−0.50 **
VO_2max	0.00	−0.21	−0.17	−0.28 *	−0.04	−0.23
VO_2max/v	−0.22	−0.35 *	−0.13	−0.39 **	−0.18	−0.45 **
VO_2max/HR	−0.16	−0.28 *	−0.20	−0.39 **	−0.05	−0.37 **
LA 4′	0.08	0.21	0.07	0.07	−0.06	0.07
LA 10′	0.16	0.17	0.10	0.10	−0.06	0.20
Index LA	−0.10	0.01	−0.01	−0.01	0.11	−0.09
Index ME	0.01	−0.21	−0.03	−0.03	0.13	0.05

Note ** $p < 0.01$, * $p < 0.05$.

3.3. Residual Statistics

A scatter plot matrix was used to assess the independence of residuals. The scatter plots depict the dispersion of points with respect to the dependent variable across various movement speeds, and that is for HR parameters (Figure 1,), VO_2max parameters (Figure 2), and lactate parameters (Figure 3).

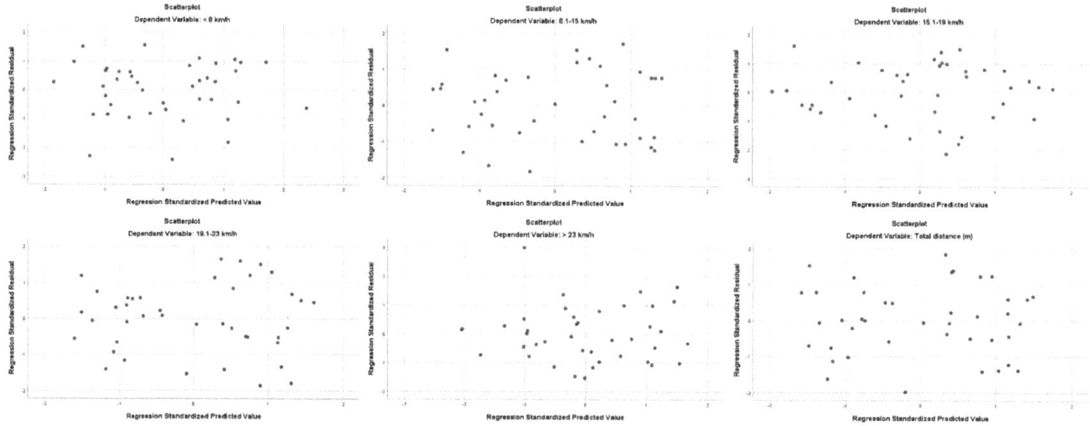

Figure 1. Scatter plot of standardized residuals; HR parameters for dependent MRP variables.

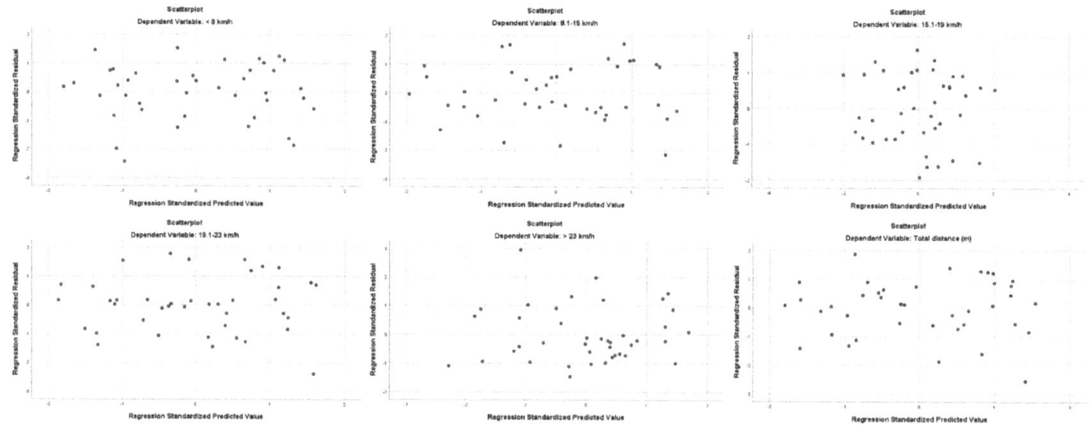

Figure 2. Scatter plot of standardized residuals; VO_2max parameters for dependent MRP variables.

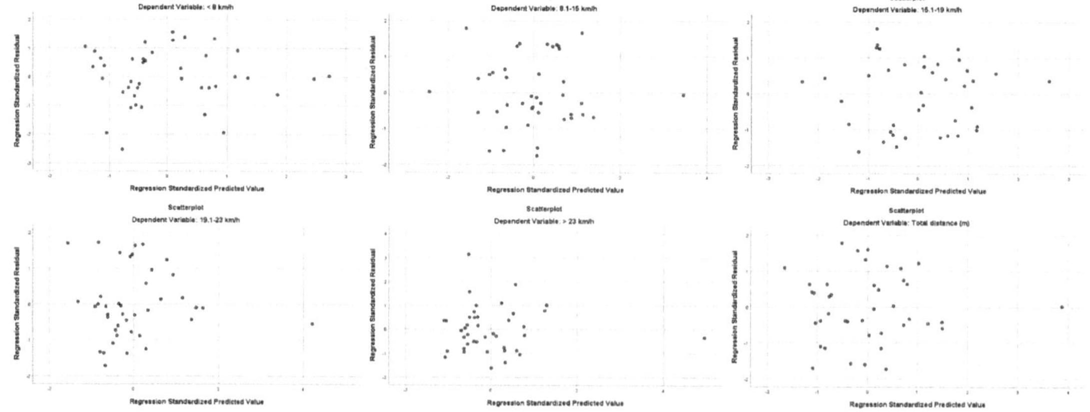

Figure 3. Scatter plot of standardized residuals; lactate parameters for dependent MRP variables.

3.4. Multiple Regression Analysis

The multiple regression results indicate that a model with four independent cardiovascular parameter variables explains a total of 54.3% of the variance in the dependent variable "total distance" (Table 6) at a significant level (p = 0.000). Based on the beta coefficients, the variables that contribute the most to the model are HRmax (0.573), HR 2′ (−0.528), and HR AT (−0.360). When considering different player movement speeds, it should be noted that cardiovascular parameters explain a total of 46.4% of the variance in the dependent variable "high-speed running" at a significant level (p = 0.000). Based on the beta coefficients, the variables that contribute the most to the model are HR 2′ (−0.551) and HRmax (0.526). Additionally, cardiovascular parameters explain a total of 33.6% of the variance in the dependent variable "jogging" at a significant level (p = 0.004), and the variable that contributes the most to the model is HR 2′ (−0.420). There were no significant models for the remaining dependent variables (walking, running, and sprinting).

Table 6. The result of multiple regression for cardiorespiratory and metabolic parameter effects on the match running performance parameters.

	<8 km/h	8.1–15 km/h	15.1–19 km/h	19.1–23 km/h	>23 km/h	Total
HR max	0.258	0.429	0.478	0.526 *	−0.114	0.573 *
HR AT	0.011	−0.311	−0.383	−0.250	−0.168	−0.360 *
HR 1′	0.111	0.087	−0.112	0.059	0.298	0.128
HR 2′	−274	−0.420 *	−0.146	−0.551 *	−0.064	−0.528 *
R	0.379	0.580	0.390	0.681	0.251	0.737
R^2	0.144	0.336	0.152	0.464	0.063	0.543
p	0.219	0.004	0.191	0.000	0.661	0.000
VO_2max	0.472	0.162	0.005	0.197	0.085	0.342
VO_2max/v	−0.272	−0.313	−0.005	−0.262	−0.248	−0.403 *
VO_2max/HR	−0.374	−0.217	−0.204	−0.391	0.034	−0.398
R	0.344	0.371	0.203	0.447	0.196	0.498
R^2	0.118	0.138	0.041	0.200	0.038	0.248
p	0.194	0.135	0.664	0.039	0.690	0.014
LA 4′	−0.500	0.793	0.367	−0.050	−0.869	0.342
LA 10′	1.216	−0.149	−0.178	0.361	1.210	0.534
Index LA	1.072	−0.329	−0.279	0.278	1.300	0.325
Index ME	0.684	0.545	−0.055	0.186	0.360	0.725
R	0.468	0.272	0.240	0.156	0.415	0.368
R^2	0.219	0.074	0.058	0.024	0.173	0.135
p	0.058	0.583	0.699	0.922	0.136	0.250

Legend: R—multiple correlation; R^2—coefficient of determination; p—statistical significance; * denotes statistical significance of $p < 0.05$.

Regression analysis also revealed that a model with four independent derived cardiorespiratory parameters explains a total of 24.8% of the variance in the dependent variable "total distance" at a significant level (p = 0.014). Based on the beta coefficients, the variable that contributes the most to the model is VO_2max/v (−0.403). It was also found that the derived cardiorespiratory parameters explain a total of 20% of the variance in the dependent variable "high-speed running" at a significant level (p = 0.039). All other models were non-significant.

Regarding lactate levels, the model was not significant for any of the dependent variables.

4. Discussion

The aim of this study was to examine the association between cardiorespiratory and metabolic parameters and match running performance (MRP) in national-level football players. Based on multiple regression analysis, the key findings were as follows: (i) cardiac parameters HRmax, HR 2′, and HR AT are associated with total running distance, with HR 2′ and HRmax also being associated with high-speed running, while HR 2′ is associated with jogging; (ii) respiratory parameter VO_2max/v is associated with total running distance; and (iii) lactate parameters are not associated with movement performance.

Upon examining cardiac parameters, it was noted that the average HRmax values among footballers in the top level of competition in Serbia were 192.90 ± 7.95 bpm, which is consistent with findings from other studies, such as 195 bpm in Greece [46], 193 bpm in Greece [47], 192.9 bpm in Belgium [48], 191.3 bpm in Croatia [49], and an HRmax of 188 bpm in Greece [50]. The average values of heart rate at the anaerobic threshold (HR AT) were 167.20 ± 8.02 bpm, which closely corresponds to the values of 169 bpm for Greek footballers [46], but they are slightly lower than the values estimated for Belgium (178.2 bpm) [48] and, especially, for Croatian footballers (182.96 bpm) [49]. However, these differences may be due to different assessment methodologies.

Our resting heart rate (RHR) values, specifically HR 1′ and HR 2′, are 170.05 and 129.44, respectively, with HR 1 representing 88% of HRmax, which aligns with the results for Champions League footballers (91% of HRmax) [51] and Scottish players (90% of HRmax) [52]. The other RHR parameter (HR 2′) is 67% of HRmax; however, it is not possible to compare this data with recent studies as there are no studies that have examined this parameter.

The average values of VO_2max are 61.15 ± 3.89 mL/kg/min, which are slightly lower than the values achieved by footballers from Spain (65.5 mL/kg/min) [53] and approximately align with professional soccer players from other countries such as Norway (63.7 mL/kg/min), England (61.6 mL/kg/min), [54], the United Kingdom (59.4 mL/kg/min) [55], the Czech Republic (59.2 mL/kg/min) [56], and slightly higher values compared to footballers from Greece (58.8 mL/kg/min) [47], Belgium (58.0 mL/kg/min) [48], Croatia (57.63 mL/kg/min) [49], and Cyprus (57.35 mL/kg/min) [57]. It is noteworthy that these values are consistent with the observation that professional soccer players' VO_2max can vary from 55 to 65 mL/kg/min [58,59]. However, it should be noted that these values can vary based on playing position, the playing style of individuals, and the team. Additionally, some authors [60,61] suggest that the VO_2max of elite players should be above 60 mL/kg/min to cope with the demands of modern football, which corresponds to the values achieved by Serbian football players in this study. Other cardiorespiratory parameters were not analyzed in other studies, making them difficult to compare.

One significant finding of this research is that heart parameters, such as HRmax, HR 2′, and HR AT, are associated with the total distance covered during a match. This relationship between heart parameters and total distance has a high degree of correlation (R2 = 54.3%), indicating that cardiac function is crucial for the endurance of football players. Unlike HRmax and HR AT, where a positive correlation was achieved, HR 2′ showed a negative correlation, meaning that a lower heart rate during recovery is associated with a greater overall distance covered. This result may suggest that the speed of recovery after intensive effort is important for the efficiency of football players during matches. In other words, players with better results in these parameters possess a higher level of physical preparedness, enabling them to efficiently execute a greater number of high-intensity movements during the game and eliminate fatigue in shorter time intervals, preparing them for subsequent exertions.

Furthermore, the research indicates that respiratory parameters, such as VO_2max/v, influence the overall distance covered. This emphasizes the importance of optimal respiratory efficiency for achieving better sports results. Concerning high-intensity running, the relationship between heart parameters and fast running has also been confirmed. HR 2′ and HRmax made the most significant contribution to the model, highlighting the role of these two variables in achieving high speeds during matches.

Recent studies have revealed a connection between cardiorespiratory parameters and MRP in football. Studies have shown that average VO_2max values are moderately correlated with the total distance covered [29] and high-intensity running in footballers [30,31]. However, conflicting results were found in a study by Metaxas et al. [32], who did not find a connection between VO_2max and MRP. In our study, although there was no direct link established between VO_2max and MRP, a moderate connection was achieved between the VO_2max model and MRP, with the greatest contribution coming from the VO_2max/v parameter. This suggests that VO_2max and HR should be further examined as they are linearly interconnected [62].

These results highlight the importance of the development of the cardiovascular and respiratory systems in professional footballers. The efficiency of the aerobic energy system, which provides about 90% of the energy during a football match, is crucial for achieving better cardiorespiratory endurance [7]. Adaptive changes, such as an increase in the dimensions of the left ventricle and improved circulation, contribute to an increase in the capacity of oxidative metabolism and overall cardiorespiratory endurance [63]. Therefore, footballers with a more efficient aerobic system can maintain a higher intensity before the onset of fatigue [64,65].

The aerobic and anaerobic system both significantly contribute to match performance [6]. The aerobic energy system plays a crucial role in recovery between high-intensity sprints [7]; however, key moments in football games occur during high-intensity activities that need to be repeated many times [4,66]. Our findings have highlighted the association between cardiorespiratory parameters and high-intensity running, as well as the total distance covered. It is clear that during high-intensity running, functional capacities must be at a higher level to ensure an adequate oxygen supply. On the other hand, football players exhibit developed capacities precisely in these areas, as they perform a large number of intense actions during a match, indicating a high rate of anaerobic energy exchange during a game. There is significant utilization of creatine phosphate, along with the accumulation of lactate [67]. In this regard, for monitoring the physiological response, in addition to heart rate frequencies and VO2, an essential parameter is the concentration of lactate in the blood [68].

When it comes to assessing lactate levels during a football match, post-game lactate levels were mostly evaluated, with lactate max values of 11.0 mmol/L in Belgium [40], 11.2 mmol/L [69], and 11.7 mmol/L [41]. These findings indicate that the rate of lactate production in muscles is high during aa game. It is considered that a fairly high concentration of lactate during a football match [70,71] represents an accumulated/balanced response to a series of high-intensity activities. These values approximately correspond to the load that football players achieved during the multistage treadmill test. Blood lactate concentration after four minutes (LA 4′) was 9.42 ± 1.73 mmol/L, while after 10 min of recovery, lactate levels dropped to 6.94 ± 1.37 mmol/L. Additionally, Index LA and Index ME were assessed, but these parameters are underutilized in recent research.

In our study, we did not find a connection between lactate parameters and movement performance. However, the authors in [72] reported that modifying the testing protocol with progressive stages and lactate analysis procedures can affect physiological parameters. So, instead of laboratory testing, a suggestion for future research would be to measure lactate concentration during effort in a football match and see if it is associated with movement performance. Also, from a methodological standpoint, there are differences in lactate concentration depending on the sampling site, and the most accurate approach would be to take a blood sample from the working muscles [73]. Authors also emphasize that the level of blood lactate concentration can be influenced by reduced glycogen reserves in skeletal muscle cells, a diet with low carbohydrate intake, or previous exhausting physical activities [74], as well as factors such as the type of muscle fibers, the activity of glycolytic and lipolytic enzymes, and the density of capillaries and mitochondria [75]. Therefore, it is clear that there are various reasons as to why lactates have not shown an association with MRP.

When it comes to MRP, it should be noted that the achieved average total distance (10,799.79 m) and distance covered at higher speeds by highly trained Serbian players are somewhat higher than those of better-ranked Croatian football players [76,77]. These values correspond to general elite footballer benchmarks, ranging between 9 and 13 km during matches, with around 5–15% of that distance covered at high running speeds [41,78,79]. It is well known that distance covered at high intensities is traditionally recognized as a key indicator of physical performance in football [15] because key match activities in football may be influenced by higher running performance, especially at higher speeds [80,81]. Thus, in this study, a connection is demonstrated between total distance and high-intensity running and cardiorespiratory endurance.

The explanation of these results is based on the observation that the cardiorespiratory endurance of footballers is a crucial factor for success in football matches. From a physiological perspective, better cardiorespiratory endurance in footballers is directly linked to the development of the cardiovascular and respiratory systems' ability to maintain oxygen delivery to actively engaged muscles during prolonged physical activity, as well as the muscles' ability to obtain the necessary energy through aerobic processes [82,83]. Accordingly, footballers who have shown better results in HR and VO2 parameters, as measures of cardiorespiratory system functioning, achieved greater distances in high-intensity activities and in the overall distance covered. The physiological explanation implies that footballers with greater cardiorespiratory system capacities are able to maintain lower heart rate values at the same running speed, as indicators of system load. In other words, even at the same running speed, the physiological load on the body varies. Our study has shown, through parameters such as HR max and HR AT, that players who achieved higher values of maximum heart rate, as well as lower values of heart rate at the anaerobic threshold, covered a greater total distance and had greater distances in high-intensity activities (above 19 km/h). On the other hand, the HR 2′ parameter indicates that footballers with lower heart rate parameters during recovery have cardiovascular system capacities to recover faster from intensive activities, which is very important as football involves alternating periods of work and rest.

It is recognized that high-intensity running is of great importance for performance in elite football [84,85], as numerous studies have shown that this parameter is discriminative between players at higher versus lower levels of competition [86,87]. High-intensity periods during football matches impose high demands on footballers' bodies, leading to the increased involvement of the anaerobic energy system, with the accumulation of lactic acid and decreased pH values in exercising muscles [71]. The cumulative effects of numerous high-intensity stimuli lead to higher concentrations of lactic acid in the blood of footballers [88]. Therefore, good aerobic fitness of players is important, as it enables better plasma flow through the system, requiring faster removal of harmful metabolic by-products [89] and thus accelerating recovery between intermittent stimuli, while good anaerobic capacity compensates for the high intensities required during play [73].

In our study, a relationship between lactate and MRP was lacking, suggesting that the methodology for assessing lactate and movement performance should be reconsidered. Specifically, from a methodological standpoint, the site of blood sampling for lactate concentration measurement and the laboratory methods used can also influence test results. The authors in [90] suggest that the most accurate approach would be to take blood samples from working muscles, which is not the case in our study. Regarding movement performance, it is noted that other factors related to the complexity of football matches can influence the achieved result. Primarily, these include the playing formation [4], opponent [90], ball possession [91], and the technical level of the footballers [92]. This indicates that some players with high physical capacities do not cover great distances due to the tactical limitations of their role in the team.

This study represents a significant contribution to understanding the impact of cardiorespiratory and metabolic parameters on the MRP of professional football players. One of the key strengths of this research is that the findings have determined which cardiovascular, respiratory, and metabolic parameters are most strongly associated with various running speeds of football players. This constitutes a major contribution to this field, as based on the analysis of previous research, it is noticeable that there is no study that has comprehensively tracked the relationship between physiological and metabolic parameters at different movement speeds. Additionally, it is important to note that this is the first study to gather valuable information about national-level football players in Serbia.

The study's limitation lies in the relatively small sample size of participants; however, one of the restricting circumstances is the challenge of recruiting a sample of national-level football players and subjecting them to detailed analyses. Furthermore, another limitation pertains to the fact that the observed football players in the overall sample were aged between 18 and 32 years, despite the physiological differences between an 18-year-old and a 32-year-old. A suggestion for future research would be to examine lactate levels in competitive conditions and analyze the given parameters based on playing positions, ideally with a large sample size of participants.

Practical Application

Recording the current physiological demands of world-class male football players holds scientific value and direct practical applications, as it is a rare occurrence due to limited access to such subjects. The practical significance of this observation lies in the realization that training these abilities should be developed to the highest possible level.

Furthermore, the direct practical application of this research is that this knowledge can assist coaches in making evidence-based decisions by providing new normative physiological data that can be used for player selection and profiling. Ultimately, these data can be valuable for coaches and fitness trainers in national-level teams to highlight the requirements of higher-level competitions and to design training sessions, which can aid players in transitioning to an elite competition.

5. Conclusions

The purpose of this study was to determine the association between cardiorespiratory and metabolic parameters and running performance in highly trained football players. Based on multiple regression analysis, the key findings were as follows: (i) cardiac parameters HRmax, HR 2′, and HR AT are associated with total running distance, with HR 2′ and HRmax also being associated with high-speed running, while HR 2′ is associated with jogging; (ii) respiratory parameter VO_2max/v is associated with total running distance; and (iii) lactate parameters are not associated with movement performance. Based on this, it can be concluded that the first two hypotheses are partially accepted, while the third hypothesis is rejected.

A detailed analysis of regression results for functional variables emphasizes the significance of heart rate at all levels, particularly at critical points (HR max, HR AT), recovery heart rate (HR 2) as an indicator of intensity and player fatigue, and the efficiency of the respiratory system (VO_2max/v) as an integral factor of functional performance. The explanation for these regression analysis results is based on the observation that functional abilities represent a significant quality/potential for expressing movement performance, a crucial condition for success in football.

This research has contributed to understanding the relationship between cardiorespiratory and metabolic parameters and running performance among highly trained football players in Serbia, and it meticulously determined which cardiovascular and metabolic parameters are associated with different running speeds. Therefore, this study, as one of the few that extensively examine the cardiorespiratory and metabolic domains and their relationship with various movement performances, has contributed to this field by elucidating which physiological parameters should be emphasized in the conditioning of football players.

Author Contributions: Conceptualization, R.R. and B.K.; methodology, R.R. and B.K.; software, M.S.; validation, M.S.; formal analysis, S.Ž.F.; investigation, B.K.; resources, B.M.; data curation, M.S. and S.Ž.F.; writing—original draft preparation, R.R., B.K. and M.S.; writing—review and editing, B.K., M.S. and B.M.; visualization, S.Ž.F.; supervision, B.K. and B.M.; project administration, R.R., S.Ž.F. and B.M. All authors have read and agreed to the published version of the manuscript.

Funding: This research received no external funding.

Institutional Review Board Statement: All procedures conducted in this study were in accordance with the Helsinki Declaration and approved by the Ethics Committee of the Faculty of Medical Sciences, University of Kragujevac (decision number: 01-15731; date: 29 December 2021).

Informed Consent Statement: Informed consent was obtained from all subjects involved in the study.

Data Availability Statement: Data are contained within the article.

Conflicts of Interest: The authors declare no conflicts of interest.

References

1. Andrašić, S.; Gušić, M.; Stanković, M.; Mačak, D.; Bradić, A.; Sporiš, G.; Trajković, N. Speed, change of direction speed and reactive agility in adolescent soccer players: Age related differences. *Int. J. Environ. Res. Public Health* **2021**, *18*, 5883. [CrossRef] [PubMed]
2. Čaprić, I.; Stanković, M.; Manić, M.; Preljević, A.; Špirtović, O.; Đorđević, D.; Spehnjak, M.; Damjan, B.; Sporiš, G.; Trajković, N Effects of plyometric training on agility in male soccer players—A systematic review. *J. Men's Health* **2022**, *18*, 147.
3. Stanković, M.; Đorđević, D.; Andrašić, S.; Tomac, Z.; Vlahović, T.; Franić, M.; Trajković, N. Gym Versus Home-Based Training During Transition Period in Adolescent Soccer Players: Effects on Physical Performance. *J. Men's Health* **2022**, *18*, 134.
4. Rampinini, E.; Coutts, A.J.; Sastagna, C. Variation in Top Level Soccer Match Performance. *J. Sports Med.* **2007**, *28*, 1018–1024 [CrossRef] [PubMed]
5. Gunglielmo, L.G. Vallidity of carminatti's test of determine physiological indices of aerobic power and capacity in soccer and futsal players. *J. Strength Cond. Res.* **2011**, *25*, 3099–3106.
6. Béres, B.; Györe, I.; Petridis, L.; Utczás, K.; Kalabiska, I.; Pálinkás, G.; Szabó, T. Relationship between biological age, body dimensions and cardiorespiratory performance in young soccer players. *Acta Gymnica* **2021**, *51*, e2021. [CrossRef]
7. Tomlin, D.L.; Wenger, H.A. The relationship between aerobic fitness and recovery from high intensity intermittent exercise. *Sports Med.* **2001**, *31*, 1–11. [CrossRef] [PubMed]
8. Higino, W.P.; de Souza Sorroche, A.; de Mattos Falqueiro, P.G.; Lima, Y.C.S.; Higa, C.L. Determination of aerobic performance in youth soccer players: Effect of direct and indirect methods. *J. Hum. Kinet.* **2017**, *56*, 109–118. [CrossRef]
9. Stankovic, M.; Djordjevic, D.; Trajkovic, N.; Milanovic, Z. Effects of High-Intensity Interval Training (HIIT) on Physical Performance in Female Team Sports: A Systematic Review. *Sports Med.-Open* **2023**, *9*, 78. [CrossRef]
10. Gabrys, T.; Stanula, A.; Szmatlan-Gabrys, U.; Garnys, M.; Charvát, L.; Gupta, S. Metabolic and cardiorespiratory responses of semiprofessional football players in repeated Ajax shuttle tests and curved sprint tests, and their relationship with football match play. *Int. J. Environ. Res. Public Health* **2020**, *17*, 7745. [CrossRef]
11. Wells, C.M.; Edwards, A.M.; Winter, E.M.; Fysh, M.L.; Drust, B. Sport-specific fitness testing differentiates professional from amateur soccer players where VO2max and VO2 kinetics do not. *J. Sports Med. Phys. Fitness* **2012**, *52*, 245. [PubMed]
12. Åstrand, P.O.; Rodahl, K. *Textbook of Work Physiology. Physiological Bases of Exercise*, 4th ed.; Human Kinetics: Champaign, IL, USA, 2003.
13. Angoorani, H.; Basharkhah, A.; Mazaherinezhad, A.; Nazari, A. Evaluation of Cardiorespiratory Fitness and Its Correlation with Team Performance, Player Position and Physical Characteristics in the Soccer Premium League of Iran. *Asian J. Sports Med.* **2021**, *12*, e109724. [CrossRef]
14. Redkva, P.E.; Paes, M.R.; Fernandez, R.; da-Silva, S.G. Correlation between match performance and field tests in professional soccer players. *J. Hum. Kinet.* **2018**, *62*, 213. [CrossRef] [PubMed]
15. Mohr, M.; Krustrup, P.; Bangsbo, J. Match performance of high-standard soccer players with special reference to development of fatigue. *J. Sports Sci.* **2003**, *21*, 519–528. [CrossRef] [PubMed]
16. Paul, D.J.; Bradley, P.S.; Nassis, G.P. Factors affecting match running performance of elite soccer players: Shedding some light on the complexity. *Int. J. Sports Physiol. Perform.* **2015**, *10*, 516–519. [CrossRef] [PubMed]
17. Modric, T.; Versic, S.; Morgans, R.; Sekulic, D. Match running performance characterizing the most elite soccer match-play. *Biol. Sport* **2023**, *40*, 949–958. [CrossRef] [PubMed]
18. Stølen, T.; Chamari, K.; Castagna, C.; Wisløff, U. Physiology of soccer: An update. *Sports Med.* **2005**, *35*, 501–536. [CrossRef] [PubMed]
19. Russell, M.; Sparkes, W.; Northeast, J.; Cook, C.J.; Love, T.D.; Bracken, R.M.; Kilduff, L.P. Changes in acceleration and deceleration capacity throughout professional soccer match-play. *J. Strength Cond. Res.* **2016**, *30*, 2839–2844. [CrossRef] [PubMed]
20. Lattier, G.; Millet, G.Y.; Martin, A.; Martin, V. Fatigue and recovery after high-intensity exercise Part II: Recovery interventions. *Int. J. Sports Med.* **2004**, *25*, 509–515. [CrossRef]
21. Stanula, A.; Gabrys, T.; Szmatlan-Gabrys, U.; Roczniok, R.; Maszczyk, A.; Pietraszewski, P. Calculating lactate anaerobic thresholds in sports involving different endurance preparation. *J. Exerc. Sci. Fitness* **2013**, *11*, 12–18. [CrossRef]
22. Tønnessen, E.; Hem, E.; Leirstein, S.; Haugen, T.; Seiler, S. Maximal aerobic power characteristics of male professional soccer players, 1989–2012. *Int. J. Sports Physiol. Perform.* **2013**, *8*, 323–329. [CrossRef] [PubMed]
23. Ostojić, S. *Fiziologija Fudbala (Physiology of Football)*; Data Status: Belgrade, Serbia, 2015.

24. Draper, N.; Brent, S.; Hale, B. The influence of sampling site and assay method on lactate concentration in response to rock climbing. *Eur. J. Appl. Physiol.* **2006**, *98*, 363–372. [CrossRef] [PubMed]
25. Noakes, T.D. The central governor model of exercise regulation applied to the marathon. *Sports Med.* **2007**, *37*, 374–377. [CrossRef] [PubMed]
26. Modric, T.; Versic, S.; Sekulic, D. Aerobic fitness and game performance indicators in professional football players; playing position specifics and associations. *Heliyon* **2020**, *6*, e05427. [CrossRef] [PubMed]
27. Doncaster, G.; Iga, J.; Unnithan, V. Influence of Cardio-Respiratory Fitness on Physical Performance in Elite Youth Soccer. *J. Phys. Fit. Med. Treat. Sports* **2018**, *4*, 1–8. [CrossRef]
28. Helgerud, J.; Engen, L.C.; Wisløff, U.; Hoff, J.A.N. Aerobic endurance training improves soccer performance. *Med. Sci. Sports Exerc.* **2001**, *33*, 1925–1931. [CrossRef] [PubMed]
29. Bangsbo, J.; Lindquist, F. Comparison of various exercise tests with endurance performance during soccer in professional players. *Int. J. Sports Med.* **1992**, *13*, 125–132. [CrossRef]
30. Krustrup, P.; Mohr, M.; Ellingsgaard, H.; Bangsbo, J. Physical demands during an elite female soccer game: Importance of training status. *Med. Sci. Sports Exerc.* **2005**, *37*, 1242–1248. [CrossRef] [PubMed]
31. Abt, G.; Lovell, R.I.C. The use of individualized speed and intensity thresholds for determining the distance run at high-intensity in professional soccer. *J. Sports Sci.* **2009**, *27*, 893–898. [CrossRef]
32. Metaxas, T.; Sendelides, T.; Koutlianos, N.; Mandroukas, K. Seasonal variation of aerobic performance in soccer players according to positional role. *J. Sports Med. Phys. Fitness* **2006**, *46*, 520.
33. Aslan, A.; Acikada, C.; Güvenç, A.; Gören, H.; Hazir, T.; Özkara, A. Metabolic demands of match performance in young soccer players. *J. Sports Sci. Med.* **2012**, *11*, 170. [PubMed]
34. McKay, A.K.; Stellingwerff, T.; Smith, E.S.; Martin, D.T.; Mujika, I.; Goosey-Tolfrey, V.L.; Sheppard, J.; Burke, L.M. Defining training and performance caliber: A participant classification framework. *Int. J. Sports Physiol. Perform.* **2021**, *17*, 317–331. [CrossRef] [PubMed]
35. Eston, R.G.; Reilly, T. *Kinanthropometry and Exercise Physiology Laboratory Manual: Exercise Physiology*; Taylor & Francis: London, UK, 2009; Volume 2.
36. Todorov, I. *Efekti Specifičnog Treninga na Kardiorespiratornu Izdržljivost i Kontraktilni Potencijal Mišića Džudista [Effects of Specific Training on Cardiorespiratory Endurance and Muscle Contractile Potential of Judoka]*; University of Nis: Nis, Serbia, 2014.
37. Kolić, L. Utjecaj Protokola Testa Hodanja s Progresivnim Opterećenjem na Pokretnom Sagu na Pokazatelje Energetskih Kapaciteta [The Influence of the Walking Test Protocol with Progressive Load on a Moving Carpet on Indicators of Energy Capacities. Ph.D Thesis, University of Zagreb, Faculty of Kinesiology, Zagreb, Croatia, 2020.
38. Von Duvillard, S.P.; Pokan, R.; Hofmann, P.; Wonisch, M.; Smekal, G.; Alkhatib, A.; Leithauser, R. Comparing blood lactate values of three different handheld lactate analyzers to YSI 1500 lactate analyzer. *Med. Sci. Sports Exerc.* **2005**, *37*, S25.
39. Vulović, R.; Radaković, R.; Peulić, A.; Nikolić, D.; Filipović, N. Method for software tracking and analysis of players motion during a football match. In *Abstract Book of: International Conference*; FSFV: Belgrade, Serbia, 2012; pp. 314–323.
40. Lago-Peñas, C.; Rey, E.; Lago-Ballesteros, J.; Casais, L.; Dominguez, E. Analysis of work-rate in soccer according to playing positions. *Int. J. Perform. Anal. Sport* **2009**, *9*, 218–227. [CrossRef]
41. Di Salvo, V.; Gregson, W.; Atkinson, G.; Tordoff, P.; Drust, B. Analysis of high intensity activity in Premier League soccer. *Int. J. Sports Med.* **2009**, *30*, 205–212. [CrossRef] [PubMed]
42. Radaković, R.; Dopsaj Vulović, R.; Leontijević, B.; Filipović, N. Reliability of motion analysis of elite football players during the match measured by the Tracking Motion software system. In *Abstract Book of: Internacional Conference Bioinformatics and Bioingeenering*; BIBE: Belgrade, Serbia, 2016.
43. Taylor, R. Interpretation of the correlation coefficient: A basic review. *J. Diagn. Med. Sonogr.* **1990**, *6*, 35–39. [CrossRef]
44. Khamis, H.J.; Kepler, M. Sample size in multiple regression: 20+ 5k. *J. Appl. Stat. Sci.* **2010**, *17*, 505.
45. Pallant, J. *Survival Manual. A Step by Step Guide to Data Analysis Using SPSS*; Allen & Unwin: Berkshire, UK, 2011.
46. Mourtziapis, A.; Alexopoulos, P.; Kaprinis, S.; Dedes, V.; Panoutsopoulos, G.; Kipreos, G. Physiological profile of Greek elite soccer players. *Int. J. Phys. Educ. Sports Health* **2020**, *7*, 201–207.
47. Metaxas, T.I. Match running performance of elite soccer players: VO2max and players position influences. *J. Strength Cond. Res.* **2021**, *35*, 162–168. [CrossRef]
48. Colosio, A.L.; Lievens, M.; Pogliaghi, S.; Bourgois, J.G.; Boone, J. Heart rate-index estimates aerobic metabolism in professional soccer players. *J. Sci. Med. Sport* **2020**, *23*, 1208–1214. [CrossRef]
49. Modric, T.; Versic, S.; Sekulic, D. Does aerobic performance define match running performance among professional soccer players? A position-specific analysis. *Res. Sports Med.* **2021**, *29*, 336–348.
50. Rousopoulos, E.; Cooke, C.; Paradisis, G.; Zacharogiannis, E.; Kouyoufa, E.P.; Till, K. The Physiological Profile of Male Professional Soccer Players: The Effect of Playing Division. *J. Biomed. Res. Environ. Sci.* **2021**, *2*, 1078–1084. [CrossRef]
51. Sassi, R.; Reilly, T.; Impellizzeri, F. A comparison of small-side games and interval training in elite professional soccer players. In *Science and Football V*; Reilly, T., Cabri, J., Araújo, D., Eds.; Routledge: Oxford, UK, 2005; pp. 352–354.
52. Owen, A.L.; Wong, D.P.; McKenna, M.; Dellal, A. Heart rate responses and technical comparison between small-vs. large-sided games in elite professional soccer. *J. Strength Cond. Res.* **2011**, *25*, 2104–2110. [CrossRef] [PubMed]

53. Casajús, J.A. Seasonal variation in fitness variables in professional soccer players. *J. Sports Med. Phys. Fitness* **2001**, *41*, 463–469. [PubMed]
54. Clark, N.A.; Edwards, A.M.; Morton, R.H.; Butterly, R.J. Season-to-season variations of physiological fitness within a squad of professional male soccer players. *J. Sports Sci. Med.* **2008**, *7*, 157. [PubMed]
55. Strudwick, A.; Doran, T.R.D. Anthropometric and fitness profiles of elite players in two football codes. *J. Sports Med. Phys. Fitness* **2002**, *42*, 239. [PubMed]
56. Botek, M.; Krejčí, J.; McKune, A.J.; Klimešová, I. Somatic, Endurance Performance and Heart Rate Variability Profiles of Professional Soccer Players Grouped According to Age. *J. Hum. Kinet.* **2016**, *54*, 65–74. [CrossRef] [PubMed]
57. Parpa, K.; Michaelides, M. Aerobic capacity of professional soccer players before and after COVID-19 infection. *Sci. Rep.* **2022**, *12*, 11850. [CrossRef]
58. Reilly, T.; Bangsbo, J.; Franks, A. Anthropometric and physiological predispositions for elite soccer. *J. Sports Sci.* **2000**, *18*, 669–683. [CrossRef]
59. Metaxas, T.I.; Koutlianos, N.; Sendelides, T.; Mandroukas, A. Preseason physiological profile of soccer and basketball players in different divisions. *J. Strength Cond. Res.* **2009**, *23*, 1704–1713. [CrossRef]
60. Reilly, T.; Williams, A.M.; Nevill, A.; Franks, A. A multidisciplinary approach to talent identification in soccer. *J. Sports Sci.* **2000**, *18*, 695–702. [CrossRef] [PubMed]
61. Almeida, A.; Santos-Silva, P.; Pedrinelli, A.; Hernandez, A. Aerobic fitness in professional soccer players after anterior cruciate ligament reconstruction. *PLoS ONE* **2018**, *13*, e0194432. [CrossRef] [PubMed]
62. Bok, D. Dinamika akutnog fiziološkog odgovora na različita opterećenja [Dynamics of acute physiological response to different loads]. In *Zbornik Radova 19. Godišnje Međunarodne Konferencije Kondicijska Priprema Sportaša, 35*; Kineziološki fakultet: Zagreb, Croatia, 2021.
63. Arsić, K.; Radovanović, D.; Arsić, D. Mechanisms of physiological adaptation to endurance training. *PONS-Med. Časopis* **2011**, *8*, 30–33.
64. Cosgrove, M.J.; Wilson, J.; Watt, D.; Grant, S.F. The relationship between selected physiological variables of rowers and rowing performance as determined by a 2000 m ergometer test. *J. Sports Sci.* **1999**, *17*, 845–852. [CrossRef] [PubMed]
65. Bentley, D.J.; McNaughton, L.R.; Thompson, D.; Vleck, V.E.; Batterham, A.M. Peak power output, the lactate threshold, and time trial performance in cyclists. *Med. Sci. Sports Exerc.* **2001**, *33*, 2077–2081. [CrossRef] [PubMed]
66. Iaia, F.M.; Ermanno, R.; Bangsbo, J. High-intensity training in football. *Int. J. Sports Physiol. Perform.* **2009**, *4*, 291–306. [CrossRef] [PubMed]
67. Laursen, P.; Buchheit, M. *Science and Application of High-Intensity Interval Training*; Human Kinetics: Champaign, IL, USA, 2019.
68. Bangsbo, J. Physiological demands of football. *Sports Sci. Exch.* **2014**, *27*, 1–6.
69. Murmu, S.K.; Chatterjee, K. Estimation of blood lactate with the progression of a football match. *Indian J. Phys. Educ. Sports Appl. Sci.* **2016**, *10*, 30–35.
70. Bangsbo, J. The physiology of football—With special reference to intense intermittent exercise. *Acta Physiol. Scand.* **1994**, *151*, 1–155.
71. Krustrup, P.; Mohr, M.; Steensberg, A.; Bencke, J.; Kjær, M.; Bangsbo, J. Muscle and blood metabolites during a soccer game: Implications for sprint performance. *Med. Sci. Sports Exerc.* **2006**, *38*, 1165–1174. [CrossRef]
72. Bentley, D.J.; Newell, J.; Bishop, D. Incremental exercise test design and analysis: Implications for performance diagnostics in endurance athletes. *Sports Med.* **2007**, *37*, 575–586. [CrossRef] [PubMed]
73. Forsyth, J.J.; Farrally, M.R. A comparison of lactate concentration in plasma collected from the toe, ear, and fingertip after a simulated rowing exercise. *Br. J. Sports Med.* **2000**, *34*, 35–38. [CrossRef] [PubMed]
74. Reilly, T.; Woodbridge, V. Effects of moderate dietary manipulations on swim performance and on blood lactate-swimming velocity curves. *Int. J. Sports Med.* **1999**, *20*, 93–97. [CrossRef] [PubMed]
75. Midgley, A.W.; McNaughton, L.R.; Jones, A.M. Training to enhance the physiological determinants of long-distance running performance: Can valid recommendations be given to runners and coaches based on current scientific knowledge? *Sports Med.* **2007**, *37*, 857–880. [CrossRef] [PubMed]
76. Modric, T.; Versic, S.; Sekulic, D.; Liposek, S. Analysis of the association between running performance and game performance indicators in professional soccer players. *Int. J. Environ. Res. Public Health* **2019**, *16*, 4032. [CrossRef] [PubMed]
77. Jerkovic, Z.; Modric, T.; Versic, S. Analysis of the associations between contextual variables and match running performance in Croatian First Division Soccer. *Sport Mont* **2022**, *20*, 125–130. [CrossRef]
78. Andrzejewski, M.; Chmura, J.; Pluta, B.; Konarski, J.M. Sprinting activities and distance covered by top level Europa league soccer players. *Int. J. Sports Sci. Coach.* **2015**, *10*, 39–50. [CrossRef]
79. Gomez-Piqueras, P.; Gonzalez-Villora, S.; Castellano, J.; Teoldo, I. Relation between the physical demands and success in professional soccer players. *J. Hum. Sport Exerc.* **2019**, *14*, 1–11. [CrossRef]
80. Andrzejewski, M.; Chmura, P.; Konefał, M.; Kowalczuk, E.; Chmura, J. Match outcome and sprinting activities in match play by elite German soccer players. *J. Sports Med. Phys. Fitness* **2018**, *58*, 785–792. [CrossRef]
81. Chmura, P.; Konefał, M.; Chmura, J.; Kowalczuk, E.; Zając, T.; Rokita, A.; Andrzejewski, M. Match outcome and running performance in different intensity ranges among elite soccer players. *Biol. Sport* **2018**, *35*, 197–203. [CrossRef]

82. Hawkins, M.N.; Raven, P.B.; Snell, P.G.; Stray-Gundersen, J.; Levine, B.D. Maximal oxygen uptake as a parametric measure of cardiorespiratory capacity. *Med. Sci. Sports Exer.* **2007**, *39*, 103–107.
83. Bradley, P.S.; Sheldon, W.; Wooster, B.; Olsen, P.; Boanas, P.; Krustrup, P. High-intensity running in English FA Premier League soccer matches. *J. Sports Sci.* **2009**, *27*, 159–168. [CrossRef] [PubMed]
84. Krustrup, P.; Zebis, M.; Jensen, J.M.; Mohr, M. Game-induced fatigue patterns in elite female soccer. *J. Strength Cond. Res.* **2010**, *24*, 437–441.
85. Mohr, M.; Krustrup, P.; Andersson, H.; Kirkendal, D.; Bangsbo, J. Match activities of elite women soccer players at different performance levels. *J. Strength Cond. Res.* **2008**, *22*, 341–349. [CrossRef] [PubMed]
86. Andersson, H.Å.; Randers, M.B.; Heiner-Møller, A.; Krustrup, P.; Mohr, M. Elite female soccer players perform more high-intensity running when playing in international games compared with domestic league games. *J. Strength Cond. Res.* **2010**, *24*, 912–919. [CrossRef]
87. Nielsen, J.J.; Mohr, M.; Klarskov, C.; Kristensen, M.; Krustrup, P.; Juel, C.; Bangsbo, J. Effects of high-intensity intermittent training on potassium kinetics and performance in human skeletal muscle. *Physiol. J.* **2004**, *554*, 857–870. [CrossRef] [PubMed]
88. Šentija, D. *Fiziologija Sporta [Physiology of Sport]*; Faculty of Kinesiology: Zagreb, Croatia, 2009.
89. Gharbi, Z.; Dardouri, W.; Haj-Sassi, R.; Chamari, K.; Souissi, N. Aerobic and anaerobic determinants of repeated sprint ability in team sports athletes. *Biol. Sport* **2015**, *32*, 207–212. [CrossRef] [PubMed]
90. Bradley, P.S.; Carling, C.; Archer, D.; Roberts, J.; Dodds, A.; Di Mascio, M.; Paul, D.; Gomez Diaz, A.; Peart, D.; Krustrup, P. The effect of playing formation on high-intensity running and technical profiles in English FA Premier League soccer matches. *J. Sports Sci.* **2011**, *29*, 821–830. [CrossRef]
91. Bradley, P.S.; Lago-Peñas, C.; Rey, E.; Gomez Diaz, A. The effect of high and low percentage ball possession on physical and technical profiles in English FA Premier League soccer matches. *J. Sports Sci.* **2013**, *31*, 1261–1270. [CrossRef]
92. Rampinini, E.; Impellizzeri, F.M.; Castagna, C.; Coutts, A.J.; Wisløff, U. Technical performance during soccer matches of the Italian Serie A league: Effect of fatigue and competitive level. *J. Sci. Med. Sport* **2009**, *12*, 227–233. [CrossRef]

applied sciences

Article

Effects of Specific Training Using a Rowing Ergometer on Sport Performance in Adolescents

Juan Gavala-González [1,2], Mª Elena Porras-García [2,3,*], José Carlos Fernández-García [2,4,*] and Mateo Real-Pérez [2]

[1] Department of Physical Education and Sports, School of Education Sciences, University of Seville, 41013 Seville, Spain; jgavala@us.es
[2] Researching in Sport Sciences: Research Group (CTS-563) of the Andalusian Research Plan, University of Málaga, 29010 Málaga, Spain; mateo.realperez@gmail.com
[3] Department of Physiology, Anatomy and Cellular Biology, University of Pablo de Olavide, 41013 Seville, Spain
[4] Department of Didactics of Languages, Arts and Sport, Andalucía-Tech, Instituto de Investigación Biomédica de Málaga (IBIMA), University of Málaga, 29016 Málaga, Spain
* Correspondence: meporgar@upo.es (M.E.P.-G.); jcfg@uma.es (J.C.F.-G.)

Abstract: The main purpose of this study was to study the effects of a specific rowing ergometer training program on the athletic performance of young adolescents (N = 56; 11.73 ± 1.4 years old) compared to a workout based on general strength training. An eight-week training program was implemented, with four sessions per week and two hours per session. The sample was divided into two groups: a control group (CG) that performed circuit training with exercises aimed at building general strength and an experimental group (EG) who focused on specifically training on a rowing ergometer (rowing machine). The data obtained in a rowing meter test over the competition distance were analyzed to obtain the average power attained (W) at the beginning of the training, at the middle (4 weeks), at the end of the training (8 weeks) and one year after the experimentation. The results show that although both forms of training improve the average W obtained in both categories, the EG subjects (+29.94 W) obtained better averages in all phases of the study compared to the CG (+5.88 W). Furthermore, this increase was greater in male rowers (+34.06 W) than in female rowers (+24.54 W). These results reveal that a specific rower rowing ergometer training program has a more significant effect than a general strength program and these effects can even be observed a year after the intervention.

Keywords: rowing; sport performance; adolescents

1. Introduction

Rowing is a strength and endurance sport in which competition performance depends on a combination of parameters involving cardiovascular endurance, muscular strength and motor skills, making it a perfect activity for adolescents who want to develop a range of physical and mental skills while enjoying a rewarding physical sport experience [1,2]. Consequently, muscular strength is a vital component of rowing, and the major role it plays in this discipline cannot be underestimated.

Muscular strength is the capacity of a muscle to exert a force through contraction, allowing it to overpower, resist or exert pressure against resistance [3,4]. Muscular strength plays a critical role in rowing because athletic performance is built over physical strength [2]. Young athletes who engage in this sport work on building strength in many muscle groups, such as those of the arms, legs, back and trunk; it is also a challenge for the cardiorespiratory system, since rowing requires a large intake of oxygen [5]. Strength in these muscle groups gives rowers the power they need to efficiently and quickly move the boat through the water [2,6,7].

One of the advantages of focusing on building muscle strength in adolescence is that it is a critical period of growth and development [3]. Research into strength training in young people has generated significant controversy in the physical fitness world over the years [8,9]. Although the earliest studies published on how strength training influences adolescents did not report positive effects for young people [10,11], there is now sufficient scientific evidence to assert that strength training in adolescents, provided it is controlled and supervised by professionals who focus on developing proper technique and ensuring individual safety, is beneficial to the health and performance of young athletes [3].

The World Health Organization's global recommendations suggest that children and adolescents should spend at least 60 min per day engaging in moderate to vigorous intensity physical activity, mainly aerobic, and engage in muscle and bone strengthening activities at least three times per week [12]. Additionally, the American College of Sports Medicine prioritizes strength training at an early age to improve musculoskeletal system function and the overall fitness level of young people through the practice of a variety of safe, effective and fun strength training activities [3].

Among the benefits of strength training in 11–13 year olds, there are studies showing how mechanical stress, induced through strength training, was beneficial for body and bone growth [8,13]. This not only corroborates the theory that suggests that, because of the low surrounding hormone levels in bone structures, adolescents cannot handle overloading during training and, therefore, may suffer alterations in the bone formation process or deformities, as some studies suggest without sufficient significant evidence [14], but it also shows us that strength training based on moderate and high-intensity exercises can be a powerful positive stimulus on bone structures [8,15]. Furthermore, regarding another controversial topic of strength training research—the high risk of injury during training—recent studies have shown that strength training at an early age helps to reduce injuries by up to 50% [3]. This suggests that the increase in physical conditioning levels enables adolescents to successfully cope with the challenges posed by the demands on the musculoskeletal system during physical and sports activities, thus reducing the injury rate [16].

Adolescents who engage in rowing-specific strength training programs not only improve their ability to perform on the water, but also help develop healthy cardiorespiratory, muscular and skeletal systems [5]. Moreover, as we have seen above, muscular strength in rowing has a direct impact on preventing injuries [6,16]. Strong muscles provide additional joint support and help stabilize the body during the repetitive motion involved in rowing. This decreases the risk of injury to joints and muscles, critical to keeping teens active and healthy throughout their rowing careers.

Another advantage of developing muscular strength through rowing is its impact on mental performance. The confidence and self-esteem of adolescents increase as they see improvements in their strength and performance. Likewise, the discipline required to stick to a consistent strength training program translates into greater determination and perseverance, valuable skills that will apply to all areas of a young person's life [17].

However, when it comes to lower-level performance, is general strength training enough to improve athletic performance? In the following experimental study, we aim to observe the influence of a controlled specific muscle strength training program on athletic performance in young people aged between 11 and 13 years. The aim of this study is to determine which training (specific rowing ergometer training program vs. a workout based on general strength training) is more beneficial for athletic performance in adolescent rowers aged 11–13 years old.

2. Materials and Methods

2.1. Subjects

A sample of students/rowers (N = 56; boys: n = 32; girls: n = 24) with a mean age of 11.73 ± 1.4 years, belonging to two categories (10–11 years old: n = 25 and 12–13 years old: n = 31), completed an eight-week training program, with four weekly sessions of two hours each one, consisting of one hour of specific training followed by an hour of rowing on the water.

The sample was divided into the following two groups:

(1) A control group (CG: n = 26) received specific training based on general strength circuit training with exercises using their own body weight at six stations (squat jump, push-up, plank, back-squat, pull-ups with elastic bands, side-plank). They performed three 30-s sets of each exercise in a rotating circuit with 30-s rests between each set.

(2) An experimental group (EG: n = 30) whose training consisted of a specific training protocol using a rowing ergometer (rowing machine model CONCEPT 2 D PM5, Concept-2, Morrisville, VT, USA) [18] consisted of two blocks of five sets of 90 s, at 18 strokes at maximum power, resting 60 s between sets and 4 min between each of the blocks. A drag factor (DF) of 140 was established (higher than what is usually set during training in the juvenile and youth categories, which is around 90–100 DF or the resistance of the water when paddling). The DF measures how quickly the fan blades slow down between each pull.

2.2. Procedure

To determine the participants' level, several tests were first performed using the rowing ergometer to find the baseline of each athlete. A pre-test measurement was taken during the first week, using the competition distance as a reference (500 m for the 10–11 years old category; 1000 m for the 12–13 years old category) where data related to the watts (W) generated in relation to the time/distance covered were obtained (all these figures are available using the rowing machine's PM5 software (https://www.vermontc2.com/tienda/monitor-pm5-rowerg/ (accessed on 1 March 2024)).

During the training protocol, a test (intermediate test) was established at 4 weeks; and a measurement (post-test) at the end of 8 weeks of training. Finally, a test was carried out one year after the experimentation in order to analyze the effects of both training programs (all measurements were taken over the same competition distance based on category and under controlled conditions).

Participants were informed about the importance of performing the tests to the best of their abilities. To avoid positively or negatively influencing the data collection, each athlete performed the test without being given any data, technical details, or external motivation. At the end of the test, information was collected from the sample.

Classification into the different groups of the study (CG vs. EG) was made considering the result obtained in the initial test, sex, category, and weight/height of the participants, understanding that, with the same categories, sex, weight, height and result in the rowing ergometer test, one subject was included in the CG, and the most similar subject according to the same criteria was included in the EG. The breakdown of the comparative groups in the study was as follows (Table 1):

Table 1. Breakdown of the groups in the study.

Category	**10–11 Years Old (N = 25)**				**12–13 Years Old (N = 31)**			
Sex	**Male**		**Female**		**Male**		**Female**	
n	**14**		**11**		**17**		**14**	
Study group	CG	EG	CG	EG	CG	EG	CG	EG
	7	7	6	5	8	9	5	9
Age (Mean ± SEM)	10.71 ± 0.28	11.14 ± 0.26	10.50 ± 0.22	10.60 ± 0.25	12.37 ± 0.18	12.50 ± 0.16	12.40 ± 0.25	12.75 ± 0.16

CG: control group; EG = experimental group; SEM (Standard Error of the Mean).

2.3. Equipment

The tests were performed on a CONCEPT 2 D PM5 rowing ergometer [18]. This model is equipped with software and various applications that can track all the rower's data (meters, strokes, watts, etc.), as well as the transformation of watts (W) to time and vice versa; it can also provide other measurements such as the average watts achieved in the test, an important factor considering that we have two groups with different competition distances (10–11 years old: 500 m, and 12–13 years old: 1000 m). This implies that if a subject completes a distance of 500 m in 2:00 min, the average watts (average of W = distance/time) will be 2:00; on the other hand, if another subject completes 1000 m in 4:00 min (double the distance and time), the average watts would also be the same.

2.4. Ethical Aspects

Once the initial selection was made, informed consent was collected from both the participating rowers and the parents/legal guardians after a discussion where the nature of the study was explained to them, clarifying that their anonymity would be maintained at all times, following the ethical considerations of Sport and Exercise Science Research [19], and with the principles included in the Declaration of Helsinki [20], which define the ethical guidelines for research on human subjects, and the University of Malaga gave the identification number registered for the Ethics Committee: 65-2020-H. During the study and afterwards, we acted under the provisions of Organic Law 3/2018 of December 5 on the Protection of Personal Data and Guarantee of Digital Rights, regarding the protection of personal data under Spanish law.

2.5. Statistical Analysis

A frequency analysis was conducted for the variables of age, sex, group, and study category. An analysis of descriptive statistics was also performed according to the experimental group to quantify the changes produced in the means obtained from the different measurements of the study. Unless otherwise indicated, data are presented as mean ± SEM (Standard Error of the Mean). To determine the influence of the category variable considering the sample group and the measurements obtained in the test performed with the rowing machine in the different phases of the study, a comparative analysis of the averages was performed (ANOVA test [groups (control vs. experimental) × test (pre-test vs. intermediate-test vs. post-test and vs. one year-test)]). Likewise, we used the same statistical procedure to determine the influence of the sex variable on the results obtained in each group ANOVA test [groups (control vs. experimental) × test (pre-test vs. intermediate-test vs. post-test and vs. one year-test) × sex (female vs. male)] and the age (ANOVA test [groups (control vs. experimental) × test (pre-test vs. intermediate-test vs. post-test and vs. one year-test) × age group (10–11 vs. 12–13 years old)]). The Holm–Sidak post hoc test was applied in all cases. Analysis of all study variables was conducted using the SPSS version 25 statistical package (SPSS, Inc., IBM, Armonk, NY, USA).

3. Results

Table 2 shows the frequency analysis of the sample. Participants were divided according to sex, group, age, and age category (Table 2).

The analysis of the descriptive statistics by sample group shows that control group subjects obtained lower averages in all phases of the study, compared to the experimental group (Table 3).

Figure 1 shows the evolution of the averages obtained by the different groups according to the phase of the study. This graph shows a positive evolution for both study groups, but it is higher in the experimental group ($dif_{pre\text{-}test/post\text{-}test}$ = +29.94 W) with respect to the control group ($dif_{pre\text{-}test/post\text{-}test}$ = +5.88 W). Statistically significant differences were found between groups ($F_{(3,216)} = 0.81$; two-way ANOVA and Holm–Sidak test).

Table 2. Frequency analysis.

		Frequency	Percentage (%)
Age (years)	10	9	16.07
	11	13	23.21
	12	18	32.14
	13	16	28.57
Sex	Male	32	57.14
	Female	24	42.85
Group	Control	26	46.42
	Experimental	30	53.57
Category	10–11 years old	25	44.64
	12–13 years old	31	55.35

Table 3. Descriptive statistics by group.

	Control (Mean ± SEM)	Experimental (Mean ± SEM)
Pre-test (W)	134.21 ± 8.99	156.89 ± 8.01
Intermediate-test (W)	137.13 ± 8.98	179.44 ± 10.56
Post-test (W)	140.10 ± 9.21	186.83 ± 10.69

[$F_{(3,216)} = 0.81$; two-way ANOVA and Holm–Sidak test]. W = watts; SEM (Standard Error of the Mean).

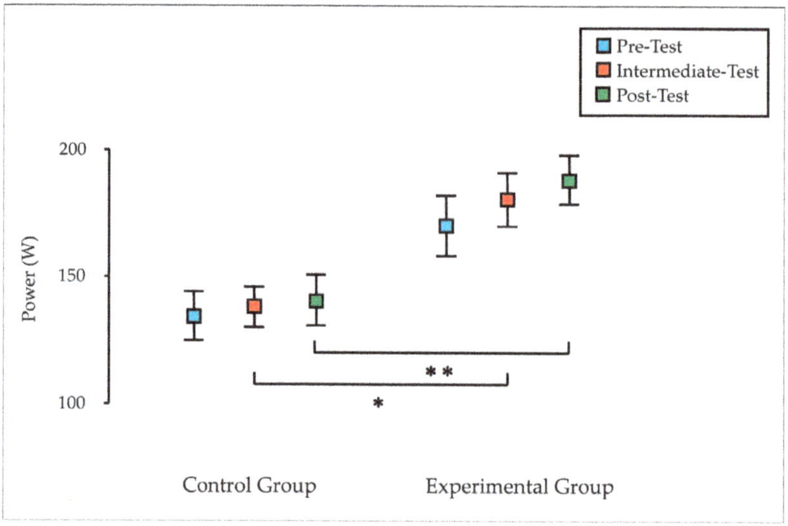

Figure 1. Evolution of the averages obtained (W) on the rowing ergometer. Statistically significant interaction between tests and groups were found [$F_{(3,216)} = 0.81$; two-way ANOVA and Holm-Sidak test; *, $p < 0.05$; **, $p < 0.001$)].

Table 4 analyzes the influence of the category to which subjects belong in the study groups. There is an improvement in the mean values obtained in the parameters of muscular strength (W), which is statistically higher in those subjects in the experimental group (EG10–11 years old: $dif_{pre/post\text{-}test} = +15.82$ W; EG12–13 years old: $dif_{pre/post\text{-}test} = +39.35$ W) than that obtained by the control groups (CG10–11 years old: $dif_{pre/post\text{-}test} = +4.56$ W; CG12–13 years old: $dif_{pre/post\text{-}test} = +7.21$ W). In addition, the measurements obtained by the 12–13-year-old subjects are statistically higher than those of the subjects aged 10–11 years old (Table 4). [$F_{(9,208)} = 0.54$; two-way ANOVA and Holm–Sidak test; $p < 0.05$]).

Table 4. Intrasubject analysis of muscle strength by group and category.

	Control Group		Experimental Group	
	10–11 Years (Mean ± SEM)	**12–13 Years (Mean ± SEM)**	**10–11 Years (Mean ± SEM)**	**12–13 Years (Mean ± SEM)**
Pre-test (W)	112.05 ± 12.13	156.38 ± 10.37	134.28 ± 11.22	171.97 ± 9.74
Intermediate-test (W)	114.45 ± 12.30	159.82 ± 9.94	144.23 ± 11.66	202.91 ± 13.31
Post-test (W)	116.61 ± 12.74	163.58 ± 9.97	150.10 ± 11.67	211.32 ± 13.35

[$F_{(9,208)}$ = 0.54; two-way ANOVA and Holm–Sidak test].

Figure 2 offers the evolution of the different values obtained by sex and the study group. Although the improvement is noticeable in both groups, there is a more prominent positive trend in the experimental groups, especially in the male group.

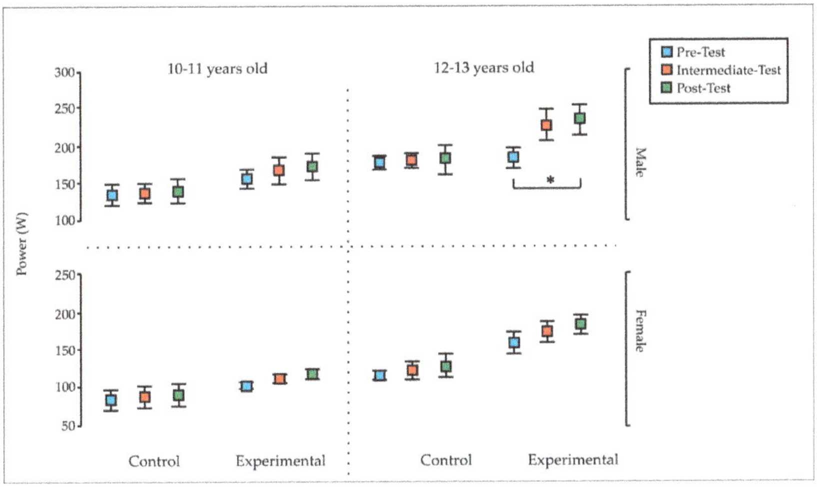

Figure 2. Evolution of the averages obtained by group and sex. CG = control group; EG = experimental group; W = watts. [$F_{(21,192)}$ = 0.45; two-way ANOVA and Holm–Sidak test; *, $p < 0.05$].

Table 5 examines how sex influences the study groups, and how the averages obtained in the experimental group are statistically higher than those obtained in the control group in both male and female cases [$F_{(9,208)}$ = 0.39; two-way ANOVA and Holm–Sidak test]. Comparing changes produced throughout the different phases of the study by sex, an improvement can be seen for both the control group (male CG: $dif_{pre/post\text{-}test}$ = +3.86 W; female CG: $dif_{pre/post\text{-}test}$ = +8.65 W), and the experimental group (male EG: $dif_{pre/post\text{-}test}$ = +34.06 W; female EG: $dif_{pre/post\text{-}test}$ = +24.54 W), although the change is statistically more pronounced in the latter (Table 5).

Table 5. Intra-subject analysis of muscle strength by group and sex.

	Control Group		Experimental Group	
	Male (Mean ± SEM)	**Female (Mean ± SEM)**	**Male (Mean ± SEM)**	**Female (Mean ± SEM)**
Pre-test (W)	159.18 ± 9.85	100.16 ± 9.55	173.97 ± 9.38	134.5 ± 11.46
Intermediate-test (W)	160.49 ± 10.08	105.27 ± 10.31	201.68 ± 13.72	150.35 ± 13.00
Post-test (W)	163.04 ± 10.51	108.81 ± 10.99	208.04 ± 13.99	159.10 ± 13.55

[$F_{(9,208)}$ = 0.39; two-way ANOVA and Holm–Sidak test]. W = watts; SEM (Standard Error of the Mean).

Finally, once eight weeks of the intervention program were completed, both groups of rowers returned to identical training sessions: four sessions/week (2 h duration: 1 h of general muscular strength exercises, and 1 h of rowing). One year after the beginning of the program, a test on the rowing machine was again performed to collect data on the subjects' performance (Figure 3).

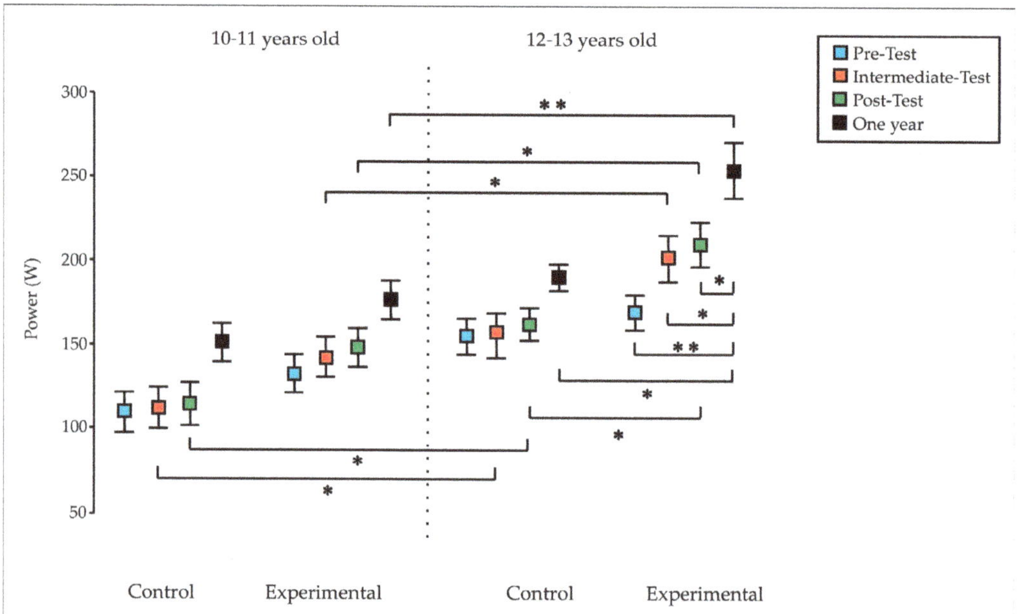

Figure 3. Evolution of the averages obtained (W) according to the group (control vs. experimental) and category (10–11 years vs. 12–13 years); and results obtained one year after the training program. [$F_{(9,208)}$ =0.54; two-way ANOVA and Holm–Sidak test; (**, $p < 0.001$; *, $p < 0.05$)]. W = watts.

Table 6 shows that the effects of specific strength training in adolescents continued to provide statistically significant differences one year later and had a positive correlation with respect to the performance of the rowing test on the rowing machine (Table 6, Figure 4).

Table 6. Intrasubject analysis of muscle strength by group and category one year after the training program.

	Control Group		**Experimental Group**	
	10–11 Years (Mean ± SEM)	**12–13 Years (Mean ± SEM)**	**10–11 Years (Mean ± SEM)**	**12–13 Years (Mean ± SEM)**
Post-test (W)	116.61 ± 12.74	163.58 ± 9.97	150.10 ± 11.67	211.32 ± 13.35
One year later (W)	152.92 ± 11.25	191.85 ± 8.286	177.83 ± 11.71	254.83 ± 16.79
$\Delta Dif_{post\text{-}test/one\ year\ later}$ (W)	+36.32	+28.26	+27.73	+43.52

[$F_{(9,208)}$ = 0.54; two-way ANOVA and Holm–Sidak test]. W = watts.

Table 7 and Figure 4 show the evolution of the different groups according to sex one year after the training program. Statistically significant differences were found after one year of training in the experimental groups (male and female) with respect to their control groups ([$F_{(9,208)}$ = 0.39; two-way ANOVA and Holm–Sidak test]).

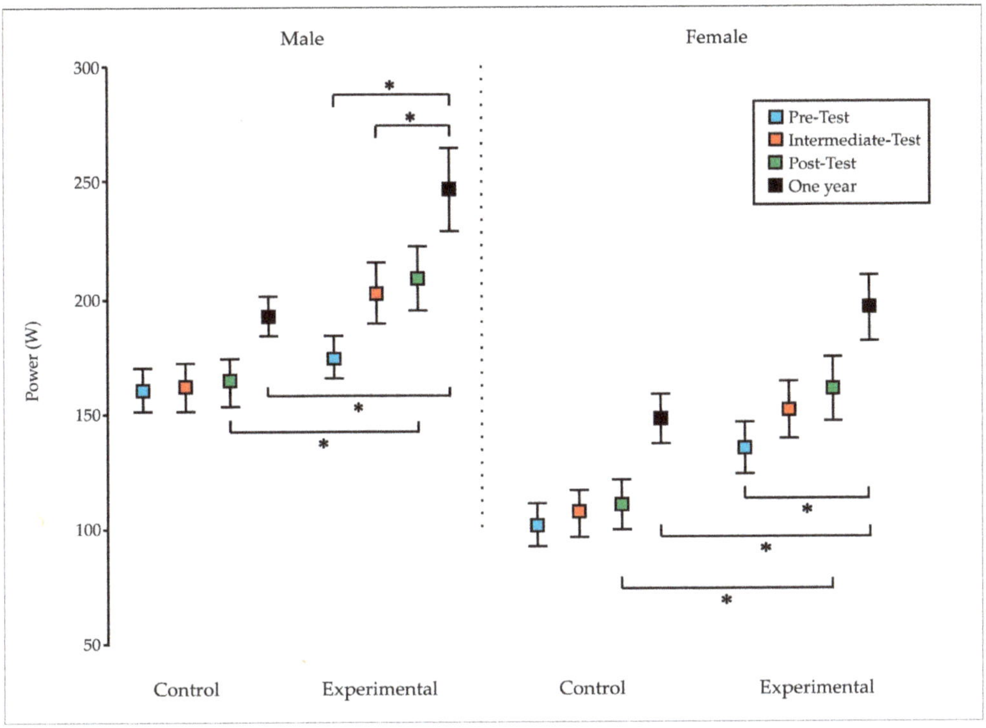

Figure 4. Evolution of the averages obtained (W) according to group and sex; and results obtained one year after the training program. [$F_{(9,208)} = 0.39$; two-way ANOVA and Holm–Sidak test; (*, $p < 0.05$)]. W = watts.

Table 7. Intra-subject analysis of muscle strength by group and sex one year after the training program.

	Control Group		Experimental Group	
	Male (Mean ± SEM)	**Female (Mean ± SEM)**	**Male (Mean ± SEM)**	**Female (Mean ± SEM)**
Post-test (W)	163.04 ± 10.51	108.81 ± 10.99	208.04 ± 13.99	159.10 ± 13.55
One year later (W)	191.47 ± 8.41	146.36 ± 10.67	246.65 ± 18.67	194.46 ± 14.37
$\Delta Dif_{post\text{-}test/one\ year\ later}$ (W)	+28.43	+37.55	+38.61	+35.36

[$F_{(9,208)} = 0.39$; two-way ANOVA and Holm–Sidak test]. W = watts.

4. Discussion

The purpose of this study was to test the effects of a specific rowing ergometer training program compared to general strength training on sport performance in adolescent rowers. After analyzing the results obtained, we were able to verify that although the results improved in both the CG and the EG following the training program, there was a greater positive and statistically significant correlation between the power achieved in the rowing ergometer test (W) and the rowing-specific strength training.

To assess the performance of rowers in both categories, we adjusted the competition course distance to match their accustomed level of challenge. This procedure allowed us to analyze the athletic performance of each participant and compare the results of both categories, and thus we set out to estimate the athletic performance of each participant to compare the results after completing the defined training program. In this sense, there are studies that show significant relationships between strength values and performance, using the rowing ergometer tests as a predictor of athletic performance in rowers [6].

If we focus on the sport of rowing in relation to muscular strength, studies analyzing the influence of aerobic capacity on athlete performance are predominantly prevalent across various disciplines, including Olympic rowing [21] with research addressing the issue of the relative contribution and demands of muscular strength and power only being very limited [2]. In this sense, recent studies have shown how important muscle strength is during the initial phase of rowing, when the athlete is subjected to high levels of acceleration while extending the upper body [2,5]. Therefore, it is important to investigate the relationship between the way we train our young athletes and their performance to encourage their athletic performance while promoting proper body development [22,23].

Accordingly, a literature review reveals the importance of strength training as a beneficial tool for the health of the target population [24]. Some examples indicate that an eight-week training program based on strength training significantly improves sit-ups, push-ups, sit and reach, standing broad jumps, as well as the height reached during the Counter Movement Jump (CMJ) test [25]. A recently published review on the influence of variables associated with muscle strength training in prepubescent youth demonstrated its efficacy, not only in increasing muscle strength values in 100% of cases, but also in significantly increasing jumping and sprinting skills. At a morphological level, strength training helps to decrease the percentage of body fat and increase lean body mass [3,26], so it is not only beneficial for maintaining an adequate body mass index, but also helps in the correct motor development of young athletes [12,27].

Lee et al. [28] conducted a study comparing various training protocols in female rowers and found greater benefits, compared to the time spent in covering 2000 m on the rowing meter, in those groups that performed higher intensity strength training based on weight lifting exercises (with equipment for five sets of 30 s and a maximum of 18 repetitions for each exercise), compared to another group that performed low repetitions (four sets with two to six repetitions per exercise). On the other hand, Thiele et al. [29] carried out a comparison with adolescent competitive female rowers who trained following a high-intensity strength–endurance training program (4 sets of 12 repetitions at 75–95% of 1-MR maximum repetition) versus a low-intensity strength–endurance training program (4 sets of 30 repetitions at 50–60% of 1-MR). In this study, they concluded that rowers improved their fitness level with high-intensity training (maximum strength, muscular power, anaerobic endurance, and speed of execution), whereas low-intensity exercises were shown to be more effective in improving specific performance in the sport of rowing. Consequently, we suggest further research is required to identify the relationship between the type of specific strength training and sport-specific performance in rowing sports.

Regarding the results obtained in this study, taking into account the gender of the rowers and the competition category, improvements were obtained in both groups after completing the training program, although more notably in the experimental group that underwent the specific training program on rowing machines.

Other studies that refer to the difference between sex in adolescent rowers concluded that boys demonstrated greater muscular power (measured in W), but also a higher score in perceived effort at all ages except between 12 and 14 years old [30], which could be associated with a greater metabolic demand at the age of puberty, although other factors should also be taken into account. In terms of differences in performance, another study found improvements in the rowing ergometer tests at the end of the program, but mostly in women [31]. This study shows that there is significant progression in both groups, although our results show better results in 12–13-year-old adolescents than in 10–11-year-old adolescents and in boys more than in girls.

Rowing training in adolescents is associated with adaptation not only of the cardiorespiratory system, including an increase in the internal diameter and size of the myocardium, but also of the skeletal muscles, triggering the processes of hypertrophy in the muscle fibers, especially in the slow twitch fibers. Additionally, a correct development program with qualified coaches can favor correct biological growth and body development, as well as the improvement of physical fitness (muscular strength, muscular endurance) [27]. According to this study, our results show that specific training programs conducted on rowing machines can help and be a useful tool for developing rowing talent, since they are highly correlated with athletic performance.

5. Conclusions

The present study has been able to confirm the positive effect of specific rowing training using a rowing ergometer on performance improvement in male and female rowers. This information contributes to clarifying the relationship between strength training and performance in young athletes, which can be highly beneficial as long as the training is supervised by qualified personnel. It's crucial to consider the importance of technique, gradual load progression, and adherence to safety standards.

As a result of this study, coaches involved in rowing with adolescents should complement water training with rowing ergometer sessions to improve muscular strength and endurance since during these ages, we have found that the effects of this type of training are noticeable even one year after experimentation.

In the future, it would be interesting to increase the sample of rowers and corroborate these results with a larger sample and with different ages to see if the same differences exist and, at the same time, to continue observing how long significant differences exist between the performance of EG and CG subjects.

Author Contributions: Conceptualization, M.R.-P. and J.G.-G.; methodology, J.G.-G. and J.C.F.-G.; software, M.E.P.-G. and M.R.-P.; validation, J.G.-G. and J.C.F.-G.; formal analysis, M.R.-P., M.E.P.-G. and J.G.-G.; investigation, M.R.-P. and J.G.-G.; resources, J.G.-G. and J.C.F.-G.; data curation, M.R.-P. and M.E.P.-G.; writing—original draft preparation, M.R.-P. and M.E.P.-G.; writing—review and editing, J.G.-G. and J.C.F.-G.; visualization, J.G.-G.; supervision, J.G.-G. and J.C.F.-G.; project administration, J.G.-G. and J.C.F.-G.; funding acquisition, J.C.F.-G. All authors have read and agreed to the published version of the manuscript.

Funding: This research received no external funding.

Institutional Review Board Statement: The study was conducted in accordance with the Declaration of Helsinki and approved by the Institutional Review Board (or Ethics Committee) of University of Málaga (protocol code 65-2020H and date of approval: 09/10/2020).

Informed Consent Statement: Informed consent was obtained from all subjects involved in the study. Written informed consent has been obtained from the patients to publish this paper.

Data Availability Statement: For privacy reasons, the data presented in this study are available upon request to the corresponding author.

Acknowledgments: We would like to thank the students/rowers (and their parents/guardians) who participated in this study. We would also like to acknowledge Patricio Rojas Aznar, an exceptional rower, student and teacher/coach.

Conflicts of Interest: The authors declare no conflicts of interest.

References

1. Maetsu, J.; Jurimae, J.; Jurimae, T. Monitoring of Performance and Training in Rowing. *Sport Med.* **2005**, *35*, 597–617.
2. Ledergerber, R.J.; Jacobs, M.W.; Roth, R.; Schumann, M. Differential Effects of Strength Determinants on Different Phases of Olympic Rowing Performance in Adolescent Athletes. *Curr. Issues Sport Sci.* **2023**, *8*, 022. [CrossRef]

3. Sánchez Pastor, A.; García-Sánchez, C.; Marquina Nieto, M.; de la Rubia, A. Influence of Strength Training Variables on Neuromuscular and Morphological Adaptations in Prepubertal Children: A Systematic Review. *Int. J. Environ. Res. Public Health* **2023**, *20*, 4833. [CrossRef] [PubMed]
4. González-Badillo, J.J.; Ribas Serna, J. *Bases de La Programación Del Entrenamiento de La Fuerza*; INDE: Barcelona, Spain, 2003.
5. Volianitis, S.; Yoshiga, C.C.; Secher, N.H. The Physiology of Rowing with Perspective on Training and Health. *Eur. J. Appl. Physiol.* **2020**, *120*, 1943–1963. [CrossRef]
6. Akça, F. Prediction of Rowing Ergometer Performance from Functional Anaerobic Power, Strength and Anthropometric Components. *J. Hum. Kinet.* **2014**, *41*, 133–142. [CrossRef] [PubMed]
7. Penichet-Tomás, A.; Pueo, B. Performance Conditional Factors in Rowing. *Retos Nuevas Tend. En Educ. Física Deport. Y Recreación* **2017**, *32*, 238–240.
8. Chen, L.; Zhang, Z.; Huang, Z.; Yang, Q.; Gao, C.; Ji, H.; Sun, J.; Li, D. Meta-Analysis of the Effects of Plyometric Training on Lower Limb Explosive Strength in Adolescent Athletes. *Int. J. Environ. Res. Public Health* **2023**, *20*, 1849. [CrossRef] [PubMed]
9. Nuzzo, J.L. Narrative Review of Sex Differences in Muscle Strength, Endurance, Activation, Size, Fiber Type, and Strength Training Participation Rates, Preferences, Motivations, Injuries, and Neuromuscular Adaptations. *J. Strength Cond. Res.* **2023**, *37*, 494–536. [CrossRef]
10. Vrijens, J. Muscle Strength Development in the Pre- and Post-Pubescent Age. *Med. Sci. Sport* **1978**, *11*, 152–158.
11. Docherty, D.; Wenger, H.A.; Collis, M.L.; Quinney, H.A. The Effects of Variable Speed Resistance Training on Strength Development in Prepubertal Boys. *J. Hum. Mov. Stud.* **1987**, *13*, 377–382.
12. Comité Nacional de Medicina del Deporte Infantojuvenil. Entrenamiento de La Fuerza En Niños y Adolescentes: Beneficios, Riesgos y Recomendaciones. *Arch. Argent. Pediatr.* **2018**, *116*, 82–91. [CrossRef]
13. Behm, D.G.; Faigenbaum, A.D.; Falk, B.; Klentrou, P. Canadian Society for Exercise Physiology Position Paper: Resistance Training in Children and Adolescents. *Appl. Physiol. Nutr. Metab.* **2008**, *33*, 547–561. [CrossRef] [PubMed]
14. Pitton, P.M. Prepubescent Strength Training: The Effects of Resistance Training on Strength Gains in Prepubescent Children. *Natl. Strength Cond. Assoc. J.* **1992**, *14*, 55. [CrossRef]
15. Paillard, T.; El Hage, R.; Al Rassy, N.; Zouhal, H.; Kaabi, S.; Passelergue, P. Effects of Different Levels of Weightlifting Training on Bone Mineral Density in a Group of Adolescents. *J. Clin. Densitom.* **2022**, *25*, 497–505. [CrossRef] [PubMed]
16. Lloyd, R.S.; Cronin, J.B.; Faigenbaum, A.D.; Haff, G.G.; Howard, R.; Kraemer, W.J.; Micheli, L.J.; Myer, G.D.; Oliver, J. National Strength and Conditioning Association Position Statement on Long-Term Athletic Development. *J. Strength Cond. Res.* **2016**, *30*, 1491–1509. [CrossRef] [PubMed]
17. Camuñas Vega, D.; Alcaide Risoto, M. La Influencia de La Práctica Deportiva En El Autoconcepto y Rendimiento Académico En Alumnos de Secundaria. *Rev. Española Educ. Física Y Deport.* **2021**, 55–67. [CrossRef]
18. Soper, C.; Hume, P.A. Rowing: Reliability of Power Output during Rowing Changes with Ergometer Type and Race Distance. *Sports Biomech.* **2004**, *3*, 237–248. [CrossRef] [PubMed]
19. Harriss, D.J.; Macsween, A.; Atkinson, G. Standards for Ethics in Sport and Exercise Science Research: 2018 Update. *Int. J. Sports Med.* **2017**, *38*, 1126–1131. [CrossRef]
20. Ebihara, A. World Medical Association Declaration of Helsinki. *Jpn. Pharmacol. Ther.* **2000**, *14*, 983–986. [CrossRef]
21. Ledergerber, R.; Jacobs, M.W.; Roth, R.; Schumann, M. Contribution of Different Strength Determinants on Distinct Phases of Olympic Rowing Performance in Adolescent Athletes. *Eur. J. Sport Sci.* **2023**, *23*, 2311–2320. [CrossRef]
22. Almeida-Neto, P.F.D.; Silva, L.F.D.; Miarka, B.; De Medeiros, J.A.; de Medeiros, R.C.D.S.C.; Teixeira, R.P.A.; Aidar, F.J.; Cabral, B.G.D.A.T.; Dantas, P.M.S. Influence of Advancing Biological Maturation on Aerobic and Anaerobic Power and on Sport Performance of Junior Rowers: A Longitudinal Study. *Front. Physiol.* **2022**, *13*, 892966. [CrossRef]
23. Almeida-Neto, P.F.D.; de Morais Ferreira, A.B.; Baxter-Jones, A.; de Medeiros, J.A.; Felipe da Silva, L.; Silva Dantas, P.M.; Cabral, B.G.D.A.T. Physiological Mechanisms of Muscle Strength and Power Are Dependent on the Years Post Obtaining Peak Height Velocity in Elite Juniors Rowers: A Cross-Sectional Study. *PLoS ONE* **2023**, *18*, e0286687. [CrossRef] [PubMed]
24. Gabbett, T. Training the Adolescent Athlete. *Sports Health Multidiscip. Approach* **2022**, *14*, 11–12. [CrossRef] [PubMed]
25. Kretschmann, R. Effects of an 8-Week after-School Resistance Program in Secondary School Students. *J. Phys. Educ. Sport* **2023**, *23*, 1376–1384. [CrossRef]
26. Manzano-Carrasco, S.; Garcia-Unanue, J.; Lopez-Fernandez, J.; Hernandez-Martin, A.; Sanchez-Sanchez, J.; Gallardo, L.; Felipe, J.L. Differences in Body Composition and Physical Fitness Parameters among Prepubertal and Pubertal Children Engaged in Extracurricular Sports: The Active Health Study. *Eur. J. Public Health* **2022**, *32* (Suppl. S1), i67–i72. [CrossRef]
27. Thiele, D.; Prieske, O.; Gäbler, M.; Granacher, U. Association between Biological Maturity, Body Constitution and Physical Fitness with Performance on a Rowing Ergometer in Elite Youth Female Rowers. *Sport. Sport.* **2023**, *37*, 116–125. [CrossRef]
28. Lee, M.; Waddell, M.; Belfry, G. A Four-Week 30 s Weight Training Intervention Improves 2000 m Rowing Ergometer Performance of Provincial to National Collegiate Female Rowers during Their Competitive Season. *Gazz. Medica Ital. Arch. Sci. Mediche* **2022**, *181*, 731–743. [CrossRef]
29. Thiele, D.; Prieske, O.; Lesinski, M.; Granacher, U. Effects of Equal Volume Heavy-Resistance Strength Training Versus Strength Endurance Training on Physical Fitness and Sport-Specific Performance in Young Elite Female Rowers. *Front. Physiol.* **2020**, *11*, 888. [CrossRef]

30. Bardin, J.; Maciejewski, H.; Diry, A.; Droit-Volet, S.; Thomas, C.; Ratel, S. Sex- and Age-related Differences in the Rating of Perceived Exertion after High-intensity Rowing Exercise during Childhood and Adolescence. *Psychophysiology* **2023**, *60*, e14296. [CrossRef]
31. Riganas, C.; Papadopoulou, Z.; Margaritelis, N.V.; Christoulas, K.; Vrabas, I.S. Inspiratory Muscle Training Effects on Oxygen Saturation and Performance in Hypoxemic Rowers: Effect of Sex. *J. Sports Sci.* **2019**, *37*, 2513–2521. [CrossRef]

applied sciences

MDPI

Review

Load Monitoring Methods for Controlling Training Effectiveness on Physical Conditioning and Planning Involvement: A Narrative Review

Anderson G. Macedo [1,2,3], Tiago A. F. Almeida [4], Danilo A. Massini [4], David M. de Oliveira [5,6], Mário C. Espada [7,8,9,10,11,*], Ricardo A. M. Robalo [7,8,9], Víctor Hernández-Beltrán [12], José M. Gamonales [12,13,14], Andréia M. S. Vilela Terra [1,2] and Dalton M. Pessôa Filho [3,4]

1 Institute of Motricity Sciences, Federal University of Alfenas (UNIFAL), Rua Gabriel Monteiro da Silva, 700, Alfenas 37130-001, MG, Brazil; andersongmacedo@yahoo.com.br (A.G.M.); andreia.silva@unifal-mg.edu.br (A.M.S.V.T.)
2 Postgraduate Program in Rehabilitation Sciences, Institute of Motricity Sciences, Federal University of Alfenas (UNIFAL), Santa Clara Campus, Avenida Jovino Fernandes Sales, Alfenas 37130-001, MG, Brazil
3 Postgraduate Program in Human Development and Technology, São Paulo State University (UNESP), Rio Claro 13506-900, SP, Brazil; dalton.pessoa-filho@unesp.br
4 Department of Physical Education, School of Sciences, São Paulo State University (UNESP), Av. Eng. Luiz Edmundo Carrijo Coube, 14-01, Vargem Limpa, Bauru 17033-360, SP, Brazil; tiagofalmeida.w@gmail.com (T.A.F.A.); dmassini@hotmail.com (D.A.M.)
5 Department of Physical Education, Federal University of Jataí (UFJ), km 195, Jataí 75801-615, GO, Brazil; profdoliveira@ufj.edu.br
6 Postgraduate Program in Animal Bioscience (PPGBA), Institute of Health Sciences (ICS), Federal University of Jataí (UFJ), Prédio da Pós-Graduação BR 364, km 195, Jataí 75801-615, GO, Brazil
7 Instituto Politécnico de Setúbal, Escola Superior de Educação, 2914-504 Setúbal, Portugal; ricardo.robalo@ese.ips.pt
8 Life Quality Research Centre (CIEQV), Instituto Politécnico de Setúbal, 2914-504 Setúbal, Portugal
9 Centre for the Study of Human Performance (CIPER), Faculdade de Motricidade Humana, Universidade de Lisboa, Cruz Quebrada-Dafundo, 1499-002 Lisboa, Portugal
10 Comprehensive Health Research Centre (CHRC), Universidade de Évora, 7004-516 Évora, Portugal
11 SPRINT Sport Physical Activity and Health Research & Innovation Center, 2001-904 Santarém, Portugal
12 Training Optimization and Sports Performance Research Group (GOERD), Faculty of Sport Science, University of Extremadura, 10005 Cáceres, Spain; vhernandpw@alumnos.unex.es (V.H.-B.); martingamonales@unex.es (J.M.G.)
13 Faculty of Education and Psychology, University of Extremadura, 06006 Badajoz, Spain
14 Programa de Doctorado en Educación y Tecnología, Universidad a Distancia de Madrid, 28400 Collado Villalba, Spain
* Correspondence: mario.espada@ese.ips.pt

Abstract: Monitoring the training load during training is important for quantifying the demand on psychological and physiological responses. This procedure is achieved through subjective and objective methods applied to the control of the level of training, to the attainment of conditioning and performance goals, and to the prevention of injuries. Training load refers to either external load, such as the variables of speed, distance, accelerations, and decelerations, or internal load, which is related to the psychological and physiological responses during an exercise session or training period (e.g., rating of perceived exertion—RPE; and heart rate—HR). To measure external load, traditional methods include pedometers, accelerometers, global positioning systems, and volume load. For internal load, methods include RPE, training monotony, strain, and impulse, HR, hormonal and biochemical markers, and training diaries and questionnaires. The current review reinforces the assumption that the methods should be combined to improve confidence with the information, mainly when assessing internal load stress during training. Moreover, training load provides an objective assessment of performance levels and involvement in different training phases, thus providing relevant information to analyse strategies for the effectiveness of conditioning progress, performance enhancement, and injury prevention.

Keywords: workload; performance; rating of perceived exertion; performance indicators

1. Introduction

The process of prescribing and periodizing a training program, whether for sports performance, fitness, or health, is systematic and complex, aiming to induce morphological, metabolic, and functional changes to enhance performance or health [1]. Given the complexity and systematic nature of the training process, rigorous monitoring is necessary to implement all planned changes effectively. Typically, assessments are conducted throughout load monitoring, which involves controlling and analyzing the athletic responses to training through less time-demanding or invasive procedures; however, these assessments are usually recommended at specific intervals (e.g., weeks or months) to ensure the effectiveness of the monitoring strategies [1]. Hence, optimizing the daily training plan according to the individual responses (e.g., performance and conditioning adjustments, fatigue and pain levels, and recovery capacity) is essential for individualizing tasks (i.e., exercise mode, intensity, and volume adjustments) and for enhancing athletic and health goals while preventing maladaptive responses and injuries [2–4].

Indeed, training load monitoring can quantify the psychological and physiological stress levels induced by single or multiple training sessions using objective and subjective methods and tools, such as the rating of perceived exertion (RPE), training impulse (TRIMP), heart rate (HR), amount of movement (accelerometers), and metabolic activation (blood lactate and oxygen uptake) and disturbance (serum levels of creatine kinase and cortisol) [3,4]. The main advantages of monitoring training load include minimizing errors in training prescription through different metrics, enabling the control of dose-response stimuli from one or more training sessions, assessing individual stress and fatigue levels, preventing undesirable overreaching, early detection of overtraining, and preventing acute and chronic injuries [2,3]. These advantages have contributed to the effectiveness of physical adaptations, performance enhancement, and injury prevention [3,4].

In sports science, training load can be classified into external and internal loads. External load refers to the training variables corresponding to the work performed during training or a set of sessions. In contrast, internal load refers to the psychological and physiological stress imposed on the body during exercise, which are crucial factors in the adaptation process to training [2,5]. Understanding these concepts is crucial for selecting the appropriate method or tool for quantification. In recent years, a growing body of scientific evidence has emerged supporting the use of these tools and strategies in sports and fitness [2,5].

Measurements of external load can be made using parameters such as distance covered, global positioning data, sprints performed, power output, and/or weight lifted [1,6]. However, more than merely understanding the methods and tools related to external load, there is a need to ensure successful monitoring. In this process, coaches play a crucial role which involves being aware of the most appropriate methods and tools for monitoring the specific external load demands of a given sport or exercise, and they must also recognize how the external load metrics may vary between individuals [5]

On the other hand, some methods for monitoring internal load include RPE, monotony, training strain, TRIMP, HR, hormonal and biochemical markers, questionnaires, and diaries [2,3]. Similar to external load, it is essential that the selected methods for monitoring internal load are appropriate for the specific sport or type of exercise practiced and that internal load responses can differ between individuals even when experiencing the same external workload [5].

Although different methods of monitoring training load can provide useful information for adjusting planning according to individual needs and goals, it is crucial to highlight the inter- and intra-individual variability when assessing external and internal load during training. Indeed, training load is influenced by factors such as training level, body composition, team position, environmental condition, and health status [7]. For example, resistance-trained individuals perform a higher number of repetitions at a given relative strength (e.g., 60% and 80% 1RM—one maximal repetition) than low or moderate-trained individuals, evidencing the influence of muscle endurance, strength, and power on external load (i.e., volume load) monitoring [8]. Similarly, displacement during soccer matches varies by player position (e.g., midfielders cover ~11.5 km, while defenders and attackers cover 10 to 10.5 km) [9]. Furthermore, RPE scores have shown differences when comparing experienced individuals regarding the level of fatigue and pain during exercise [5,7], as well as the athletes who train at a target similar HR zone might show differences indifferently perceived and metabolic responses (e.g., RPE and blood lactate concentration) if the mode of exercise differs (e.g., cycling vs. running: 12.8 ± 0.4 vs. 11.6 ± 0.3, and 6.2 ± 0.3 vs. 2.9 ± 0.3 mmol/L), due to the differences in the level of muscle activation and fiber type II recruitment (both higher in cycling than running) [10].

Understanding, selecting, and applying methods and tools for monitoring external and internal load in physical training programs is crucial for controlling and improving training planning. Therefore, this study aimed to present and describe the use of the main tools and methods for assessing internal and external load to assist in the monitoring of the level of responses to the planning (according to the expected level of training) or the analysis of the planning (rethink the strategies according to the proposal of training, i.e., whether sports performance or healthcare). The search for this revision was not constrained to a given period and was conducted in the Embase, ESPORTDiscuss, LILACS, PEDro, PubMed, and SciELO electronic databases, covering studies published until 30 May 2024. The search used the terms "training load" OR "internal load" OR "external load" OR "training monitoring" OR "planning" OR "sport performance" OR "athletic enhancement" OR "health improvement" OR "humans". Manual searches were conducted in the references of eligible articles in the PubMed, Scopus, and Google Scholar databases to add other relevant titles. Seventy-eight references were selected among the titles screened.

2. External Load Monitoring

The external load can be monitored by quantifying the parameters performed during the training session, such as distance covered, sprints performed, power output, number of repetitions, and/or weight lifted [2,3]. Quantifying individual sessions or the cumulative load across sessions allows coaches to assess the external load applied to the individual, whether in a training program for performance or for fitness [3]. However, some of these methods for quantifying external load monitoring may involve calculations and require technological instruments, ranging from simpler devices like pedometers to more complex ones like accelerometers or global positioning systems (GPS). In addition, the choice of methods may vary depending on the type of sport (e.g., team, individual, endurance, strength, or power) [2,3]. Moreover, utilizing two or more methods can be beneficial for monitoring external load and identifying variables that influence performance [2,5]. For example, monitoring the swimming velocity and stroke rate can support coaches regarding metabolic pace and swimming efficiency, informing about the swimmer's skill and conditioning levels [11]. In this way, GPS and accelerometers have been considered tools with accuracy in assessing swimming velocity and stroke rate due to the correlation to data from kinematics analysis [12] For example, stroke counting with accelerometer and video analysis correlated in breaststroke ($r > 0.98$) and butterfly ($r > 0.99$), as well as the measurements of velocity with GPS, and video analysis showed an acceptable standard error in freestyle (0.13 m/s) and breaststroke (0.12 m/s) swimming. Hence, in other sports in which displacement velocity and motion rate are important variables to infer the level and progress in conditioning and performance (e.g., running and cycling velocity, step rate and length in running, and rotation per minute in cycling), the information from different variables of external loads might reduce mistakes while planning and evaluating training [5,13].

2.1. Time–Motion Analysis

For many sports and even for fitness, time–motion analysis is important for performance and training programs. Methods for time–motion analysis include pedometers, accelerometers, and GPS [2,3,7,14].

2.1.1. Pedometers and Accelerometers

Pedometers are simple instruments used to measure the steps taken by individuals during exercise, such as walking or running [15]. These devices are programmed to detect vertical movement of the hip, providing an approximate estimate of the horizontal distance covered during exercise [16]. Although pedometer use in monitoring the total number of steps during physical activity has been correlated with other devices, such as accelerometers (i.e., r = 0.86), the high mean difference in steps measured by these devices (accelerometers > pedometers) suggests a poor convergent validity of the pedometer [17]. However, the high correlation between pedometer and accelerometer regarding the counts of steps per a given unit of time suggests that pedometers can be considered a feasible method for providing individual feedback on time spent at different categories of step intensities (light, moderate, and vigorous), as were estimated using an accelerometer [17].

It is important to note that the pedometer only registers steps when the body moves vertically; therefore, pedometers cannot independently discriminate intensity levels during the movement, exercise mode, duration, distance, physical activity level, or the tolerance. However, when combined with other devices (e.g., stopwatch, pace tracker, accelerometer, and GPS) or additional information (e.g., age, body composition, height, weight, RPE, heart rate, and oxygen uptake), pedometers can estimate these variables with reasonable accuracy [7,14,18]. For example, the amount of steps per day determined with a pedometer correlates positively with conditioning tests (e.g., 6 min walk, r = 0.69), exercise tolerance (e.g., time in treadmill test, r = 0.41) and cardiorespiratory function (peak VO_2, r = 0.22), and negatively with index of obesity (body mass index, r = −0.27) and aging (e.g., age, r = −0.21) [18]. Although pedometers are simpler instruments compared to devices such as accelerometers or GPS, an important application as a step counter device is the monitoring of the quantity of movement to achieve a recommended level of daily physical activity [15,17]. Despite the low accuracy in measuring steps during walking and running, pedometers should not be dismissed as a tool for monitoring light to moderate aerobic activity, especially when other methods are unavailable. In such cases, pedometers can help individuals without training supervision to follow the World Health Organization 2020 guidelines on physical activity [19]. Consequently, because of the aforementioned limitations and the possibility of applying pedometers in controlling exercise for health purposes, it may be better recommended for training to enhance conditioning levels for a healthy lifestyle than athletic performance.

On the other hand, accelerometers offer a greater range of information compared to pedometers [14,16,20]. For more than two decades, this instrument has been used in performance and fitness training programs [11,12]. The accelerometer provides a wide range of data that facilitate monitoring external load, including distance covered, session duration, intensity times within the training session, HR, energy expenditure, sleep duration and quality, body temperature, and more [16,20]. Moreover, monitoring step frequency with accelerometers presented high correlations with measurements of running velocity (r^2 = 0.80), and when taking into account the effect of leg length and mass on the step frequency and displacement, the energy expenditure can be estimated accurately during walking (r^2 = 0.84) and running (r^2 = 0.86) [21]. Thus, accelerometers are considered suitable tools for controlling training load and adjusting planning according to individual goals, since data from external (distance, speed, and power) and internal (estimating energy demand) loads can be assessed and combined to enhance the analysis of training effects on health and performance [16,20].

All this information assists coaches and athletes in understanding the intensity of training sessions and making informed decisions about the progression of training variables [13,14,20]. The use of accelerometers is widespread in both team and individual sports and endurance activities [14,20].

2.1.2. Global Positioning Systems (GPS)

GPS is widely used for measuring external load, especially in team sports [22]. These devices are integrated with satellites, providing information about distance, speed, and acceleration. For example, GPS measurements of player displacement during a specific test on an Australian football field were compared with data from computer-based tracking (CBT) analysis and a trundle wheel pedometer. The results showed a high correlation between GPS and CBT data (r = 0.99), and both methods were strongly correlated with the pedometer (r = 0.99) despite a slight overestimation of the distances traveled compared to the actual values [23]. Therefore, when combined with accelerometers, GPS can offer a comprehensive range of data about player movement during sports performance [24–27].

An important aspect of using GPS in team sports is the ability of this device to quantify specific demands according to players' positions, which is essential information to adjust training in line with player needs. Additionally, this instrument aids in categorizing athletes by better individualizing the workload within the training program [28]. The literature has investigated the validity and reliability of GPS in various team sports such as rugby, soccer, and American football [28]. For example, in soccer, which is characterized by technical–tactical complexity that defines match performance, the external load is usually measured using GPS for tracking positioning and understanding factors contributing to successful performance, such as high-speed running, player load, accelerations, and decelerations during matches [29]. In rugby, GPS devices can provide information on the specific match demands according to the player's position, thereby enabling better planning of training tasks aligned with the physical demands of official match requirements [30].

However, the validity and reliability of GPS can be influenced by factors such as duration, speed, type of activity, and different devices used. For example, studies have shown that GPS accuracy can decline at higher speeds or in complex environments (e.g., the standard error for the estimate of the velocity is 0.7% during walking, but can attain 5.6% during running, as well as the coefficient of variation for the measurement of the velocity tending to be lower (<5.3%) with a higher sampling rate) [22,24,31]. Furthermore, while GPS provides reports with various data points, many coaches and athletes may still struggle with interpreting or relating these parameters effectively for monitoring external load (e.g., the control of the velocity—ranging from 2 to 20 km/h—correlated with r = 0.99 with the stopwatch record, as well as distance measures improving with longer duration, showing the coefficient of variation being reduced from ~32 to 4% in distances ranging from 10 to 140 m) [22,31]. In addition, the use of inertial devices to analyze training load in different sports modalities has increased over the past decade, with GPS being the most commonly used technology [26,27,31].

Although GPS provides a significant amount of information for monitoring external load, one of its limitations is the use of speed zones for athletes [17]. Consequently, the combination of GPS with accelerometers has become common in team sports, not only to complement the information limited by GPS but also because accelerometers provide additional complementary data [27,28,31]. The combined use of GPS and accelerometers enables coaches to better interpret performance, conditioning, and physical fitness, especially in team sports, allowing for more effective monitoring of external load throughout the training program [28,31].

2.2. *Power Meters and Linear Encoder*

The measurements of power meters, including power output, acceleration, speed, cadence, average power, and peak power, among others, can be used for monitoring and quantifying external load [2,31]. These parameters are particularly important for sports like cycling and provide coaches with information on adaptation and performance related to the training program [31]; power meters can inform about exercise power at different exercise intensities due to the high correlation with power increment during incremental tests in cycling (r = 0.992 to 0.997) [32]. Power parameters can be recorded during tests, training, or competition by specific measurement instruments and analyzed later using software [2]. While power meter measurements are valid, the expected power output may vary depending on the conditions or location of the meter [31,32].

The linear encoder is a sensor device that measures linear position and velocity during exercises and can be attached to barbells or body segments [33]. When combined with an external constant load or synchronized with load measuring devices (such as strain gauges), mechanical power during the movement can also be assessed, allowing the monitoring of external load during strength and/or power training [34]. Indeed, linear encoder sensors have provided reliable measurements of power and velocity variables during strength training and are recommended to simplify the testing and monitoring of training routines for athletes and non-athletes [35].

2.3. Repetition Method and Volume Load

The repetition method is a simple tool for measuring the total number of repetitions and volume (i.e., when combined with the number of sets) performed in an exercise, session, week, or training cycle. Due to its simplicity, absolute volume load is often more suitable for measuring external load and monitoring the balance between exercise intensity and volume in resistance training [36]. Volume load is a method for quantifying external load by calculating the product of load and volume during resistance training (load in kg × number of sets × number of repetitions). This method allows for the determination of the exercise volume load, and the sum of the volume loads of the exercises in a session quantifies the total volume load [36,37].

While absolute volume load is widely used, it has some limitations, particularly regarding differences in movement force–velocity profile and endurance between individuals with varying levels of strength. A more effective way to compare volume load between two individuals is a calculation using the number of sets × number of repetitions × % 1RM (in arbitrary units), which is better for comparing volume load between two individuals [37].

Lastly, a recommended strategy for determining the intensity of a session or exercise in resistance training is to divide the volume load (session or exercise) by the number of repetitions performed (session or exercise), providing the average load (kg) lifted per repetition [37]. In addition, movement velocity is another variable of exercise intensity, which, in combination with the load lifted, can be useful for monitoring the level of exertion when planning training to develop muscle power (i.e., the ability to increase work per time) [34]. In practical terms, velocity is indeed a costly variable to be measured accurately [35], and power measurements are restricted to laboratory conditions. While this information can provide valuable insights for external load analysis, there is still not easy applicability to real-world training management [7].

3. Internal Load Monitoring

The literature has shown a wide range of methods for monitoring internal load, primarily including HR, RPE, monotony, strain training, TRIMP, physiological markers, and the use of diaries and questionnaires. Among these methods, HR is the most commonly used response to measure and quantify the internal load of players during training sessions and matches, due to the functional meaning of this variable [5,38]. However, combining these methods is often recommended for a more comprehensive understanding of training internal load [2,3].

An example of the enhanced potential of combining two or more internal load methods to analyze the physiological demand imposed with training is evident in studies reporting a low association between cognitive perception of effort (e.g., RPE) and metabolic responses (e.g., blood lactate accumulation) [3,4,7]. Therefore, despite the assumption that individuals can monitor physiological stress using perception, studies have shown that physiological variables, rather than perceptual ones, can better distinguish the training demands of similar exercise modes that are planned differently [5,6,13].

In addition, it is interesting to consider the variability in responses to training (i.e., conditioning and performance adjustments), which can be observed when comparing different individuals experiencing the same training load (i.e., inter-individual trainability) and when comparing the same individual across different seasons (i.e., intra-individual trainability) [13]. These variabilities indicate that individuals not only respond and adapt differently to training, but their responses also oscillate over time, regardless of sex, age, and conditioning level [5,13], ratifying the importance of monitoring internal loads to avoid untoward outcomes with training [38].

3.1. Rating of Perceived Exertion (RPE)

The RPE score is a commonly used and cost-effective scale for monitoring internal load demands during training, supported by solid scientific evidence showing correlations with exercise intensity, HR, and lactate concentrations [7]. The RPE scale involves the practitioner pointing to the descriptor (perceived effort intensity) and then the corresponding number. Initially proposed in 1974 by Borg [39], the scores of efforts ranged from 6 to 20 points, which was the former index to rate the post-exercise level of exertion perceptually from a "very, very light—6" to a "very, very hard and maximal—19 or 20" [40]. Over the years, other scales, such as the category ratio (CR-10) and the session RPE (sRPE), have also been introduced [41–43].

The RPE scale proposed by Borg reflects the exerciser's subjective intensity of effort during or immediately after exercise. This RPE scale was initially based on HR during running, with 6 corresponding to resting HR (60 beats per minute) and 20 to maximum effort, which would be (200 beats per minute) [39]. This correspondence was investigated in sedentary and athletic individuals, either to discriminate the exercise intensity or the demand upon the cardiocirculatory system. For example, the 6–20 RPE scale was considered a reliable tool for prescribing and self-regulating high-intensity interval training (HIIT) in the sedentary population. This was an assumption postulated after no significant differences were shown in HR responses to HIIT sessions prescribed and regulated by the HR reserve method and RPE at low-intensity interval planning (~50% of HR reserve or 9–11 points on the RPE scale: 135 $\pm$ 15 bpm vs. 138 $\pm$ 20 bpm), and at high-intensity intervals (~85% of HR reserve or 15–17 points on the RPE scale: 168 $\pm$ 15 bpm vs. 170 $\pm$ 18 bpm) [44].

The application of the RPE scale in sports and fitness has also been used in the CR-10 [39,45]. The CR-10 scale has a narrower numeric range, with 0 representing rest and 10 representing maximum effort. In contrast to the 6–20 scale, the CR-10 features twice the intensity range of the previous scale, but its application is similar to that of the 6–20 RPE scale [5,41,46].

In 2001, Foster and colleagues introduced the sRPE scale. Unlike the other RPE scales (6–20 and CR-10), which assess the perceived intensity of effort during or immediately after exercise, the sRPE scale evaluates the perceived intensity of effort over the entire training session [5]. Originally, this scale was meant to be applied only 30 min after the conclusion of the training session. To use this scale, the individual should be familiarized with it and select the descriptor followed by the corresponding number representing the perceived effort intensity during the training session, where 0 represents rest, and 10 maximum effort [43]. The use of sRPE to monitor training is a reasonably accurate measure of internal load in different exercises, regardless of mode and intensity, such as resistance training, high-intensity interval training, or plyometric training [13].

Indeed, the literature has evidenced that applying the sRPE scale 10 min after the conclusion of the training session does not significantly differ from applying it after 30 min [47], despite the initial recommendation for a longer waiting period. The sRPE, developed by Foster, has proven reliability concerning HR zones, with strong correlations reported between HR zones and sRPE (r = 0.75 to r = 0.90) [38]. Moreover, another study involving soccer players also demonstrated a strong correlation between sRPE and HR zones (r = 0.54 to r = 0.85) [5,42]. Typically, sRPE is combined with other factors such as exercise duration, HR, or blood lactate levels to provide a better understanding of the internal load experienced by the individual [7,13].

The literature has demonstrated that training session load can be calculated using arbitrary units by multiplying the training session duration (exercise time, recovery intervals, warm-up, and cool-down) by the sRPE [42,48]. However, for resistance training sessions, arbitrary units are quantified by multiplying the sRPE by the total number of repetitions in the session. It is worth noting that there is currently no standardized classification of session load for this type of training [49,50]. Calculating arbitrary units for a training session is essential for applying the concepts of monotony and training strain.

However, some factors such as individual experience, training level, training specificity, fibre distribution, environmental conditions, and psychological states, affect RPE reports, hence limiting its use for monitoring internal load, regardless of its wide scientific support [13].

3.2. Monotony and Training Strain

Training monotony reflects the variability of the training load, and depending on this variability, the adaptive responses to training can be either positive or negative [51]. A 7 to 10-day period is typically used to calculate training monotony, with calculations often based on a 7-day window. Initially, the average of arbitrary units for the sessions within the analyzed period (e.g., 7 days) is calculated by averaging the daily load (i.e., sRPE multiplied by session duration) in arbitrary units. This value is then divided by the standard deviation of the average weekly load (i.e., the sum of daily loads over a week) to determine the monotony index, from which the strain index can be assessed by multiplying the weekly load by the monotony [51–53].

For example, if a training session lasts 120 min and is reported as 6 (on RPE scale ranging from 0–10), the daily load is 720, which can be considered heavy training [50]. Therefore, if the next planned sessions demand slight variation in RPE (e.g., 5 to 7) but not in session duration, the weekly load can total 2160 arbitrary units with three sessions per week. The monotony also tends to approach high values (e.g., average load in a week = 720 divided by the standard deviation of the weekly load = 97.98, resulting in 7.3 arbitrary units), which indicates a higher strain (e.g., weekly load multiplied by the standard-deviation of the weekly load, resulting in 15.873 arbitrary units).

Thus, when analyzing sRPE, monotony, and strain responses to training, information regarding an exacerbated demand on a single training stimulus can be obtained, supporting training plan revision to avoid unsatisfactory results [51–53]. Therefore, monitoring sRPE, weekly load, monotony, and strain during physical sports practice can be essential for controlling the demands required based on the specific modality practiced.

3.3. Training Impulse (TRIMP)

TRIMP is a widely used method for assessing training load and can identify the time spent at each training intensity [3,52,53]. Bannister and Calvert [53] were the first to present the TRIMP model to quantify internal training load. Subsequently, other TRIMP models were introduced using different physiological parameters for TRIMP calculations [3,53,54].

The TRIMP method by Edwards [55] involves multiplying the duration that individuals spend within designated intensity zones during the training session. These zones of intensities are determined according to the percentage of maximum HR elicited during exercise (Zone 1: 50–60%; Zone 2: 60–70%; Zone 3: 70–80%; Zone 4: 80–90%; and Zone 5: 90–100%). The TRIMP method proposed by Lucia et al. [56] is based on ventilatory thresholds and is divided into three phases or zones: Phase I, representing low intensity below the ventilatory threshold; Phase II, indicating moderate intensity between the ventilatory threshold and the respiratory compensation point; and Phase III, signifying high intensity above the respiratory compensation point. In the TRIMP model, each phase is assigned a coefficient multiplied by the training duration within each zone, resulting in the TRIMP score [57,58].

Lastly, the Bannister and colleagues modified TRIMP model, known as Stagno's TRIMP, relates blood lactate levels to HR zones [41]. It is important to note that all TRIMP models were initially developed for endurance sports, and further research is needed to address the applicability to sports demanding other physical abilities (e.g., power, and anaerobic capacity).

3.4. Physiological Markers

Physiological markers for monitoring training internal load can be used to detect fatigue levels, physiological stress, and training recovery [2,3,5]. Among the physiological markers, HR is the commonly used method by athletes and exercise practitioners. This variable primarily assesses whether an individual can tolerate the training load and the recovery process.

The most applied HR analyses for monitoring internal load are HR recovery (HRR) and HR variability (HRV) [2,3,59]. Every time an exercise is completed, there is an immediate rapid reduction in HR. Decreases in HRR can indicate fatigue, detraining, an inability to withstand the training load, or undesirable overreaching [60,61]. HR recovery corresponds to the decline in HR after the end of the exercise. Typically, this recovery interval can vary from 30 to 120 s after the session's conclusion, with 60 s being the commonly used duration [61]. HR recovery can be expressed in two ways: absolute HRR (the number of heartbeats recovered within a certain period) and relative difference (the relative difference between the average HR in the final 30 s of exercise and the rate 60 s after exercise completion) [5,61,62].

Similar to HRR, the HRV has been used to obtain insights about an individual's positive or negative adaptations to physical training [63,64]. HRV involves measuring the intervals between cardiac beats. A reliable method for its measurement is the natural logarithm (Ln rMSSD) of the differences between intervals (R-R), calculated for 10 to 60 s [63]. For HRV monitoring, it is recommended to measure it at least three times a week over a prolonged period to obtain adaptive responses to training. A reduction in HRV may indicate that the individual is experiencing a negative response to training, while an increase in HRV suggests that the individual is experiencing positive adaptations [61,63]. Monitoring HR through HRR or HRV can provide important information about an individual's training adaptations. However, monitoring should not solely rely on HR and should be complemented by other methods and tools, such as RPE or lactate concentrations, to enhance the reliability of internal load assessments [3,61,63].

Saliva samples that monitor hormonal markers can provide information about an individual's health status and prevent overtraining [64,65]. Hormones measured in saliva, such as testosterone, cortisol, or the testosterone/cortisol ratio, seem to have implications for detecting overreaching or overtraining states [38,66]. Testosterone is an anabolic hormone that plays a role in growth and protein synthesis, as well as in psychological aspects contributing to performance [65]. Cortisol, on the other hand, is crucial for metabolism as it increases substrate availability to muscles and regulates immune system function. Increased levels of cortisol after physical exercise or competition are expected due to exercise-induced stress [64], which is further supported by a high correlation between cortisol levels and exercise intensity ($r = 0.86$) [66]. Due to its crucial importance, cortisol is one of the most measured hormones for training monitoring, especially among athletes [47,65].

The testosterone/cortisol ratio is an interesting tool for monitoring sports since it reflects the balance between anabolism and catabolism states. A high ratio suggests anabolic adaptations, while a low ratio may be detrimental as it indicates a catabolic state [65]. Hormonal monitoring can be valuable for managing training loads and the individual's recovery process [64,67]. Blood samples are also used for biochemical analyses, providing information to assess an individual's training status. Among the primary biochemical markers for exercise monitoring is creatine kinase. Due to the ease of collecting and examining this enzyme, serum creatine kinase (CK) activity has become an important marker widely used in sports and fitness, with increases in CK activity indicating structural muscle damage at the level of the sarcolemma and Z-disks [68,69]. Therefore, this biochemical marker has been used to assess muscle damage since its levels increase acutely in response to training loads [69]. Other muscle enzymes, such as serum lactate dehydrogenase (LDH), myoglobin, and troponin, can also be measured to indicate the extent of muscle damage with excessive exercise training [69]. For instance, LDH activity is a marker of cell damage, with increases helping to assess adaptation to training, while myoglobin release indicates degradation of protein structures within muscle and correlates with neutrophil response induced by stress [69]. In addition, cardiac and skeletal muscle troponins are released with high-intensity exercise, indicating disruption of the actin–myosin structure [69]. Given these molecules' structural and functional importance, they are considered valuable markers for monitoring the effects of training load on muscle tissue.

Immunological and inflammation markers can be used to assess physiological stress in response to training load. Excessive training can lead to immunosuppression and inflammation, increasing the individual's risk of illness [70]. Several immunological and inflammatory markers are associated with physical exercise and sports; among them, cytokines play a significant role in acute and chronic responses to physical training. The most commonly measured cytokines include interleukin-6 (IL-6), interleukin-8 (IL-8), interleukin-10 (IL-10), and interleukin-1ß (IL-1β) [71,72]. Hence, cytokines are molecules that modulate inflammation and immune responses. According to Suzuki [71], increases in interleukin IL-1ra, IL-6, IL-8, and IL-10 appear to be more closely related to exercise intensity (physiological load/stress) than to muscle damage. Furthermore, long-duration exercise tends to elicit a significantly higher response of these cytokines compared to short-duration intensive exercise. Even with the complexity of the cytokine network, the pro-inflammatory cytokines (e.g., IL-1β, IL-6, IL-8, TNF-α) and the anti-inflammatory cytokines, also with immunosuppressive function (e.g., IL-1ra, IL-10, and IL-4), contribute to muscle injury and susceptibility to infections. Therefore, the inflammatory cytokines, neutrophils, and macrophages can be markers of exhaustive exercise-induced muscle tissue damage [71].

3.5. Questionnaires and Diaries

Athletes and exercise practitioners frequently use questionnaires and training diaries as simple and cost-effective tools to gain insights into training loads for individual or upcoming sessions. These tools collect subjective data; thus, it is important to complement the information with data from objective methods for monitoring training loads (i.e., physiological or performance metrics) to improve accuracy [5,72,73]. Among the primary questionnaires and diaries, the following stand out: the training diary, profile of mood states (POMS), recovery–stress questionnaire for athletes (RESTQ-Sport), and total quality recovery (TQR). These tools can be applied to athletes, trained individuals, or those beginning their exercise journey [72–74].

In training diaries, the individual describes everything that occurred during the training session, such as difficulties, pain, and more, and is used more commonly by athletes than by physical exercise practitioners [72,73]. The POMS questionnaire consists of 65 items that assess six mood states: vigorous activity, anxiety-tension, dejection-depression, anger-hostility, fatigue–inertia, and confusion–bewilderment [56,58]. The RESTQ-Sport comprises 76 questions divided into 19 scales, of which 7 assess overall stress, 5 evaluate overall recovery, 3 assess sport-related stress, and 4 evaluate specific recovery issues [72,75]. Lastly, the TQR assesses the individual's recovery over the last 24 h by asking "how do you feel now?" on a scale from 6 to 20, where 6 means "not recovered at all" and 20 means "completely recovered" and is widely used between training sessions [72]. The TQR in its modified form with a 0–10 scale can also be found and used [76].

4. Practical Considerations for Training Load Monitoring

When applying and using methods for monitoring training load, it is essential to take into account several key points: the method's validity and reliability with scientific evidence, having a good understanding of how to apply the chosen method, using methods or tools that are relevant to the training and specific sport, providing feedback to the practitioner based on the collected data, and being capable of interpreting the data collected through the utilized methods [1]. Table 1 summarizes the methods covered, specifying the type of load, application methods, and the sports and fitness disciplines in which each method can be used. Figure 1 suggests practical approaches for the methods discussed in this article for monitoring training load in sports and fitness.

Table 1. Training load monitoring methods characteristics.

Method	Load Monitoring	Evaluated Parameters	Application	Sports and Fitness Modalities
Accelerometers	External load	Time-motion analysis	During exercise or competition, assess HR, distance covered, and energy expenditure.	In individual or team sports.
GPS	External load	Time-motion analysis	During exercise or competition, assess distance, speed, and changes of direction, and provide performance insights for players in different positions.	Mainly in team sports.
Power Metrics	External load	Power output analysis	During exercise or competitions.	Mainly in cycling
Linear encoder	External load	Measurement of linear position and velocity during exercises	Used for assessing a single exercise of a session	Mainly in resistance exercise and power training
Method Repetitions	External load	Quantification of the number of repetitions of exercise or session.	Used for assessing a single exercise or the entire session.	Mainly in resistance exercise and power training.
Volume Load	External load	Absolute: Quantification of the product: number of sets × number of repetitions × load (kg). Relative: Quantification of the product: number of sets × number of repetitions × % 1RM	Used for assessing a single exercise or the entire session, representing the sum of the set of exercises.	Mainly in resistance exercise and power training.
RPE	Internal load	Subjective perceived effort intensity of the exercise by the individual.	The RPE (6–20 or CR-10) assesses subjective intensity during or immediately after exercise. The sRPE (0–10) measures the subjective effort intensity of the training session.	In individual or team sports.
TRIMP	Internal load	Identify the time spent at each training intensity.	It is determined by multiplying the duration that individuals remained within intensity zones during the session. These zones are based on different physiological factors (HR, ventilatory threshold, and blood lactate)	Usually in individual sports, especially in endurance sports.
HRR and HRV	Internal load	Recovery and adaptation	The recovery interval following the sessions lasted for 60 s, with this duration being predominantly employed for HRR and HRV analyses.	In individual or team sports.
Hormonal and Biochemical Markers	Internal load	Fatigue control, recovery, and adaptation.	Collection of saliva post-exercise and during the recovery process between sessions, as well as assessment of chronic exercise adaptation through hormonal concentration measurements. Blood collection for acute or chronic exercise recovery and adaptation assessment.	In individual or team sports, encompasses both strength and endurance exercises.
POMS, RESTQ-Sport, and TQR	Internal load	Recovery and fatigue.	Subjective information through questionnaires.	In individual or team sports.

Abbreviations: HR, Heart rate; RPE, Rating of perceived exertion; TRIMP, Training impulse; HRR, Heart rate recovery; HRV, Heart rate variability; POMS, Profile of mood states; RESTQ-Sport, Recovery–stress questionnaire for athletes; TQR, Total quality recovery.

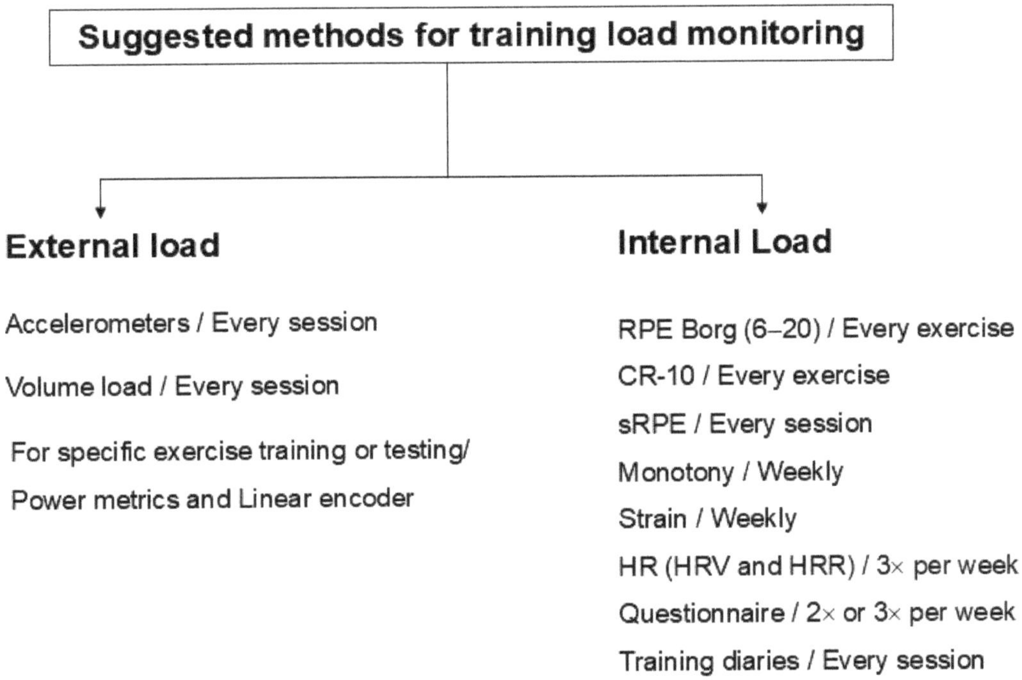

Figure 1. Training load monitoring suggested methods.

5. Final Considerations

Training load monitoring methods are essential for tracking physical training adaptations and reducing the risk of injuries and overtraining. Despite the separate approach in the literature to external and internal load methods, not only are both methods important but also several measurements as well and should be monitored to quantify better psychological and physiological stress induced by training in individuals. The choice of method may vary depending on the athlete's sport, financial resources, or practicality.

The large number of variables recorded by monitoring devices during training sessions and official matches provides the opportunity to understand the athlete's demands and make decisions regarding training management and injury risk assessment.

Analyzing athletes' physical demands through monitoring systems will allow team technical staff to personalize training loads and determine the intensities at which athletes must perform tasks during training sessions to improve sports performance. Thus, it will also help to reduce the number of injuries associated with overload. Therefore, it is essential to use the different types of existing monitoring systems.

Author Contributions: Conceptualization, A.G.M., T.A.F.A., D.A.M., M.C.E., V.H.-B., J.M.G. and D.M.P.F.; methodology, A.G.M., T.A.F.A., D.A.M. and D.M.d.O.; writing—review and editing, A.G.M., T.A.F.A., D.A.M., D.M.d.O., M.C.E., R.A.M.R., V.H.-B., J.M.G., A.M.S.V.T. and D.M.P.F.; visualization, A.M.S.V.T., M.C.E., R.A.M.R., V.H.-B., J.M.G. and D.M.P.F.; supervision, M.C.E., V.H.-B., J.M.G. and D.M.P.F. All authors have read and agreed to the published version of the manuscript.

Funding: A.G.M. would like to thank CAPES—Brazil (CAPES—Finance Code 001) for the partial financial support. The author T.A.F.A. would also like to thank the scholarships granted by the Coordination of Superior Level Staff Improvement, in the scope of the Program CAPES-PrInt (number 88887.310463/2018-00) and International Cooperation Project (number 88887.310796/2018-00), scholarship number 88887.580265/2020-00. This study was supported by the São Paulo Research Foundation (FAPESP), under Grant 2017/23717-9, Portuguese Foundation for Science and Technology,

I.P. under Grant UID04045/2020, and Instituto Politécnico de Setúbal. Also, the research was partially funded by the GOERD of the University of Extremadura and the Research Vicerectory of Universidad Nacional. This study was partially supported by the funding for research groups (GR21149) granted by the Government of Extremadura (Employment and Infrastructure Office—Consejería de Empleo e Infraestructuras), with the contribution of the European Union through the European Regional Development Fund (ERDF) by the Optimisation of Training and Sports Performance Research Group (GOERD) of the Faculty of Sports Sciences of the University of Extremadura. Also, this research was partially funded by the project entitled "Scientific-technological support to analyze the training load in basketball teams according to gender, players' level and period of the season" (PID2019-106614GBI00), financed by MCIN/AEI/10.13039/501100011033.

Institutional Review Board Statement: Not applicable.

Informed Consent Statement: Not applicable.

Data Availability Statement: Not applicable.

Conflicts of Interest: The authors declare no conflicts of interest.

References

1. Gibson, A.; Wagner, D.; Heyward, V. *Advanced Fitness Assessment and Exercise Prescription*; Human Kinetics: Champaign, IL, USA, 2019.
2. Bourdon, P.C.; Cardinale, M.; Murray, A.; Gastin, P.; Kellman, M.; Varley, M.C.; Gabbett, T.J.; Coutts, A.J.; Darren, J.; Gregson, W.; et al. Monitoring athlete training loads: Consensus statement. *Int. J. Sports Physiol. Perform.* **2017**, *12*, S161–S170. [CrossRef] [PubMed]
3. Halson, S.L. Monitoring training load to understand fatigue in athletes. *Sports Med.* **2014**, *44*, 139–147. [CrossRef] [PubMed]
4. Haller, N.; Blumkaitis, J.C.; Streep, T.; Shmuttermains, A.; Lorenz, A.; Pearker, S.; Neuberger, E.; Kranzinger, C.; Kranzinger, S.; O'Brien, J.; et al. Comprehensive training load monitoring with biomarkers, performance testing, local positioning data, and questionaries—First results elite youth soccer. *Front. Physiol.* **2022**, *13*, 1000898. [CrossRef] [PubMed]
5. McGuigan, M. *Monitoring Training and Performance in Athletes*; Human Kinetics: Champaign, IL, USA, 2017.
6. Hamlin, M.J.; Wilkes, D.; Elliot, C.A.; Lizamore, C.A.; Kathiravel, Y. Monitoring training loads and perceived stress in young elite university athletes. *Front. Physiol.* **2019**, *10*, 34–39. [CrossRef] [PubMed]
7. Foster, C.; Rodríguez-Marroyo, J.A.; Koning, J.J. Monitoring training loads: The past, the present, and the future. *Int. J. Sports Physiol. Perform.* **2017**, *12*, 22–28. [CrossRef]
8. Shimano, T.; Kraemer, W.J.; Spiering, B.A.; Volek, J.S.; Hatfield, D.L.; Silvestre, R.; Vingren, J.L.; Fragala, M.S.; Maresh, C.M.; Fleck, S.J.; et al. Relationship between the number of repetitions and selected percentages of one repetition maximum in free weight exercises in trained and untrained men. *J. Strength Cond. Res.* **2006**, *20*, 819–823. [CrossRef]
9. Bradley, P.S.; Di Mascio, M.; Peart, D.; Olsen, P.; Sheldon, B. High-intensity activity profiles of elite soccer players at different performance levels. *J. Strength Cond. Res.* **2010**, *24*, 2343–2351. [CrossRef]
10. Kodesh, E.; Law, P.; Haddad, F.; Stehli, A.; Falk, B.; Radom-Aizik, S. Leukocytes and lactate responses to cycling and running at the same target heart rate. *Eur. J. Sport Sci.* **2024**, *24*, 606–613. [CrossRef]
11. Almeida, T.A.F.; Espada, M.C.; Massini, D.A.; Macedo, A.G.; Castro, E.A.; Ferreira, C.C.; Reis, J.F.; Pessôa Filho, D.M. Stroke and physiological relationships during the incremental front crawl test: Outcomes for planning and pacing aerobic training. *Front. Physiol.* **2023**, *14*, 1241948. [CrossRef]
12. Beanland, E.; Main, L.C.; Aisbett, B.; Gastin, P.; Netto, K. Validation of GPS and accelerometer technology in swimming. *J. Sci. Med. Sport* **2014**, *17*, 234–238. [CrossRef]
13. Borresen, J.; Lambert, M.I. The quantification of training load, the training response and the effect on performance. *Sports Med.* **2009**, *39*, 779–795. [CrossRef] [PubMed]
14. Sato, K.; Sands, W.A.; Stone, M.H. The reliability of accelerometry to measure weightlifting performance. *Sports Biomech.* **2012**, *11*, 524–531. [CrossRef] [PubMed]
15. Basset, D.R.; Toth, L.P.; LaMunion, S.R.; Crouter, S.E. Step counting: A review of measurement considerations and health-related applications. *Sports Med.* **2017**, *47*, 1303–1315. [CrossRef] [PubMed]
16. Gomez-Carmona, C.D.; Bastida-Castillo, A.; Ibáñez, S.J.; Pino-Ortega, J. Accelerometry as a method for external workload monitoring in invasion team sports. A systemic review. *PLoS ONE* **2020**, *15*, e0236643. [CrossRef]
17. Tudor-Locke, C.; Ainsworth, B.E.; Thompson, R.W.; Matthews, C.E. Comparison of pedometer and accelerometer measures of free-living physical activity. *Med. Sci. Sports Exerc.* **2002**, *34*, 2045–2051. [CrossRef]
18. Tudor-Locke, C.; Williams, J.E.; Reis, J.P.; Pluto, D. Utility of pedometers for assessing physical activity. *Sports Med.* **2004**, *34*, 281–291. [CrossRef]
19. Bull, F.C.; Al-Ansari, S.S.; Biddle, S.; Borodulin, K.; Buman, M.P.; Cardon, G.; Carty, C.; Chaput, J.-P.; Chastin, S.; Chou, R.; et al. World Health Organization 2020 guidelines on physical activity and sedentary behavior. *Br. J. Sports Med.* **2020**, *54*, 1451–1462. [CrossRef]

20. Clevenger, K.A.; Montoye, A.H.K.; Van Camp, C.A.; Straht, S.J.; Pfeiffer, K.A. Methods for estimation physical and energy expenditure using raw accelerometry data or novel analytical approaches: A repository, framework, and reporting guidelines. *Physiol. Meas.* **2022**, *43*, 6579. [CrossRef]
21. Wixted, A.J.; Thiel, D.V.; Hahn, A.G.; Gore, C.J.; Pyne, D.B.; James, D.A. Measurement of energy expenditure in elite athletes using MEMS-based triaxial accelerometers. *IEEE Sens. J.* **2007**, *7*, 481–488. [CrossRef]
22. Jennings, D.; Cormack, S.; Coutts, A.J.; Boyd, L.; Aughey, R.J. The validity and reliability of GPS units for measuring distance in team sport specific running patterns. *Int. J. Sports Physiol. Perform.* **2010**, *5*, 328–341. [CrossRef]
23. Edgecomb, S.J.; Norton, K.I. Comparison of global positioning and computer-based tracking systems for measuring player movement distance during Australian football. *J. Sci. Med. Sport* **2006**, *9*, 25–32. [CrossRef]
24. Varley, M.; Aughey, R. Validity and reliability of GPS for measuring instantaneous velocity during acceleration, deceleration, and constant motion. *J. Sports Sci.* **2012**, *30*, 121–127. [CrossRef]
25. Espada, M.C.; Gamonales, J.M.; Verardi, C.E.L.; Pessôa Filho, D.M.; Ferreira, C.C.; Robalo, R.A.M.; Dias, A.A.P.; Hernández-Beltrán, V.; Santos, F.J. The effect of pitch size manipulation during small sided-games performed by different age category football players: A pilot study. *J. Mens. Health* **2023**, *19*, 1–10. [CrossRef]
26. Santos, F.; Clemente, F.M.; Sarmento, H.; Ferreira, C.; Figueiredo, T.; Hernández-Beltrán, V.; Gamonales, J.M.; Espada, M. External load of different format small-sided games in youth football players in relation to age. *Int. J. Sports Sci. Coach.* **2024**, *19*, 2024–2034. [CrossRef]
27. Rago, V.; Brito, J.; Figueiredo, P.; Costa, J.; Barreira, D.; Krustrup, P.; Rebelo, A. Methods to collect and interpret external training load using microtechnology incorporating GPS in professional football: A systemic review. *Res. Sports Med.* **2020**, *28*, 437–458. [CrossRef]
28. Cummins, C.; Orr, C.R.; O'Connor, H. Global positioning system (GPS) and microtechnology sensors in team sports: A systemic review. *Sports Med.* **2013**, *43*, 1025–1042. [CrossRef]
29. Costa, J.A.; Rago, V.; Brito, P.; Figueiredo, P.; Sousa, A.; Abade, E.; Brito, J. Training in women soccer players: A systematic review on training load monitoring. *Front. Phychol.* **2022**, *13*, 943857. [CrossRef]
30. Bridgeman, L.A.; Gill, N.D. The use of global positioning and accelerometer systems in age-grade and senior rugby union: A systematic review. *Sports Med-Open* **2021**, *7*, 15. [CrossRef]
31. Schutz, Y.; Chambaz, A. Could a satellite-based navigation system (GPS) be used to assess the physical activity of individuals on earth? *Eur. J. Clin. Nutr.* **1997**, *51*, 338–339. [CrossRef]
32. Iglesias-Pino, J.; Herrero-Molleda, A.; Saavedra-García, M.Á.; García-López, J. Concurrent validity and reliability of two portable power meters (Power2Max vs. PowerTap) to measure different types of efforts in cycling. *Sensors* **2023**, *23*, 7745. [CrossRef]
33. Martín-San Agustín, R.; Sánchez-Barbadora, M.; García-Vidal, J.A. Validity of an inertial system for measuring velocity, force, and power during hamstring exercises performed on a flywheel resistance training device. *PeerJ* **2020**, *8*, e10169. [CrossRef]
34. Bollinger, L.M.; Brantley, J.T.; Tarlton, J.K.; Baker, P.A.; Seay, R.F.; Abel, M.G. Construct validity, test-retest reliability, and repeatability of performance variables using a flywheel resistance training device. *J. Strength Cond. Res.* **2020**, *34*, 3149–3156. [CrossRef]
35. Illera-Domínguez, V.; Fernández-Valdés, B.; Gisbert-Orozco, J.; Ramirez-Lopez, C.; Nuell, S.; González, J.; Weakley, J. Validity of a low-cost friction encoder for measuring velocity, force and power in flywheel exercise devices. *Biol. Sport* **2023**, *40*, 805–811. [CrossRef]
36. Haff, G.G. Quantifying workloads in resistance training: A brief review. *UK Strength Cond. Assoc. J.* **2010**, *19*, 31–40.
37. Hernández-Beltrán, V.; Ibáñez, S.J.; Espada, M.C.; Gamonales, J.M. Analysis of the external and internal load in wheelchair basketball considering the game situation. *Appl. Sci.* **2024**, *14*, 269. [CrossRef]
38. Foster, C. Monitoring training in athletes with reference to overtraining syndrome. *Med. Sci. Sports Exerc.* **1998**, *30*, 1164–1168. [CrossRef]
39. Borg, G.A.; Noble, B.J. Perceived exertion. *Exerc. Sport Sci. Rev.* **1974**, *2*, 131–153. [CrossRef]
40. Borg, G.A. Psychophysical scaling with application in physical work and the perception of exertion. *Scand. J. Work Environ. Health* **1990**, *16*, 55–58. [CrossRef]
41. Borg, G.A. Psychophysical bases of perceived exertion. *Med. Sci. Sports Exerc.* **1982**, *14*, 377–381. [CrossRef]
42. Foster, C.; Heiman, K.M.; Esten, P.L.; Brice, G.; Porcari, J.P. Differences in perceptions of training by coaches and athletes. *S. Afr. J. Sports Med.* **2001**, *8*, 3–7.
43. Foster, C.; Florhaug, J.A.; Franklin, J.; Krovatin, L.A.; Parker, S.; Doles, P. A new approach to monitoring exercise training. *J. Strength Cond. Res.* **2001**, *15*, 109–115.
44. Ciolac, E.G.; Mantuani, S.S.; Neiva, C.M.; Verardi, C.E.L.; Pessôa Filho, D.M.; Pimenta, L. Rating of perceived exertion as a tool for prescribing and self-regulating interval training: A pilot study. *Biol. Sport* **2015**, *32*, 103–108. [CrossRef]
45. Borg, G.A. *Borg's Perceived Exertion and Pain Scales*; Human Kinetics: Champaign, IL, USA, 1998.
46. Sing, F.C.; Foster, C.; Tod, D.; Mcguigan, M.R. Monitoring different types of resistance training using session rating perceived exertion. *Int. J. Sports Physiol. Perform.* **2007**, *2*, 34–35. [CrossRef]
47. Akubat, I.; Barret, S.; Abt, G. Integrating the internal and external training loads in soccer. *Int. J. Sports Physiol. Perform.* **2014**, *9*, 457–462. [CrossRef]

48. Foster, C.; Daines, L.; Hector, L.; Synder, A.C.; Welsh, R. Athletic performance in relation to training load. *Wis. Med. J.* **1996**, *95*, 370–374.
49. Day, M.L.; Mcguigan, M.R.; Brince, G.; Foster, C. Monitoring exercise intensity during resistance training using the session RPE scale. *J. Strength Cond. Res.* **2004**, *18*, 355–358. [CrossRef]
50. Sweet, T.W.; Foster, C.; McGuigan, M.R.; Brice, G. Quantitation of resistance training using of the session perceived exertion method. *J. Strength Cond. Res.* **2004**, *18*, 796–802. [CrossRef]
51. McGuigan, M.R.; Foster, C. A new approach to monitoring resistance training. *J. Strength Cond. Res.* **2004**, *26*, 42–47. [CrossRef]
52. Banister, E.W.; Calvert, T.W. Planning for future performance: Implications for long term training. *Can. J. Appl. Sport Sci.* **1980**, *5*, 170–176. [PubMed]
53. Banister, E.; Carter, J.B.; Zarkadas, P.C. Training theory and taper: Validation in triathlon athletes. *Eur. J. Appl. Physiol. Occup. Physiol.* **1999**, *79*, 182–191. [CrossRef]
54. Morton, R.H.; Fitz-Clarke, J.R.; Banister, E.W. Modeling human performance in running. *J. Appl. Physiol.* **1999**, *69*, 1171–1177. [CrossRef] [PubMed]
55. Edwards, S. *The Heart Rate Monitor Book*; Feet Fleet Press: Sacramento, CA, USA, 1992.
56. Lucia, A.; Hoyos, J.; Perez, M.; Chicharro, L. Heart rate and performance parameters in elite cyclists: A longitudinal study. *Med. Sci. Sports Exerc.* **2000**, *32*, 1777–1782. [CrossRef] [PubMed]
57. Gardiner, C.; Navalta, J.W.; Carryer, B.; Aguiar, C.; Rodriguez, J.P. Training impulse and its impact on load management in collegiate and professional soccer players. *Technologies* **2023**, *11*, 79. [CrossRef]
58. Daanen, H.A.; Lamberts, R.P.; Kallen, V.L.; Jin, A.; Van Meeteren, N.L.U. A systematic review on heart-rate recovery to monitor changes in training status in athletes. *Int. J. Sports Physiol. Perform.* **2012**, *7*, 251–260. [CrossRef] [PubMed]
59. Borresen, J.; Lambert, M.I. Autonomic control of heart rate during and after exercise. Measurements and implications for monitoring training status. *Sports. Med.* **2008**, *38*, 633–646. [CrossRef]
60. Lamberts, R.P.; Stwart, B.; Capostagno, B.; Noakes, T.D.; Lambert, M.I. Heart rate recovery as a guide to monitor fatigue and predict changes in performance parameters. *Scand. J. Med. Sci. Sports* **2010**, *20*, 449–457. [CrossRef]
61. Plews, D.J.; Laursen, P.B.; Kilding, A.E.; Buchheit, M. Evaluating training adaptation with heart-rate measures: A methodological comparison. *Int. J. Sports Physiol. Perform.* **2013**, *8*, 688–691. [CrossRef]
62. Plews, D.J.; Laursen, P.B.; Stanley, J.; Holts, M. Training adaptation and heart rate variability in elite endurance athletes: The door to effective monitoring. *Sports Med.* **2013**, *43*, 773–781. [CrossRef]
63. Buccheit, M. Monitoring training status with HR measures: Do all roads lead Rome? *Front. Physiol.* **2014**, *5*, 73. [CrossRef]
64. Papacosta, E.; Nassis, G.P. Saliva as a tool for monitoring steroid, peptide and immune markers in sport and exercise science. *J. Sci. Med. Sport* **2010**, *14*, 424–434. [CrossRef]
65. Springham, M.; Newton, U.R.; Strudwick, A.J.; Waldron, M. Selected immunoendocrine measures for monitoring responses to training and match load in professional association football: A Review of the evidence. *Int. J. Sports Physiol. Perform.* **2022**, *17*, 1654–1663. [CrossRef] [PubMed]
66. Port, K. Serum and saliva cortisol responses and blood lactate accumulation during incremental exercise testing. *Int. J. Sports Med.* **1991**, *12*, 490–494. [CrossRef] [PubMed]
67. Neves, R.S.; Da Silva, M.A.R.; Rezende, M.A.C.; Caldo-Silva, A.; Pinheiro, J.; Santos, A.M.C. Salivary markers responses in the post-exercise and recovery period: A systematic review. *Sports* **2023**, *11*, 137. [CrossRef] [PubMed]
68. Saw, A.E.; Main, L.C.; Gastin, P.B. Monitoring the athlete training response: Subjective self-reported measures trump commonly used objective measures: A systemic review. *Br. J. Sports Med.* **2016**, *50*, 281–291. [CrossRef] [PubMed]
69. Brancaccio, P.; Lippi, G.; Maffulli, N. Biochemical markers of muscular damage. *Clin. Chem. Lab. Med.* **2010**, *48*, 757–767. [CrossRef]
70. Nieman, D.C.; Pence, B.D. Exercise immunology: Future direction. *J. Sport Health Sci.* **2020**, *9*, 432–445. [CrossRef]
71. Suzuki, K. Cytokine response to exercise and its modulation. *Atioxidants* **2018**, *7*, 17. [CrossRef]
72. Kellmann, M. *Enhancing Recovery: Preventing Underperformance in Athletes*; Human Kinetics: Champaign, IL, USA, 2002.
73. Davis, H.; Orzeck, T.; Keelan, P. Psychometric item evaluations of the recovery-stress questionnaire for athletes. *Psych. Sport Exerc.* **2007**, *8*, 917–938. [CrossRef]
74. Morgan, W.P.; Brow, D.R.; Raglin, J.S.; Oconnor, P.; Cllickson, K.A. Psychological monitoring of overtraining and staleness. *Br. J. Sports Med.* **1987**, *2*, 107–114. [CrossRef]
75. Kenta, G.; Hassmen, P. Overtraining and recovery. A conceptual model. *Sports Med.* **1999**, *26*, 1–16. [CrossRef]
76. Sikorski, E.M.; Wilson, J.M.; Lowery, R.P.; Joy, J.M.; Laurent, S.M.; Hesson, D.; Marshall, A.N.; Averbuch, B.; Gilchrist, P. Changes in perceived recovery status scale following high-volume muscle damaging resistance exercise. *J. Strength Cond. Res.* **2013**, *27*, 2079–2085. [CrossRef] [PubMed]

applied sciences

MDPI

Review

Boost Your Brainpower: 24 Daily Sleep Hacks for Active Lifestyles

Gian Mario Migliaccio [1,2,†], Gloria Di Filippo [3,†], Federica Sancassiani [4], Johnny Padulo [5,‡] and Luca Russo [6,*,‡]

1 Department of Human Sciences and Promotion of the Quality of Life, San Raffaele Rome Open University, 00166 Rome, Italy; gianmario.migliaccio@uniroma5.it
2 Maxima Performa, Athlete Physiology, Psychology and Nutrition Unit, 20126 Milan, Italy
3 Department of Psychology, Niccolò Cusano University, 00166 Rome, Italy; gloria.difilippo@unicusano.it
4 Department of Medical Sciences and Public Health, University of Cagliari, 09124 Cagliari, Italy; federicasancassiani@yahoo.it
5 Department of Biomedical Sciences for Health, Università degli Studi di Milano, 20133 Milan, Italy; johnny.padulo@unimi.it
6 eCampus University, 22060 Novedrate, Italy
* Correspondence: luca.russo2@uniecampus.it
† These authors contributed equally to this work.
‡ These authors contributed equally to this work.

Abstract: Sleep is a fundamental biological process that plays a pivotal role in the health and performance of physically active individuals (PAI). Sleep deprivation or poor sleep quality can negatively impact recovery capacity, concentration, coordination, and muscular strength, thereby compromising physical performance and increasing the risk of injuries. Objectives: This narrative literature review aims to examine the scientific evidence on the importance of sleep hygiene for the health and performance of PAI. A search was conducted for studies published on PubMed, Scopus, and Web of Science. Studies that investigated the effect of sleep hygiene on health and performance variables in athletes were included. The literature analysis highlighted that good sleep hygiene, adequate sleep duration (7–9 h per night), high sleep quality, and a regular sleep routine are associated with a range of benefits for the health and performance of PAI, including: (1) improved post-training recovery; (2) reduced risk of injuries; (3) enhanced concentration and attention; (4) improved coordination and muscle strength; (5) better mood and mental well-being; (6) reduced risk of chronic diseases. Sleep hygiene is a key factor for the health and performance of PAI. Implementing a comprehensive and personalized sleep hygiene routine can lead to significant improvements in the quality and quantity of sleep, with positive effects on physical and mental health, and overall well-being of PAI.

Keywords: sleep hygiene; physical activity; training; health; recovery; injuries; concentration; coordination; muscle strength; mood; mental well-being; chronic diseases

1. Introduction

Achieving high-level international objectives for athletes as well as conducting a physically active everyday life matching work, family, and training for physically active individuals (PAI) require both athletes and PAI to maintain a high standard of recovery, which allows for the maximization of adaptations from the substantial volume of training they undergo [1]. In this context, the role of sleep in maintaining, supporting, and optimizing cognitive and physical performance during and after training sessions is paramount [2]. However, athletes as well as PAI in the most common situation of everyday life are highly susceptible to sleep inadequacies, characterized by habitually short sleep of less than 7 h per night, along with poor sleep quality, primarily due to high fragmentation [3]. A study conducted with professional athletes observed lower sleep quality and sleep hygiene compared to a peer age group, and difficulty falling asleep post-competition [4]. Under this light, sleep hygiene procedures must be considered fundamental. Sleep hygiene encompasses a series of behavioral and environmental practices designed to optimize sleep quality, which can significantly influence athletic performance. Originally developed for the treatment of insomnia, sleep hygiene has found significant applications in the sports context to optimize athletic performance [5]. During sleep hygiene training, PAI can be educated on a series of optimal practices, such as avoiding stimulants, implementing physical exercise routines, and creating a favorable sleep environment [6]. Sleep disorders represent an increasing area of concern in sports and exercise science. In this context, 'disorders' encompass a spectrum of sleep-related disturbances, with the six main ones highlighted as insomnia, circadian rhythm disorders, sleep-related breathing disorders, hypersomnia/narcolepsy, parasomnias, and restless legs syndrome/periodic limb movement disorder [7,8].

However, within athlete and PAI populations, other parameters have been incorporated into the definitions of sleep disorders, including prolonged sleep onset latency, excessive wakefulness after sleep onset, short total sleep time, low sleep efficiency, or poor sleep quality based on subjective and/or objective assessments, which can affect general health, injury risk, and career longevity [9]. Athletes and PAI may suffer from these conditions and might not be aware of them unless they are specifically assessed and enrolled in a sleep hygiene program. Sleep hygiene education is considered an economical and readily accessible lifestyle intervention that can limit sleep deprivation, thereby maximizing performance in the athlete population [6].

The implementation of sleep hygiene practices does not necessarily require direct supervision by a sports medicine physician, potentially increasing its accessibility for physically active individuals (PAI) who may be reluctant to seek medical intervention. Information on sleep hygiene can be easily disseminated through various channels, such as print materials or online platforms. However, it is important to note that PAI with undiagnosed sleep disorders might misuse sleep hygiene practices such as going to sleep late due to training in the late evening or waking up very early in the morning to train or not following the guidelines for correct physical activity [10,11]. In such cases, it is crucial to direct them towards treatments that are more specific.

Sleep deprivation is a widespread issue among PAI, who often fail to achieve the recommended 7–9 h of sleep per night, achieving a lesser amount compared to non-PAI [12]. This trend has been observed across various types of sports, both individual and team, and in both strength and endurance disciplines.

A comprehensive evaluation and expansion of the current evidence base supporting sleep hygiene recommendations in the context of physical exercise are necessary to elucidate their efficacy, particularly considering the different phases of the 24 h cycle: before sleep, during sleep, and after sleep. With a particular focus on application in PAI, this review aims to focus on identifying conceptual and methodological areas for direct implementation into a 24 h cycle routine that fosters behaviors conducive to improving both the quantity and quality of sleep in PAI. This includes specific strategies for each of the three phases, such as relaxation techniques and reducing blue light exposure before sleep, maintaining an optimal sleep environment throughout the night, and waking practices that facilitate the transition from sleep to full activity.

The goal will be reached by examining critically the empirical evidence for the individual components of sleep hygiene recommendations, identifying the issues caused by sleep deprivation, with a particular focus on variations in behaviors and needs related to the three distinct phases of the sleep–wake cycle: the pre-sleep, during-sleep, and post-sleep phases. This literature review aims to identify knowledge gaps in our current understanding of sleep hygiene recommendations within the physical exercise context and propose a structured sleep periodization framework that takes into account the diverse needs related to the three phases of the sleep–wake cycle. This periodized approach aims to optimize physical performance through improved sleep management, adapting sleep hygiene strategies to circadian rhythms and the specific needs of PAI at various stages of their daily routine.

2. Materials and Methods

For the review, we conducted bibliographic searches on PubMed/Medline to identify studies published from 2000 to 2024, using MeSH keywords such as "Sleep Deprivation", "Athletes", "Sleep Hygiene", "Physical Exercise", and "Athletic Performance", along with additional terms like "sleep extension", "sleep quality", "jet lag", and "circadian rhythm", in English, without limitations related to gender or age. We also manually examined the bibliographies of selected articles to verify their relevance. Studies that did not involve athletes or were focused on individuals with sleep-related pathologies, as well as those that did not consider sleep as the main outcome measure or that were animal studies, were excluded from our analysis. The search yielded two hundred and nine studies, of which one hundred and one were deemed relevant and thus subject to further examination. The selected studies presented a great heterogeneity, preventing an aggregated synthesis of the data. Most were small-scale studies with $\leq$20 participants or small cohort groups; hence, a descriptive review was opted for. The PAI in the studies participated in endurance disciplines, strength sports, and activities with combined physiology and were both men and women.

3. Pre-Sleep Phase

The initial phase of sleep is a crucial element for physical performance and can be a significant source of emotional stress for PAI [13,14]. While some individuals among the younger population can fall asleep quickly, with the time required increasing with age from 2 to 20 min [15], PAI may encounter considerable difficulties in reaching the sleep state, taking a significant amount of time to enter the REM phase due to an increase in epinephrine following intense exercise [16]. For PAI, the results demonstrate an increase in slow-wave sleep, a reduction in REM sleep, and a prolonged REM sleep latency, especially pronounced in the first 3 h after sleep onset. These changes in sleep architecture are associated with increased morning energy levels and perceived sleep quality. One proposed mechanism for the delayed REM sleep is increased aminergic neurotransmitter levels and sympathetic activity, supported by the observation that athletes with higher norepinephrine levels exhibited greater REM latency following intense exercise [17]. This issue can generate a negative psychological impact, such as frustration, and have adverse consequences on athletic performance the following day [18].

However, the adoption of specific behavioral precautions and the modification of certain habits can facilitate the process of falling asleep, placing greater emphasis on factors often overlooked [19]. A common mistake is the tendency to underestimate the efficacy of behavioral interventions, opting instead for pharmacological or external solutions [20]. This approach, although it may offer temporary relief, does not address the underlying cause of the problem and can lead to side effects. After the treatment ends, individuals tend to return to their initial state, which is often related to a misalignment between the circadian rhythm and unhealthy lifestyle habits [21].

3.1. Adherence to the Circadian Rhythm

The circadian rhythm, a biological cycle of approximately 24 h, regulates a series of physiological, cognitive, and behavioral changes in the organism [22]. One of the primary functions of this rhythm is to prepare the body for a state conducive to sleep [23]. This state is modulated by the endogenous biological clock, responsible for the secretion of specific hormones that induce states of sleep or wakefulness. Athletes should maintain a consistent sleep schedule by synchronizing their body with the sleep phase, facilitating the achievement of an optimal state of sleep at a predefined time, favored by the correct sleep pressure. However, there is no universal sleep schedule; congruence with one's own chronotype can be assessed through the observation of spontaneous awakening in the absence of external stimuli such as an alarm clock [24].

In the case of a chronotype misalignment, which could compromise daily commitments such as school or work, the most effective strategy is simply to advance the bedtime [25]. Given the rigid structure of social and sporting commitments, the waking time is often fixed; therefore, the only margin for maneuver to align sleep with the chronotype is to modify the bedtime. This can be carried out gradually, by advancing the sleep time by 5–10 min a week [26].

3.2. *Promotion of a Dark Environment*

Ambient lighting has a significant impact on the human circadian rhythm through the activation of specific photoreceptors which transmit signals to the central nervous system via the retina and the optic nerve [27]. These photoreceptors, divided into cones and rods, remain functional regardless of the state of the eyelids [28]. The rods, in particular, exhibit a sensitivity to light up to 4000 times higher than that of the cones, enabling orientation in low-light conditions [29].

The entry of light through the eyelids can generate ambiguous signals to the brain, compromising the regulation of melatonin and sleep, and, consequently, compromising its effectiveness in facilitating sleep [30]. Light exposure, even at low intensities such as 3 lux, can have implications for sleep quality and circadian rhythmicity. Recent human studies have demonstrated that exposure to light at night levels of 5–10 lux during sleep may influence sleep physiology and daytime brain function, with effects on mood and depression susceptibility [31]. Notably, light at night intensities around 3 lux are achievable not only from installed emergency lighting in public spaces but also from display screens of clocks, alarms, televisions, and electronic devices. Therefore, even minimal light sources in the sleeping environment, including electronic displays, can potentially disrupt sleep quality and biological rhythmicity.

These findings underscore the importance of minimizing light exposure during sleep, particularly from artificial sources, to maintain optimal sleep–wake cycles and associated physiological processes. Maintaining a sleep environment that is as dark as possible is therefore crucial to ensure optimal melatonin release.

3.3. *Airplane Mode*

Deactivating electronic devices such as televisions, tablets, and smartphones before nighttime rest is a practice recommended for improving sleep quality [32]. This advice, which might seem like mere parental guidance, is actually supported by robust scientific evidence. Prolonged interaction with tablets or smartphones, exceeding 8 h per day or even just for 30 min before the rest period, can have a negative impact on subsequent sleep [33]. However, simply turning off the device's screen may not be sufficient. It is crucial to place the device at a significant distance from the resting place to optimize sleep quality [34]. For example, it is suggested that electronic devices like televisions should be positioned at least 6 feet (2 m) away from the sleeping area [35]. Merely, activating "airplane mode" may not be adequate; it is more effective to completely turn off the device or place it in silent mode at a reasonable distance from the bed. Even in the case of a device with alerting properties, it can be suggested to position it far from the bed.

3.4. *Limitation of Technology*

The practice of reading can have a positive impact on sleep quality, as long as it is not carried out on electronic devices such as smartphones or tablets [36]. Reading traditional books, preferably under yellow-toned light, can improve sleep quality by up to 22% compared to the sleep quality of non-readers [37]. Additionally, reading in environments with dim lighting can double these benefits. However, it is important to note that the genre of reading can affect sleep quality; individuals who are emotionally reactive to certain stories might experience a delay in falling asleep [38]. E-books without backlighting might have a lesser impact, but the emission of LED lights can alter melatonin secretion, potentially affecting circadian rhythms and cognitive performance [39].

3.5. Training Schedules

It is noteworthy that physical activity, both intense and moderate, has a positive effect on sleep quality [40]. However, for PAI engaging in intense physical activities, it is advisable to conclude workouts at least two hours before sleep to avoid negative interferences with sleep quality [41]. Furthermore, the intense and white lighting typical of sports fields and gyms can inhibit the release of melatonin, further compromising sleep quality [42].

3.6. Stress Reduction

Falling asleep can be hindered by high mental activity, including anxious thoughts and worries [43]. In the prehistoric era, the sympathetic nervous system's response was activated only in the presence of immediate threats, while the hectic pace of modern life and constant exposure to variable stimuli maintain a high chronic activation of the sympathetic system, leading to elevated stress levels and sleep disorders [44]. Mindfulness and meditation techniques have shown potential benefits in improving sleep quality, although the scientific evidence is still limited [45].

3.7. Activation of the Parasympathetic System

For the improvement of sleep quality, breathing directly influences the ease of falling asleep, the reduction in the frequency of nocturnal awakenings, and the optimization of sleep efficiency [46]. These benefits have been observed in subjects, including those suffering from insomnia, who practiced slow and rhythmic breathing exercises for a period of 20 min before sleep [47]. Slow and deep breathing, increasingly supported by scientific evidence, involves a respiratory rate that varies between 4 and 10 breaths per minute (0.07–0.16 Hz), as opposed to the typical 10–20 breaths per minute (0.16–0.33 Hz) of the average human, which can have a close relationship with athletic performance [48].

This breathing mode, when combined with proper sleep hygiene and relaxation techniques, has proven particularly effective in facilitating falling asleep and re-sleeping, quickly synchronizing the heart rate with the respiratory rhythm [49]. Breathing techniques that maintain a rhythm of 0.1 Hz, corresponding to about six breaths per minute, have shown promising results in activating the parasympathetic nervous system, which acts in opposition to the sympathetic system, thereby promoting physical relaxation, better emotional control, and psychological well-being [50].

3.8. Maintenance of Sleep Regularity

The regularity of the circadian rhythm is a crucial element for maintaining quality sleep and, consequently, for overall health [21]. Although our ancestors relied on natural cycles of light and darkness to regulate sleep, modern life has introduced a number of factors that can disrupt this natural rhythm. For example, going to bed at different times each night can cause a form of "social jet-lag", with negative effects on both sleep quality and overall health [51].

This irregular behavior can lead to chronic sleep delay and increased variability, both associated with negative health outcomes; therefore, establishing a regular nighttime routine is imperative.

3.9. Body Weight Management

To optimize sleep quality, body weight and dietary habits can have a significant impact on sleep quality. For instance, a heavy meal consumed shortly before going to bed can disrupt sleep cycles and compromise rest quality [52]. This assertion is supported by research from Crispim et al. (2007), who demonstrated that late-night high-fat meals can negatively impact sleep quality and architecture [53]. Some foods, such as refined carbohydrates, may have a sedative effect but can also cause a glycemic spike, followed by an insulin response and potential nocturnal hunger, which could lead to nighttime awakenings [54].

This effect has been demonstrated in a study by Afaghi et al. (2007), which found that high-glycemic-index carbohydrate meals consumed 4 h before bedtime decreased sleep onset latency [55]. An ideal diet to promote quality sleep should include whole grains, nuts, dairy, fruits, and vegetables [56]. Furthermore, St-Onge et al. (2016) observed that low fiber intake and high saturated fat and sugar intake were associated with lighter, less restorative sleep with more arousals [57]. Additionally, it is important to consider that digesting a meal can take 2 to 3 h, during which sleep may be compromised [58]; Ormsbee et al. (2016) observed that protein consumption 30 min before bedtime increased overnight metabolism, suggesting prolonged digestive activity [59]. Going to bed during the digestion process might cause discomfort or nausea and further slow down digestion [60]. Kinsey and Ormsbee (2015) reviewed the effects of nighttime eating on sleep, appetite, and metabolism, providing further evidence for the complex relationship between late-night eating and sleep quality [61].

3.10. Impact of Music on Sleep Quality

Music has been identified as a non-pharmacological tool for improving sleep quality [62]. Nilsson (2009) observed a significant reduction in cortisol levels in patients listening to relaxing music [63], while Salimpoor et al. (2011) found that pleasurable music triggers dopamine release in the brain [64]. Several studies have demonstrated that music can reduce cortisol levels, the stress hormone, and promote the release of dopamine, a neurotransmitter associated with pleasure [65]. Lai and Li (2011) demonstrated that older adults listening to relaxing music at bedtime for 45 min over 3 weeks showed significant improvements in sleep quality, including longer sleep duration and less sleep disturbance [66]. These effects can contribute to better quality sleep by reducing alertness and enhancing feelings of well-being. Additionally, music can have a calming effect on the autonomic nervous system, leading to slower breathing, a lower heart rate, and reduced blood pressure [67].

There is no unanimous consensus on the type of music most effective for improving sleep quality; however, it has been suggested that selecting tracks with a beats per minute (BPM) between 60 and 80 could be particularly effective as it may synchronize with the resting heart rate [68]. Huang et al. (2016) found that music with a tempo of 60–80 BPM was most effective in reducing anxiety and improving sleep quality in patients [69]. At the same time, it is worth noting that familiar and repetitive music can trigger involuntary musical imagery that worsens sleep quality [70]. Scullin et al. (2021) found that individuals who frequently listen to music are more likely to experience 'earworms' at night, which can interfere with sleep quality [70].

3.11. Bath or Hot Shower

Pre-sleep bathing or showering can positively impact sleep, particularly in athletes [71]. A meta-analysis by Haghayegh et al. (2019) demonstrated that bathing 1–2 h before bedtime in water of 40–42.5 °C significantly improves sleep quality and reduces sleep onset latency [72]. This effect is attributed to heat loss induced by vasodilation [72].

Furthermore, maintaining warm feet during sleep in a cool environment through the use of bed socks has been associated with shortened sleep onset latency, increased total sleep time, and reduced awakenings throughout the night [73,74]. Ko and Lee (2018) found that wearing bed socks significantly enhanced sleep quality and reduced sleep onset time in adults sleeping in cool conditions [73]. A meta-analysis by Jiang et al. (2024) further corroborated that foot thermal therapy can improve various aspects of sleep quality, particularly in older adults [74].

3.12. Melatonin, Herbs, and Tryptophan

Melatonin is known as the "sleep hormone" and has various applications, including in the treatment of jet lag and some sleep disorders [75]. A meta-analysis by Liira et al. (2014)

found that melatonin slightly improves sleep quality, but the evidence is of low quality [76], and the effectiveness of taking exogenous melatonin in shift workers is still a subject of debate [77].

Herbs such as Valerian and Chamomile are often used as sleep aids, but scientific research has not yet provided solid evidence of their effectiveness [78]. The systematic review by Shinjyo et al. (2020) found limited evidence supporting Valerian's efficacy for sleep improvement [78]. Similarly, Hieu et al. (2019) conducted a meta-analysis on Chamomile's effects on sleep quality, showing modest benefits [79].

Other plants like passionflower, lavender, lemon balm, magnolia bark, and ashwagandha have shown potential, but results are mixed [80,81]. Herbal teas, however, have shown positive signs in improving sleep quality [82].

Tryptophan is an essential amino acid that acts as a precursor to serotonin, a neurotransmitter that regulates mood, sleep, and appetite [83]. A deficiency in tryptophan can lead to low levels of serotonin, causing conditions such as depression, anxiety, and insomnia [84]. Tryptophan is involved in the production of serotonin and melatonin, which regulate sleep–wake cycles [85]. Sutanto et al. (2022) conducted a meta-analysis demonstrating that tryptophan supplementation can improve sleep quality, particularly sleep latency and sleep efficiency [86].

To improve sleep quality, it is advisable to follow a diet rich in tryptophan. Foods such as tuna, salmon, chicken, beans, pumpkin seeds, almonds, bananas, yogurt, milk, and cheese are good sources of tryptophan [87]. The absorption of tryptophan is facilitated when consumed with complex carbohydrates [87].

3.13. Avoiding Alcohol

Contrary to popular belief, alcohol is not a good sleep inducer. While it may reduce sleep latency and increase NREM sleep in the first half of the night, in the second half, it suppresses REM sleep, leading to a "REM rebound" with altered dreaming [88–91]. Alcohol abstinence can also disrupt sleep homeostasis, increasing nighttime awakenings [90].

4. During-Sleep Phase

4.1. Environmental Temperature and Sleep

The environmental temperature of the sleeping area can significantly impact sleep quality. The National Sleep Foundation suggests a bedroom temperature of 16–19 °C (60–66 °F) to promote sleep [92]. Lowering body temperature can facilitate sleep induction and minimize energy expenditure [93].

4.2. Sleeping Positions

The position in which one sleeps can affect sleep quality and overall health. The National Sleep Foundation states that sleeping on one's back is generally best for health, but only 8% of people adopt this position [94].

Sleeping on the side is the most common position and can promote better airflow. It is often recommended for people who snore or have sleep-related breathing issues such as obstructive sleep apnea and can also alleviate neck and back pain [95].

Sleeping on the back can be comfortable for some people, especially those with back pain. However, it may intensify snoring and acid reflux [96].

Sleeping on the stomach is less common and can increase pressure on the spine, causing neck and back pain. It can also make breathing more difficult [96].

4.3. Mattress and Pillow

The comfort of the mattress and pillow is crucial for good sleep quality. A medium-firm mattress is generally recommended for comfort and spinal alignment [97]. Regarding pillows, the use of an orthopedic memory foam pillow is suggested to maintain a constant temperature and reduce neck pain related to sleep [98,99].

4.4. Electromagnetic Waves

Environmental electromagnetic fluctuations can affect sleep quality. Devices such as cell phones, Wi-Fi routers, and household appliances are often responsible for electromagnetic fields that can cause sleep disturbances and other health issues [100,101]. Alterations in electromagnetic fields can also affect the circadian rhythm [102].

4.5. Environmental Noise

Noise, especially in urban areas, can have a negative impact on sleep quality. It can cause physiological changes such as variations in heart rate and blood flow [103]. Eliminating environmental noise can improve sleep quality and reduce the latency of sleep onset [104].

4.6. Wearing an Eye Mask or Earplugs

Using an eye mask can have beneficial effects on memory, alertness, and cognitive function the next day even though it does not show immediate effects on sleep itself [105]. The use of earplugs can extend the duration of deep sleep (N3), especially for those who are not bothered by them [106].

4.7. Avoiding Interruptions

Nighttime interruptions leading to fragmentation can be caused by various factors, both physiological and pathological, resulting in increased objective sleepiness, decreased psychomotor performance in tasks involving short-term memory, increased reaction time, or vigilance [107]. For physiological causes, such as the need to drink or eat, it is advisable to regulate water and food intake throughout the day. For instance, limit fluid intake after 19:00 and avoid simple sugars at dinner to prevent glycemic spikes that can induce nocturnal hunger.

5. Post-Sleep Phase

5.1. Watching the Sun

Exposure to sunlight in the morning can have beneficial effects on our sleep–wake cycle by blocking residual melatonin production and activating cortisol [108]. This practice suppresses melatonin production during the day and increases cortisol levels, improving alertness, concentration, and efficiency in daily activities [108,109]. This is particularly useful for those who have experienced sleep deprivation as it helps to regulate the cycle of light and darkness exposure, improving cognitive performance and mood through the production of serotonin [110].

5.2. Not Sleeping during the Day

Avoiding prolonged afternoon sleep is crucial to maintaining a good sleep–wake cycle. A nap of over an hour can negate the "sleep pressure" accumulated during the day, making it difficult to fall asleep the following night and compromising sleep quality [111]. Instead, a "power nap" of about 20 min can provide an ideal balance, improving alertness without negatively affecting nighttime sleep [112]. Elite athletes show significantly shorter sleep latencies, suggesting that napping behavior may reflect the ability to fall asleep on demand rather than drowsiness resulting from sports-related sleep debts [111].

5.3. Engaging in Physical Exercise

Physical exercise is a powerful ally in improving sleep quality. Not only does it help reduce stress and anxiety, but it also contributes to regulating melatonin levels, the hormone that promotes sleep. Although not apparently specific for athletes, consistent activity of about 60 min four or five times a week has been shown to be effective even for patients with insomnia [113,114].

5.4. Limiting Caffeine

Caffeine is a stimulant that can interfere with sleep up to 8.8 h after consumption. To avoid sleep problems, it is recommended not to consume caffeine after 14:00–14.30 if going to bed at 23:00 [115]. Anyway, caffeine-sensitive people might need to discontinue caffeine consumption any time after noon.

6. Discussion

The literature review underlines that adherence to specific recommendations across the three phases of the sleep–wake cycle—the pre-sleep, during-sleep, and post-sleep phases—can significantly enhance both sleep quality and quantity. These improvements are associated with positive outcomes in the athletic performance, physical and mental health, and overall well-being of physically active individuals (PAI).

The pre-sleep phase involves several critical strategies for optimizing sleep conditions. Maintaining consistent sleep schedules aligns circadian rhythms with environmental cues, facilitating sleep initiation and quality enhancement. Minimizing exposure to blue light emissions from electronic devices and reducing technology use before bedtime are crucial for promoting melatonin production and sleep induction. Stress management techniques, including mindfulness, meditation, and controlled breathing exercises, are recommended to facilitate the transition to sleep. Furthermore, engaging in non-stimulating activities, such as reading physical books and listening to calming music, in conjunction with avoiding intense physical exercise proximal to bedtime, can contribute to improved sleep onset. Dietary considerations, weight management, and the judicious use of aromatherapy or supplements (e.g., melatonin and specific herbs) may also be beneficial, albeit under appropriate medical supervision.

The sleep environment is a critical factor in sleep quality. Optimal bedroom temperature (cool) and comfortable sleeping arrangements, including medium-firm mattresses and appropriate pillows, are essential for minimizing discomfort and pain. Reduction of electromagnetic exposure and environmental noise, coupled with the use of sleep aids such as eye masks and earplugs, can significantly enhance sleep quality by mitigating disturbances.

Post-sleep behaviors also play a crucial role in regulating sleep patterns and overall health. Morning exposure to natural light assists in resetting the circadian rhythm, while nutritious breakfast consumption and adequate hydration throughout the day support energy levels and improve subsequent sleep quality. Consistent physical activity during daytime hours further promotes both daytime alertness and nighttime sleep readiness.

In summary, our findings underscore the importance of comprehensive management of the sleep environment and sleep hygiene behaviors in optimizing the restorative effects of sleep, thereby enhancing physical readiness and performance. While this review primarily addresses physically active individuals, it is noteworthy that these practices may be beneficial for both sedentary and active adults. Finally, it is important to acknowledge that, in cases of severe or persistent sleep disturbances, a multifaceted approach incorporating pharmacological interventions, such as benzodiazepines, may be warranted [91]. However, a comprehensive discussion of pharmacological treatments is beyond the scope of this review.

7. Limitation

We acknowledge several limitations in our review. While the suggestions we have reported are applicable to a healthy population and athletes, we cannot definitively demonstrate that they can improve performance. This is an objective that future studies will need to address. We also found that the available data were not always able to provide answers that could demonstrate differences by sex and age. We recognize that a subsequent meta-analysis will be necessary to establish greater scientific consistency on this topic, and can also collect hygiene rules extended to 24 h. It is important to note that we found that the scientific consistency regarding athletic performance for many of the provided suggestions is currently lacking.

8. Conclusions

Despite these limitations, we believe our comprehensive literature review on evidence-based protocols for sleep hygiene provides valuable insights for both athletes and the general population. The hygiene rules and suggestions we have outlined are based on current scientific evidence and offer a solid foundation for improving sleep quality. While the direct link to athletic performance enhancement requires further investigation, we emphasize the importance of good sleep hygiene for overall health and well-being. We intend this review to serve as a reference point for healthy individuals seeking to optimize their sleep patterns and potentially support their athletic endeavors. We suggest that future research should focus on addressing the identified gaps, particularly regarding age and gender differences, and establishing more concrete connections between sleep hygiene practices and athletic performance.

Author Contributions: Conceptualization, G.M.M.; methodology, L.R., G.D.F. and F.S.; software, J.P.; validation, G.M.M., J.P. and L.R.; formal analysis, L.R.; investigation, G.M.M.; resources, J.P.; data curation, L.R.; writing—original draft preparation, G.M.M., G.D.F. and F.S.; writing—review and editing, L.R.; visualization, G.M.M.; supervision, J.P.; project administration, G.M.M., J.P. and L.R. All authors have read and agreed to the published version of the manuscript.

Funding: This research received no external funding.

Conflicts of Interest: The authors declare no conflicts of interest.

References

1. Malhotra, R.K. Sleep, Recovery, and Performance in Sports. *Neurol. Clin.* **2017**, *35*, 547–557. [CrossRef] [PubMed]
2. Samuels, C. Sleep, Recovery, and Performance: The New Frontier in High-Performance Athletics. *Phys. Med. Rehabil. Clin. N. Am.* **2009**, *20*, 149–159. [CrossRef] [PubMed]
3. Walsh, N.P.; Halson, S.L.; Sargent, C.; Roach, G.D.; Nédélec, M.; Gupta, L.; Leeder, J.; Fullagar, H.H.; Coutts, A.J.; Edwards, B.J.; et al. Sleep and the athlete: Narrative review and 2021 expert consensus recommendations. *Br. J. Sports Med.* **2021**, *55*, 356–368. [CrossRef]
4. Cameron, A.F.M.; Perera, N.; Fulcher, M. Professional Athletes Have Poorer Sleep Quality and Sleep Hygiene Compared with an Age-Matched Cohort. *Clin. J. Sport Med.* **2021**, *31*, 488–493. [CrossRef] [PubMed]
5. Cunha, L.A.; Costa, J.A.; Marques, E.A.; Brito, J.; Lastella, M.; Figueiredo, P. The Impact of Sleep Interventions on Athletic Performance: A Systematic Review. *Sports Med. Open* **2023**, *9*, 58. [CrossRef]
6. Vitale, K.C.; Owens, R.; Hopkins, S.R.; Malhotra, A. Sleep Hygiene for Optimizing Recovery in Athletes: Review and Recommendations. *Int. J. Sports Med.* **2019**, *40*, 535–543. [CrossRef]
7. Chaiard, J.; Weaver, T.E. Update on Research and Practices in Major Sleep Disorders: Part I. Obstructive Sleep Apnea Syndrome. *J. Nurs. Sch.* **2019**, *51*, 500–508. [CrossRef] [PubMed]
8. Chaiard, J.; Weaver, T.E. Update on Research and Practices in Major Sleep Disorders: Part II—Insomnia, Willis-Ekbom Disease (Restless Leg Syndrome), and Narcolepsy. *J. Nurs. Sch.* **2019**, *51*, 624–633. [CrossRef] [PubMed]
9. Creado, S.A.; Advani, S. Sleep Disorders in the Athlete. *Psychiatr. Clin. N. Am.* **2021**, *44*, 393–403. [CrossRef]
10. Chennaoui, M.; Arnal, P.J.; Sauvet, F.; Léger, D. Sleep and exercise: A reciprocal issue? *Sleep Med. Rev.* **2015**, *20*, 59–72. [CrossRef] [PubMed]
11. Bull, F.C.; Al-Ansari, S.S.; Biddle, S.; Borodulin, K.; Buman, M.P.; Cardon, G.; Carty, C.; Chaput, J.-P.; Chastin, S.; Chou, R.; et al. World Health Organization 2020 guidelines on physical activity and sedentary behaviour. *Br. J. Sports Med.* **2020**, *54*, 1451–1462. [CrossRef] [PubMed]
12. Abrams, R.M. Sleep Deprivation. *Obstet. Gynecol. Clin. N. Am.* **2015**, *42*, 493–506. [CrossRef]
13. Nédélec, M.; Halson, S.; Abaidia, A.-E.; Ahmaidi, S.; Dupont, G. Stress, Sleep and Recovery in Elite Soccer: A Critical Review of the Literature. *Sports Med.* **2015**, *45*, 1387–1400. [CrossRef] [PubMed]
14. Walters, P.H. Sleep, the athlete, and performance. *Strength Cond. J.* **2002**, *24*, 17–24. [CrossRef]
15. Monk, T.H.; Buysse, D.J.; Rose, L.R.; Hall, J.A.; Kupfer, D.J. The sleep of healthy people—A diary study. *Chronobiol. Int.* **2000**, *17*, 49–60. [CrossRef] [PubMed]
16. Netzer, N.C.; Kristo, D.; Steinle, H.; Lehmann, M.; Strohl, K.P. REM sleep and catecholamine excretion: A study in elite athletes. *Eur. J. Appl. Physiol.* **2001**, *84*, 521–526. [CrossRef] [PubMed]
17. Zapalac, K.; Miller, M.; Champagne, F.A.; Schnyer, D.M.; Baird, B. The effects of physical activity on sleep architecture and mood in naturalistic environments. *Sci. Rep.* **2024**, *14*, 5637. [CrossRef] [PubMed]

18. Bonnar, D.; Bartel, K.; Kakoschke, N.; Lang, C. Sleep Interventions Designed to Improve Athletic Performance and Recovery: A Systematic Review of Current Approaches. *Sports Med.* **2018**, *48*, 683–703. [CrossRef] [PubMed]
19. Bird, S.P. Sleep, Recovery, and Athletic Performance. *Strength Cond. J.* **2013**, *35*, 43–47. [CrossRef]
20. Tamrat, R.; Huynh-Le, M.-P.; Goyal, M. Non-Pharmacologic Interventions to Improve the Sleep of Hospitalized Patients: A Systematic Review. *J. Gen. Intern. Med.* **2014**, *29*, 788–795. [CrossRef] [PubMed]
21. Baron, K.G.; Reid, K.J. Circadian misalignment and health. *Int. Rev. Psychiatry* **2014**, *26*, 139–154. [CrossRef] [PubMed]
22. Vitaterna, M.H.; Takahashi, J.S.; Turek, F.W. Overview of Circadian Rhythms. *Alcohol Res. Health* **2001**, *25*, 85. [PubMed] [PubMed Central]
23. Adan, A.; Archer, S.N.; Hidalgo, M.P.; di Milia, L.; Natale, V.; Randler, C. Circadian Typology: A Comprehensive Review. *Chronobiol. Int.* **2012**, *29*, 1153–1175. [CrossRef] [PubMed]
24. Hirshkowitz, M. Normal human sleep: An overview. *Med. Clin. N. Am.* **2004**, *88*, 551–565. [CrossRef] [PubMed]
25. Montaruli, A.; Castelli, L.; Mulè, A.; Scurati, R.; Esposito, F.; Galasso, L.; Roveda, E. Biological Rhythm and Chronotype: New Perspectives in Health. *Biomolecules* **2021**, *11*, 487. [CrossRef] [PubMed]
26. Roenneberg, T.; Wirz-Justice, A.; Merrow, M. Life between Clocks: Daily Temporal Patterns of Human Chronotypes. *J. Biol. Rhythm.* **2003**, *18*, 80–90. [CrossRef] [PubMed]
27. Moore, R.Y. Suprachiasmatic nucleus in sleep–wake regulation. *Sleep Med.* **2007**, *8* (Suppl. 3), 27–33. [CrossRef] [PubMed]
28. Molday, R.S.; Moritz, O.L. Photoreceptors at a glance. *J. Cell Sci.* **2015**, *128*, 4039–4045. [CrossRef] [PubMed]
29. Ingram, N.T.; Sampath, A.P.; Fain, G.L. Why are rods more sensitive than cones? *J. Physiol.* **2016**, *594*, 5415–5426. [CrossRef] [PubMed]
30. Kozaki, T.; Kubokawa, A.; Taketomi, R.; Hatae, K. Effects of day-time exposure to different light intensities on light-induced melatonin suppression at night. *J. Physiol. Anthropol.* **2015**, *34*, 27. [CrossRef]
31. Obayashi, K.; Saeki, K.; Kurumatani, N. Bedroom Light Exposure at Night and the Incidence of Depressive Symptoms: A Longitudinal Study of the HEIJO-KYO Cohort. *Am. J. Epidemiol.* **2017**, *187*, 427–434. [CrossRef] [PubMed]
32. Chinoy, E.D.; Duffy, J.F.; Czeisler, C.A. Unrestricted evening use of light-emitting tablet computers delays self-selected bedtime and disrupts circadian timing and alertness. *Physiol. Rep.* **2018**, *6*, e13692. [CrossRef] [PubMed]
33. Christensen, M.A.; Bettencourt, L.; Kaye, L.; Moturu, S.T.; Nguyen, K.T.; Olgin, J.E.; Pletcher, M.J.; Marcus, G.M. Direct Measurements of Smartphone Screen-Time: Relationships with Demographics and Sleep. *PLoS ONE* **2016**, *11*, e0165331. [CrossRef] [PubMed]
34. Carter, B.; Rees, P.; Hale, L.; Bhattacharjee, D.; Paradkar, M.S. Association Between Portable Screen-Based Media Device Access or Use and Sleep Outcomes. *JAMA Pediatr.* **2016**, *170*, 1202–1208. [CrossRef] [PubMed]
35. Pigeon, W.R. Creating otpimal sleep and circadian rhythm environment. In *Encyclopedia of Sleep and Circadian Rhythms*, 2nd ed.; Elsevier: Amsterdam, The Netherlands, 2023; pp. 95–101. [CrossRef]
36. Grønli, J.; Byrkjedal, I.K.; Bjorvatn, B.; Nødtvedt, Ø.; Hamre, B.; Pallesen, S. Reading from an iPad or from a book in bed: The impact on human sleep. A randomized controlled crossover trial. *Sleep Med.* **2016**, *21*, 86–92. [CrossRef] [PubMed]
37. Finucane, E.; O'brien, A.; Treweek, S.; Newell, J.; Das, K.; Chapman, S.; Wicks, P.; Galvin, S.; Healy, P.; Biesty, L.; et al. Does reading a book in bed make a difference to sleep in comparison to not reading a book in bed? The People's Trial—An online, pragmatic, randomised trial. *Trials* **2021**, *22*, 873. [CrossRef] [PubMed]
38. Sella, E.; Palumbo, R.; di Domenico, A.; Borella, E. How emotions induced by reading influence sleep quality in young and older adults. *Aging Ment. Health* **2023**, *27*, 1812–1820. [CrossRef] [PubMed]
39. Cajochen, C.; Frey, S.; Anders, D.; Späti, J.; Bues, M.; Pross, A.; Mager, R.; Wirz-Justice, A.; Stefani, O. Evening exposure to a light-emitting diodes (LED)-backlit computer screen affects circadian physiology and cognitive performance. *J. Appl. Physiol.* **2011**, *110*, 1432–1438. [CrossRef] [PubMed]
40. Vanderlinden, J.; Boen, F.; van Uffelen, J.G.Z. Effects of physical activity programs on sleep outcomes in older adults: A systematic review. *Int. J. Behav. Nutr. Phys. Act.* **2020**, *17*, 11. [CrossRef] [PubMed]
41. Kredlow, M.A.; Capozzoli, M.C.; Hearon, B.A.; Calkins, A.W.; Otto, M.W. The effects of physical activity on sleep: A meta-analytic review. *J. Behav. Med.* **2015**, *38*, 427–449. [CrossRef] [PubMed]
42. Gooley, J.J.; Chamberlain, K.; Smith, K.A.; Khalsa, S.B.S.; Rajaratnam, S.M.W.; van Reen, E.; Zeitzer, J.M.; Czeisler, C.A.; Lockley, S.W. Exposure to room light before bedtime suppresses melatonin onset and shortens melatonin duration in humans. *J. Clin. Endocrinol. Metab.* **2011**, *96*, E463–E472. [CrossRef] [PubMed]
43. Harvey, A. A cognitive model of insomnia. *Behav. Res. Ther.* **2002**, *40*, 869–893. [CrossRef] [PubMed]
44. Miki, K.; Yoshimoto, M. Sympathetic nerve activity during sleep, exercise, and mental stress. *Auton. Neurosci.* **2013**, *174*, 15–20. [CrossRef] [PubMed]
45. Rusch, H.L.; Rosario, M.; Levison, L.M.; Olivera, A.; Livingston, W.S.; Wu, T.; Gill, J.M. The effect of mindfulness meditation on sleep quality: A systematic review and meta-analysis of randomized controlled trials. *Ann. N. Y. Acad. Sci.* **2019**, *1445*, 5–16. [CrossRef] [PubMed]
46. Tsai, H.J.; Kuo, T.B.J.; Lee, G.; Yang, C.C.H. Efficacy of paced breathing for insomnia: Enhances vagal activity and improves sleep quality. *Psychophysiology* **2015**, *52*, 388–396. [CrossRef] [PubMed]
47. Laborde, S.; Hosang, T.; Mosley, E.; Dosseville, F. Influence of a 30-Day Slow-Paced Breathing Intervention Compared to Social Media Use on Subjective Sleep Quality and Cardiac Vagal Activity. *J. Clin. Med.* **2019**, *8*, 193. [CrossRef]

48. Migliaccio, G.M.; Russo, L.; Maric, M.; Padulo, J. Sports Performance and Breathing Rate: What Is the Connection? A Narrative Review on Breathing Strategies. *Sports* **2023**, *11*, 103. [CrossRef] [PubMed]
49. Zaccaro, A.; Piarulli, A.; Laurino, M.; Garbella, E.; Menicucci, D.; Neri, B.; Gemignani, A. How Breath-Control Can Change Your Life: A Systematic Review on Psycho-Physiological Correlates of Slow Breathing. *Front. Hum. Neurosci.* **2018**, *12*, 353. [CrossRef] [PubMed]
50. Noble, D.J.; Hochman, S. Hypothesis: Pulmonary Afferent Activity Patterns during Slow, Deep Breathing Contribute to the Neural Induction of Physiological Relaxation. *Front. Physiol.* **2019**, *10*, 468017. [CrossRef] [PubMed]
51. Feliciano, E.M.C.; Rifas-Shiman, S.L.; Quante, M.; Redline, S.; Oken, E.; Taveras, E.M. Chronotype, Social Jet Lag, and Cardiometabolic Risk Factors in Early Adolescence. *JAMA Pediatr.* **2019**, *173*, 1049–1057. [CrossRef] [PubMed]
52. Blumfield, M.L.; Bei, B.; Zimberg, I.Z.; Cain, S.W. Dietary disinhibition mediates the relationship between poor sleep quality and body weight. *Appetite* **2018**, *120*, 602–608. [CrossRef] [PubMed]
53. Crispim, C.A.; Zalcman, I.; Dáttilo, M.; Padilha, H.G.; Edwards, B.; Waterhouse, J.; Tufik, S.; de Mello, M.T. The influence of sleep and sleep loss upon food intake and metabolism. *Nutr. Res. Rev.* **2007**, *20*, 195–212. [CrossRef] [PubMed]
54. Roberts, S.; Desbrow, B.; Grant, G.; Anoopkumar-Dukie, S.; Leveritt, M. Glycemic response to carbohydrate and the effects of exercise and protein. *Nutrition* **2013**, *29*, 881–885. [CrossRef] [PubMed]
55. Afaghi, A.; O'Connor, H.; Chow, C.M. High-glycemic-index carbohydrate meals shorten sleep onset. *Am. J. Clin. Nutr.* **2007**, *85*, 426–430. [CrossRef] [PubMed]
56. Godos, J.; Grosso, G.; Castellano, S.; Galvano, F.; Caraci, F.; Ferri, R. Association between diet and sleep quality: A systematic review. *Sleep Med. Rev.* **2021**, *57*, 101430. [CrossRef] [PubMed]
57. St-Onge, M.-P.; Roberts, A.; Shechter, A.; Choudhury, A.R. Fiber and Saturated Fat Are Associated with Sleep Arousals and Slow Wave Sleep. *J. Clin. Sleep Med.* **2016**, *12*, 19–24. [CrossRef]
58. Kim, S.; DeRoo, L.A.; Sandler, D.P. Eating patterns and nutritional characteristics associated with sleep duration. *Public Health Nutr.* **2011**, *14*, 889–895. [CrossRef]
59. Ormsbee, M.J.; Gorman, K.A.; Miller, E.A.; Baur, D.A.; Eckel, L.A.; Contreras, R.J.; Panton, L.B.; Spicer, M.T. Nighttime feeding likely alters morning metabolism but not exercise performance in female athletes. *Appl. Physiol. Nutr. Metab.* **2016**, *41*, 719–727. [CrossRef] [PubMed]
60. Uçar, C.; Özgöçer, T.; Yıldız, S. Effects of late-night eating of easily—Or slowly—Digestible meals on sleep, hypothalamo-pituitary-adrenal axis, and autonomic nervous system in healthy young males. *Stress Health* **2021**, *37*, 640–649. [CrossRef] [PubMed]
61. Kinsey, A.W.; Ormsbee, M.J. The Health Impact of Nighttime Eating: Old and New Perspectives. *Nutrients* **2015**, *7*, 2648–2662. [CrossRef] [PubMed]
62. Wang, C.-F.; Sun, Y.-L.; Zang, H.-X. Music therapy improves sleep quality in acute and chronic sleep disorders: A meta-analysis of 10 randomized studies. *Int. J. Nurs. Stud.* **2014**, *51*, 51–62. [CrossRef]
63. Nilsson, U. Soothing music can increase oxytocin levels during bed rest after open-heart surgery: A randomised control trial. *J. Clin. Nurs.* **2009**, *18*, 2153–2161. [CrossRef] [PubMed]
64. Salimpoor, V.N.; Benovoy, M.; Larcher, K.; Dagher, A.; Zatorre, R.J. Anatomically distinct dopamine release during anticipation and experience of peak emotion to music. *Nat. Neurosci.* **2011**, *14*, 257–262. [CrossRef] [PubMed]
65. Moraes, M.M.; Rabelo, P.C.; Pinto, V.A.; Pires, W.; Wanner, S.P.; Szawka, R.E.; Soares, D.D. Auditory stimulation by exposure to melodic music increases dopamine and serotonin activities in rat forebrain areas linked to reward and motor control. *Neurosci. Lett.* **2018**, *673*, 73–78. [CrossRef]
66. Lai, H.-L.; Li, Y.-M. The effect of music on biochemical markers and self-perceived stress among first-line nurses: A randomized controlled crossover trial. *J. Adv. Nurs.* **2011**, *67*, 2414–2424. [CrossRef] [PubMed]
67. Ellis, R.J.; Thayer, J.F. Music and Autonomic Nervous System (Dys)Function. *Music Percept.* **2010**, *27*, 317–326. [CrossRef] [PubMed]
68. Cordi, M.J.; Ackermann, S.; Rasch, B. Effects of Relaxing Music on Healthy Sleep. *Sci. Rep.* **2019**, *9*, 9079. [CrossRef] [PubMed]
69. Huang, C.-Y.; Chang, E.-T.; Lai, H.-L. Comparing the effects of music and exercise with music for older adults with insomnia. *Appl. Nurs. Res.* **2016**, *32*, 104–110. [CrossRef] [PubMed]
70. Scullin, M.K.; Gao, C.; Fillmore, P. Bedtime Music, Involuntary Musical Imagery, and Sleep. *Psychol. Sci.* **2021**, *32*, 985–997. [CrossRef] [PubMed]
71. Tai, Y.; Obayashi, K.; Yamagami, Y.; Yoshimoto, K.; Kurumatani, N.; Nishio, K.; Saeki, K. Hot-water bathing before bedtime and shorter sleep onset latency are accompanied by a higher distal-proximal skin temperature gradient in older adults. *J. Clin. Sleep Med.* **2021**, *17*, 1257–1266. [CrossRef] [PubMed]
72. Haghayegh, S.; Khoshnevis, S.; Smolensky, M.H.; Diller, K.R.; Castriotta, R.J. Before-bedtime passive body heating by warm shower or bath to improve sleep: A systematic review and meta-analysis. *Sleep Med. Rev.* **2019**, *46*, 124–135. [CrossRef] [PubMed]
73. Ko, Y.; Lee, J.-Y. Effects of feet warming using bed socks on sleep quality and thermoregulatory responses in a cool environment. *J. Physiol. Anthr.* **2018**, *37*, 13. [CrossRef] [PubMed]
74. Jiang, C.-S.; Chen, K.-M.; Belcastro, F. Effects of Temperature, Duration, and Heating Height of Foot Thermal Therapy on Sleep Quality of Older Adults: A Systematic Review and Meta-Analysis. *J. Integr. Complement. Med.* **2024**, *30*, 250–260. [CrossRef] [PubMed]

75. Claustrat, B.; Leston, J. Melatonin: Physiological effects in humans. *Neurochirurgie* **2015**, *61*, 77–84. [CrossRef] [PubMed]
76. Liira, J.; Verbeek, J.H.; Costa, G.; Driscoll, T.R.; Sallinen, M.; Isotalo, L.K.; Ruotsalainen, J.H. Pharmacological Interventions for Sleepiness and Sleep Disturbances Caused by Shift Work. *Cochrane Database Syst. Rev.* **2014**, *8*, CD009776. [CrossRef] [PubMed]
77. Pereira, N.; Naufel, M.F.; Ribeiro, E.B.; Tufik, S.; Hachul, H. Influence of Dietary Sources of Melatonin on Sleep Quality: A Review. *J. Food Sci.* **2020**, *85*, 5–13. [CrossRef] [PubMed]
78. Shinjyo, N.; Waddell, G.; Green, J. Valerian Root in Treating Sleep Problems and Associated Disorders—A Systematic Review and Meta-Analysis. *J. Evid. Based Integr. Med.* **2020**, *25*, 2515690X20967323. [CrossRef] [PubMed]
79. Hieu, T.H.; Dibas, M.; Dila, K.A.S.; Sherif, N.A.; Hashmi, M.U.; Mahmoud, M.; Trang, N.T.T.; Abdullah, L.; Nghia, T.L.B.; Y, M.N.; et al. Therapeutic efficacy and safety of chamomile for state anxiety, generalized anxiety disorder, insomnia, and sleep quality: A systematic review and meta-analysis of randomized trials and quasi-randomized trials. *Phytother. Res.* **2019**, *33*, 1604–1615. [CrossRef] [PubMed]
80. Borrás, S.; Martínez-Solís, I.; Ríos, J.L. Medicinal Plants for Insomnia Related to Anxiety: An Updated Review. *Planta Med.* **2021**, *87*, 738–753. [CrossRef]
81. Guadagna, S.; Barattini, D.F.; Rosu, S.; Ferini-Strambi, L. Plant Extracts for Sleep Disturbances: A Systematic Review. *Evid. Based Complement. Altern. Med.* **2020**, *2020*, 3792390. [CrossRef] [PubMed]
82. Baek, Y.; Kim, H.; Mun, S.; Lee, S. Three-Component Herbal Tea Alleviates Prolonged Fatigue and Improves Sleep Quality: A Randomized Controlled Pilot Study. *Explore* **2018**, *14*, 420–423. [CrossRef] [PubMed]
83. Kikuchi, A.M.; Tanabe, A.; Iwahori, Y. A systematic review of the effect of L-tryptophan supplementation on mood and emotional functioning. *J. Diet. Suppl.* **2021**, *18*, 316–333. [CrossRef] [PubMed]
84. Jenkins, T.A.; Nguyen, J.C.D.; Polglaze, K.E.; Bertrand, P.P. Influence of Tryptophan and Serotonin on Mood and Cognition with a Possible Role of the Gut-Brain Axis. *Nutrients* **2016**, *8*, 56. [CrossRef] [PubMed]
85. Zagajewski, J.; Drozdowicz, D.; Brzozowska, I.; Hubalewska-Mazgaj, M.; Stelmaszynska, T.; Laidler, P.M.; Brzozowski, T. Conversion L-tryptophan to melatonin in the gastrointestinal tract: The new high performance liquid chromatography method enabling simultaneous determination of six metabolites of L-tryptophan by native fluorescence and UV-VIS detection. *J. Physiol. Pharmacol.* **2012**, *63*, 613–621. [PubMed]
86. Sutanto, C.; Loh, W.W.; Kim, J.E. The Impact of Tryptophan Supplementation on Sleep Quality: A Systematic Review, Meta-Analysis and Meta-Regression. *Nutr. Rev.* **2022**, *80*, 306–316. [CrossRef] [PubMed]
87. Bourre, J.M. Effects of nutrients (in food) on the structure and function of the nervous system: Update on dietary requirements for brain. Part 2: Macronutrients. *J. Nutr. Health Aging* **2006**, *10*, 376.
88. Kleitman, N. *Sleep and Wakefulness*; University of Chicago Press: Chicago, IL, USA, 1939.
89. Ebrahim, I.O.; Shapiro, C.M.; Williams, A.J.; Fenwick, P.B. Alcohol and Sleep I: Effects on Normal Sleep. *Alcohol. Clin. Exp. Res.* **2013**, *37*, 539–549. [CrossRef] [PubMed]
90. Thakkar, M.M.; Sharma, R.; Sahota, P. Alcohol disrupts sleep homeostasis. *Alcohol* **2015**, *49*, 299–310. [CrossRef] [PubMed]
91. Silva, A.S.M.; de Mendonça, F.M.R.; de Mendonça, G.P.R.R.; Souza, L.C.; Galvão, L.P.; Paiva, H.S.; Périco, C.d.A.M.; Torales, J.; Ventriglio, A.; Castaldelli-Maia, J.M. Benzodiazepines and Sleep Architecture: A Systematic Review. *CNS Neurol. Disord. Drug Targets* **2023**, *22*, 172–179. [CrossRef] [PubMed]
92. Harding, E.C.; Franks, N.P.; Wisden, W. Sleep and thermoregulation. *Curr. Opin. Physiol.* **2019**, *15*, 7–13. [CrossRef] [PubMed]
93. Basner, M.; Smith, M.G.; Jones, C.W.; Ecker, A.J.; Howard, K.; Schneller, V.; Cordoza, M.; Kaizi-Lutu, M.; Park-Chavar, S.; Stahn, A.C.; et al. Associations of bedroom PM2.5, CO2, temperature, humidity, and noise with sleep: An observational actigraphy study. *Sleep Health* **2023**, *9*, 253–263. [CrossRef] [PubMed]
94. Ohayon, M.; Wickwire, E.M.; Hirshkowitz, M.; Albert, S.M.; Avidan, A.; Daly, F.J.; Dauvilliers, Y.; Ferri, R.; Fung, C.; Gozal, D.; et al. National Sleep Foundation's sleep quality recommendations: First report. *Sleep Health* **2017**, *3*, 6–19. [CrossRef] [PubMed]
95. Cary, D.; Briffa, K.; McKenna, L. Identifying relationships between sleep posture and non-specific spinal symptoms in adults: A scoping review. *BMJ Open* **2019**, *9*, e027633. [CrossRef] [PubMed]
96. Skarpsno, E.S.; Mork, P.J.; Nilsen, T.I.L.; Holtermann, A. Sleep positions and nocturnal body movements based on free-living accelerometer recordings: Association with demographics, lifestyle, and insomnia symptoms. *Nat. Sci. Sleep* **2017**, *9*, 267–275. [CrossRef] [PubMed]
97. Caggiari, G.; Talesa, G.R.; Toro, G.; Jannelli, E.; Monteleone, G.; Puddu, L. What type of mattress should be chosen to avoid back pain and improve sleep quality? Review of the literature. *J. Orthop. Traumatol.* **2021**, *22*, 51. [CrossRef] [PubMed]
98. Gordon, S.J.; Grimmer-Somers, K.; Trott, P. Pillow use: The behaviour of cervical pain, sleep quality and pillow comfort in side sleepers. *Man. Ther.* **2009**, *14*, 671–678. [CrossRef] [PubMed]
99. Jeon, M.Y.; Jeong, H.; Lee, S.; Choi, W.; Park, J.H.; Tak, S.J.; Choi, D.H.; Yim, J. Improving the Quality of Sleep with an Optimal Pillow: A Randomized, Comparative Study. *Tohoku J. Exp. Med.* **2014**, *233*, 183–188. [CrossRef] [PubMed]
100. Chen, S.-H.; Chin, W.-C.; Huang, Y.-S.; Chuech, L.S.; Lin, C.-M.; Lee, C.-P.; Lin, H.-L.; Tang, I.; Yeh, T.-C. The effect of electromagnetic field on sleep of patients with nocturia. *Medicine* **2022**, *101*, e29129. [CrossRef] [PubMed]
101. Dieudonné, M. Electromagnetic hypersensitivity: A critical review of explanatory hypotheses. *Environ. Health* **2020**, *19*, 48. [CrossRef] [PubMed]
102. Martel, J.; Chang, S.-H.; Chevalier, G.; Ojcius, D.M.; Young, J.D. Influence of electromagnetic fields on the circadian rhythm: Implications for human health and disease. *Biomed. J.* **2023**, *46*, 48–59. [CrossRef] [PubMed]

103. Kawada, T. Noise and Health—Sleep Disturbance in Adults. *J. Occup. Health* **2011**, *53*, 413–416. [CrossRef] [PubMed]
104. Muzet, A. Environmental noise, sleep and health. *Sleep Med. Rev.* **2007**, *11*, 135–142. [CrossRef] [PubMed]
105. Greco, V.; Bergamo, D.; Cuoccio, P.; Konkoly, K.R.; Lombardo, K.M.; Lewis, P.A. Wearing an eye mask during overnight sleep improves episodic learning and alertness. *Sleep* **2023**, *46*, zsac305. [CrossRef] [PubMed]
106. Demoule, A.; Carreira, S.; Lavault, S.; Pallanca, O.; Morawiec, E.; Mayaux, J.; Arnulf, I.; Similowski, T. Impact of earplugs and eye mask on sleep in critically ill patients: A prospective randomized study. *Crit. Care* **2017**, *21*, 284. [CrossRef] [PubMed]
107. Bonnet, M.H.; Arand, D.L. Clinical effects of sleep fragmentation versus sleep deprivation. *Sleep Med. Rev.* **2003**, *7*, 297–310. [CrossRef] [PubMed]
108. Leproult, R.; Colecchia, E.F.; L'hermite-Balériaux, M.; van Cauter, E. Transition from Dim to Bright Light in the Morning Induces an Immediate Elevation of Cortisol Levels. *J. Clin. Endocrinol. Metab.* **2001**, *86*, 151–157. [CrossRef] [PubMed]
109. Ostrin, L.A. Ocular and systemic melatonin and the influence of light exposure. *Clin. Exp. Optom.* **2018**, *102*, 99–108. [CrossRef] [PubMed]
110. Gabel, V.; Maire, M.; Reichert, C.F.; Chellappa, S.L.; Schmidt, C.; Hommes, V.; Viola, A.U.; Cajochen, C. Effects of Artificial Dawn and Morning Blue Light on Daytime Cognitive Performance, Well-being, Cortisol and Melatonin Levels. *Chronobiol. Int.* **2013**, *30*, 988–997. [CrossRef] [PubMed]
111. Gupta, L.; Morgan, K.; North, C.; Gilchrist, S. Napping in high-performance athletes: Sleepiness or sleepability? *Eur. J. Sport Sci.* **2021**, *21*, 321–330. [CrossRef] [PubMed]
112. Milner, C.E.; Cote, K.A. Benefits of napping in healthy adults: Impact of nap length, time of day, age, and experience with napping. *J. Sleep Res.* **2009**, *18*, 272–281. [CrossRef] [PubMed]
113. Dolezal, B.A.; Neufeld, E.V.; Boland, D.M.; Martin, J.L.; Cooper, C.B. Interrelationship between Sleep and Exercise: A Systematic Review. *Adv. Prev. Med.* **2017**, *2017*, 1364387. [CrossRef] [PubMed]
114. Li, S.; Li, Z.; Wu, Q.; Liu, C.; Zhou, Y.; Chen, L.; Lan, W.; Li, Y.; Han, S.; Chen, Z. Effect of exercise intervention on primary insomnia: A meta-analysis. *J. Sports Med. Phys. Fit.* **2021**, *61*, 857–866. [CrossRef] [PubMed]
115. Gardiner, C.; Weakley, J.; Burke, L.M.; Roach, G.D.; Sargent, C.; Maniar, N.; Townshend, A.; Halson, S.L. The effect of caffeine on subsequent sleep: A systematic review and meta-analysis. *Sleep Med. Rev.* **2023**, *69*, 101764. [CrossRef] [PubMed]

applied sciences

MDPI

Review

Analyses of Physical and Physiological Responses during Competition in Para-Footballers with Cerebral Palsy: A Systematic Review

Santiago Álvarez-Hernández [1], Daniel Castillo [2,*], José Gerardo Villa-Vicente [3], Javier Yanci [4], Diego Marqués-Jiménez [2] and Alejandro Rodríguez-Fernández [3]

1 Faculty of Sciences of Physical Activity and Sports, University of León, 24007 León, Spain; salvah01@estudiantes.unileon.es
2 REDAFLED Researh Group, Faculty of Education, University of Valladolid, 42004 Soria, Spain; diego.marques@uva.es
3 VALFIS Research Group, Institute of Biomedicine (IBIOMED), Faculty of Sciences of Physical Activity and Sports, University of León, 24007 León, Spain; jg.villa@unileon.es (J.G.V.-V.); alrof@unileon.es (A.R.-F.)
4 Society, Sports and Physical Exercise Research Group (GIKAFIT), Department of Physical Education and Sport, Faculty of Education and Sport, University of Basque Country (UPV/EHU), 01007 Vitoria-Gasteiz, Spain; javier.yanci@ehu.eus
* Correspondence: daniel.castillo@uva.es

Abstract: Background: Classification of athletes in cerebral palsy (CP) football is a key action that aims to promote the participation of all players by minimizing the impact of their physical disabilities on the outcome of the competition by establishing sports classes. As such, a new research line has been included in the classification process at an international level; that is, the analysis of locomotor demands during competition helps classifiers to understand the para-footballers' profile. Therefore, the main aim of this systematic review was to summarize the physical and physiological responses of players with CP in different sport classes during competition. Methods: A bibliographic search was conducted using PubMed, SCOPUS, and Web Of Science databases following Preferred Reporting Items for Systematic Reviews and Meta-analyses guidelines using the PICOS strategy. Results: Six studies meeting inclusion criteria analyzing physical (i.e., total distances, distances at different speeds, high-intensity and short-term actions, change of directions, etc.) and physiological (heart rate (HR), time spent at different zones of maximum HR, etc.) responses. Findings revealed that para-footballers with CP and minimal impairment impact covered greater total and distance above 23.04 km·h^{-1} and achieved higher maximum speeds during match-play. Notably, no significant differences in physiological responses were observed based on classification. Conclusions: The research suggests that para-footballers with CP and lower physical impairment may exhibit enhanced performance in terms of distance covered and speed during gameplay, highlighting their potential competence in the sport. In addition, the limited number of studies examining the physiological response of para-footballers prevents conclusive results and differentiating between classification groups.

Keywords: para-sport; official matches; performance; exercise; impairment

1. Introduction

Football (soccer) for people with cerebral palsy (CP) is a para-sport regulated globally by the International Federation of Cerebral Palsy Football (IFCPF). It is a discipline practiced by football players with central neurological injuries such as CP, head trauma, or stroke [1]. The institution which establishes the rules of the game is the Fédération Internationale de Football Association (FIFA), but the IFCPF has included some modifications such as, the match lasts two equal periods of 30 min separated by a half-time of 15 min, the field dimensions are reduced to 70 m × 50 m with 2 × 5 m goals, the offside rule does not apply, and throw-ins are put into play by rolling the ball on the ground [1].

Classification of athletes in para-sports, particularly in CP football, is a key action that aims to promote the participation of all players by minimizing the impact of their physical disabilities on the outcome of the competition by establishing sports classes [2–4]. These sport classes were called C5, C6, C7, and C8 in the first classification system [5] and later FT5 (usually diplegic), FT6 (usually ataxia or athetosis), FT7 (usually hemiplegic), and FT8 (minimal impairment). The new classification system developed by IFCPF, based on scientific knowledge published to date [6,7], reduces the classes to three profiles (FT1, FT2, and FT3), providing a new setup for competition and including a new minimum disability criterion and new assessment methods. The new structure of sports classes for players with CP is organized as follows: (1) based on the level of the impairment impacting on sport-specific football skills (FT1 = severe impairment; FT2 = moderate impairment, or FT3 = minimal impairment), and (2) the type of disability and/or affected limbs, i.e., (A) bilateral spasticity (spastic diplegia), (B) athetosis/dystonia (dyskinesia or ataxia), or (C) unilateral spasticity (spastic hemiplegia) [1]. The goal of this system is to address the issue of "cut-off points", i.e., when the classifiers must decide if a para-footballer has a moderate or mild form of spastic diplegia, athetosis/ataxia or spastic hemiplegia, in contrast with mild forms of these types of disability [8]. During the classification process, medical professionals or physiotherapists carry out the physical evaluation through a battery test to determine the degree of spastic hypertonia, dyskinesia and/or ataxia. In addition, sport technical classifiers perform the technical evaluation through tests to assess basic physical skills (coordination, balance, agility, strength, power, speed) and football-related skills from the individual point of view (ball kicks, passes, and shots, dribbles and controls, and the goalkeeper's technique) and collective (in reduced games) to assign a sport class [1].

Over the last decade, there has been a considerable increase in the number of football players with CP, as well as the number of events organized at the regional, national, and international levels. Currently, 88 countries worldwide actively participate in CP football. Additionally, there are 93 male teams (compared to 84 in 2020) and 94 female teams (compared to 28 in 2020), according to data Worldwide Participation of IFCPF. The rise of this para-sport has also been reflected in the scientific context, with a large increase in publications on football with CP [8–10]. Research into CP football has extensively explored various aspects, including specifying the anthropometric and performance characteristics of the players [11], assessing physical performance through functional tests [10,12–15], and assessing the validity and reliability of different tests [6,16,17]. Specifically, it has been shown that football players with CP exhibit lower distances covered (total, high intensity, and sprint distance) than non-disability players [18] in match-play. However, they covered a greater total distance (4%), more distance walking (38%), and more distance in medium-intensity running (5%), and maintained a similar maximum velocity (0.4%) to conventional F7 players [19]. Additionally, significant differences have been found between match demands and small-sided game demands (2vs2+Goalkeeper, pitch size 27 × 19 m) in football players with CP [20]. Understanding both the profiles of para-footballers with CP and the specifics of relevant tests is essential. Additionally, knowledge of their responses during match-play is crucial for effective training planning. The availability of this information would not only aid classifiers in making informed decisions during the classification process but also assist coaches in optimizing training for competitions.

Based on the aforementioned information, the main aim of this systematic review was to summarize the physical and physiological responses encountered by para-footballers with CP during the competition according to sport classes.

2. Materials and Methods

This systematic review was carried out according to the Preferred Reporting Items for Systematic Reviews and Meta-Analysis (PRISMA) adapted to the guidelines for conducting systematic reviews in Sports Sciences [21]. Due to the specific requirements in each area of knowledge, some modifications to the PRISMA declaration are necessary [22,23] to improve the quality of the main findings. In this study, a review of the scientific literature was carried out to analyze the physical and physiological responses of para-footballer players with CP during competition.

2.1. Search Strategy

The search and selection process for this systematic review was carried out through three specialized electronic databases in the field of Physical Activity and Sport Sciences: PubMed, SCOPUS, and Web Of Science. All records found were exported in a comma-separated values (CSV) format to a Microsoft® Excel document and in Research Information Systems (RIS) formats (PubMed and Web of Science), and directly (SCOPUS) to MENDELEY, the bibliographic manager used in this review. Keywords and their synonyms ("football", "soccer", "para-football", "football-7-a-side", "match", "competition", "performance", "activity", "cerebral palsy " and "cerebral paralysis") were entered in various combinations using boolean operators, selected using the PICOS search strategy (i.e., Population, Intervention, Comparator, Outcomes, Study design). Additionally, the bibliography (references) section of the selected articles was manually reviewed to detect potentially eligible articles not captured by the electronic searches. The final search strategy was carried out using the following combination of terms: ("football*" OR "soccer" OR "para-football*" OR "football-7-a-side") AND ("match" OR " competition" OR "performance" OR "activity") AND ("cerebral palsy" OR "cerebral paralysis").

A time restriction between 2000 and 2023 was established for the selection of studies. This search process was carried out independently by two authors (S.A.-H. and A.R.-F.), and in cases that generated discrepancies, a third author (D.C.) was consulted. The search was carried out on 31 January 2023.

The results obtained in the different databases were exported in a CSV sheet for later analysis in Microsoft® Excel (Microsoft Corporation, Readmon, WA, USA), where the articles were classified by title, author/s, date of publication, and database. This classification made it possible to detect duplicate/triplicate records (n = 45). A review of the title, abstract, and list of references for each of the studies was carried out to filter them and detect potentially relevant articles to include in the review. Subsequently, the complete versions of the included articles were reviewed to detect those that met the inclusion criteria established according to the PICOS strategy (Population: para-footballers with cerebral palsy; Intervention: data registered during an official match; Outcome: measures of physical and physiological responses; study design: an observational and descriptive design) (Table 1). Additionally, those studies that were not written in English, as well as conferences, abstracts, letters to the editor, errata, narrative reviews, systematic reviews, and meta-analyses, were excluded from our review.

Table 1. Description of the inclusion and exclusion criteria according to the PICOS search strategy.

PICOS	Inclusion Criteria	Exclusion Criteria
Population	Para-footballers with cerebral palsy	Footballers without cerebral palsy and para-athletes for other sports than soccer
Intervention	Data during an official match	Data during simulated match or small sided games
Comparator	-	-
Outcome	Measures of physical and physiological responses	Another nature responses
Study design	An observational and descriptive design	-

The following data was extracted from the selected studies: (a) author(s) and year of publication; (b) number of participants; (c) sex; (d) age; (e) number of observations; (f) competition; (g) sport class. In addition, the following variables were recorded for locomotor responses: total distance covered and distance covered at different intensity ranges in absolute and relative values, maximum speed reached, accelerations, decelerations, changes of direction, player load, and metabolic power. The following variables were used for physiological responses: average heart rate (HRm), maximum heart rate (HRmax), and time spent in different intensity ranges relative to HRmax.

2.2. Quality Assessment

The methodological quality assessment of the studies was determined following the indications of Palucci Vieira et al. [24] and was adapted from previous studies [25,26] on sport physical performance and data collection during soccer matches involving football players without disabilities (Table 2). The nine questions were: Q1 = Study objective(s) is/are clearly set out (Yes = 2; Maybe = 1; No = 0); Q2 = Demographic data (no information = 0 point; only age/age group was informed = 1 point; maturity offset also measured = 2 points); Q3 = Game rules (0–1 item described = 0 point; 2–3 items described = 1 point; 4–5 items described = 2 points; items: match duration, field size, players a-side, match type, whether rolling substitute policy was adopted); Q4 = Reliability/validity of the time-motion system/equipment is not stated, mentioned (i.e., a citation of previous studies) or measured under local conditions where data collections took place (Measured = 2; Mentioned = 1; No stated = 0); Q5 = Dependent variables defined (Yes = 2; Maybe = 1; No = 0); Q6 = Duration of players recordings/inclusion criteria is clearly indicated (Yes = 2; Maybe = 1; No = 0); Q7 = Statistics are appropriate (Yes = 2; Maybe = 1; No = 0); Q8 = Results are detailed (description of mean, standard deviation and null hypothesis significance test [p-value] = 1 point; also included effect size/magnitude-based inferences = 2 points); Q9 = Conclusions are insightful, clear, practical applications, and future directions (Yes = 2; Maybe = 1; No = 0). Subsequently, a sum of the points obtained in each question for each study was made, varying the rating between 0 (minimum points) and 18 (maximum points). Finally, the results obtained were converted into a percentage (0% minimum and 100% maximum). Studies were considered to have a high level of bias when they did not achieve a score > 75% [24].

Table 2. Sample information and scores assigned to each study for the nine quality (Q) questions.

Reference	*n*	Sex	Age	Sport Class	Observations *n*	T	Q1 (0–2)	Q2 (0–2)	Q3 (0–2)	Q4 (0–2)	Q5 (0–2)	Q6 (0–2)	Q7 (0–2)	Q8 (0–2)	Q9 (0–2)	Total (Σ)	Score (%)
Boyd et al. [27]	40	M	22.0 (7.0)	C5/6, C7, and C8	47	I	2	1	1	0	2	2	2	1	2	13	72.2
Gamonales et al. [28]	12	N	29.6 (9.1)	FT1	65	N	2	1	2	0	2	0	2	2	2	13	72.2
			32.0 (3.8)	FT2													
			37.5 (7.7)	FT3													
Henríquez et al. [29]	87	M	25.3 (6.4)	FT1, FT2, and FT3	92 (46 [a], 46 [b])	I	2	1	0	0	2	2	2	2	2	13	72.2
Reina et al. (2021) [30]	259	N	25.46 (6.15)	FT1, FT2, and FT3	259	I	2	1	1	0	2	2	2	2	2	14	77.8
Reina et al. (2020) [31]	48	M	23.0 (7.0)	FT5/6, FT7, and FT8	N	I	2	1	0	1	2	2	2	2	2	14	77.8
Yanci et al. (2018) [32]	42	M	23.0 (6.0)	FT5/6, FT7, and FT8	62	I	2	1	0	0	2	2	2	2	2	13	72.2
				Mean (SD)			2.0 (0.0)	1.0 (0.0)	0.7 (0.8)	0.3 (0.7)	2.0 (0.0)	1.2 (0.9)	2.0 (0.0)	1.8 (0.3)	2.0 (0.0)	13.2 (0.6)	73.5 (3.7)

Note: *n* = players; M = male; N = not specified; T = type; I = international tournament; N = national tournament; [a] = moderate altitude group; [b] = sea level group; SD = standard deviation.

3. Results

Figure 1 shows the study identification and selection process. A total of 167 studies were identified in an initial search of PubMed (n = 38), SCOPUS (n = 64), and Web of Science (n = 65) databases. It was found that there were 45 duplicate (or triplicate) records. Thus, the search decreased to 90 results. After reading abstracts, 71 records were excluded because they were articles in which footballers with CP did not participate, did not analyze match-play responses (physical or physiological), or did not fit the topic. Afterwards, a detailed reading of the 19 resulting studies was made, with 10 of them excluded because they were articles written in other languages (Portuguese and Korean). They did not analyze physical or physiological responses during match-play, or they analyzed these variables in training sessions or assessed functional tests. Therefore, a total of 81 records were excluded, and finally, 6 of these studies were included in the systematic review.

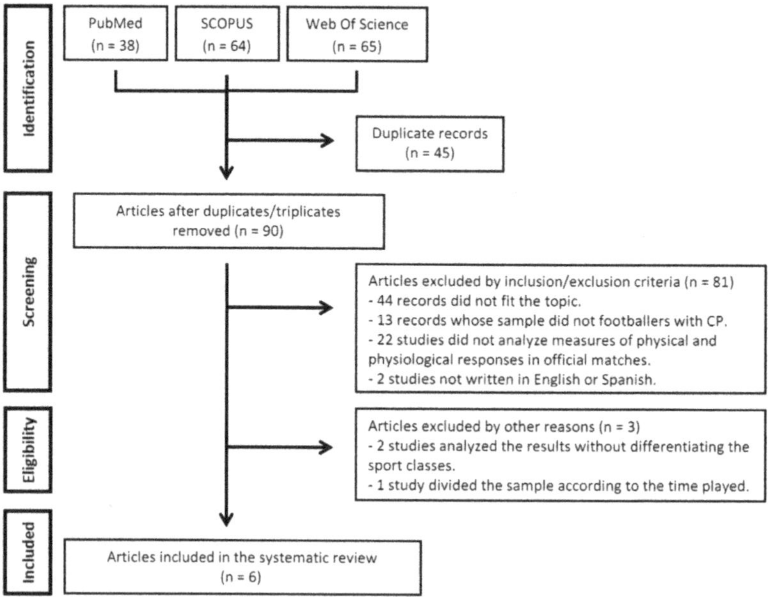

Figure 1. Diagram flow of the review.

The results of methodological quality and risk of bias in the studies included in the review are shown in Table 1; the mean score is 73.5 ± 3.7%. The highest value, 77.8%, was reported in two studies [30,31], while 66.6% of the studies reached a methodological quality of 72.2% (n = 4) [27–29,32].

All the studies fit the inclusion and exclusion criterion analyzing physical responses [27–32], but only one the physiological responses [27]. Three studies attended to the new classification FT1 to FT3 [28–30] and three to the old classifications C5/6, C7 to C8 [27], and FT5/6 to FT8 [29,31]. The number of participants in the studies analyzed was 488, of whom 4 belonged to C5/6, 29 to C7, 7 to C8, 9 to FT5/6, 32 to FT7, 7 to FT8, 64 to FT1, 238 to FT2, and 56 to FT3; of the remaining 42, it is not known how many correspond to each FT, since the authors determine and quantify the sample (8 from FT5, 3 from FT6, 42 from FT7, and 9 from FT8) by the total number of individual observations, $n = 62$ [32]. Four studies determined the sex of the sample (all male) and only two did not determine it [27,28,30,31], but they were men observing the city and the year of the competitions.

Tables 3 and 4 shows the total and distance covered at different speed ranges by players with PC during match-play, expressed in absolute and relative terms, respectively. The speed ranges to classify the distance covered were diverse: between 17.64–23.04

km·h^{-1}, above 23.04 km·h^{-1} [27], between 0.6–6 km·h^{-1}, 6–12 km·h^{-1}, 12–18 km·h^{-1}, 18–21 km·h^{-1}, 21–24 km·h^{-1}, above 24 km·h^{-1} [28], below 0.4 km/h, between 0.4–3 km·h^{-1}, 3–9 km·h^{-1}, 9–13 km·h^{-1} [29,30,32], 13–18 km·h^{-1}, and above 18 km·h^{-1} [29,30,32].

Table 3. Results for measures of total and distance covered at different speed ranges extracted from literature research of studies on para-footballers with cerebral palsy.

Variables	SC	Boyd et al. [27]
Total distance (m)	C5/6	5642 ± 674
	. C7	5532 ± 814
	C8	6343 ± 551
	TOTAL	5839 ± 668
Distance between 17.64–23.04 km/h (m)	C5/6	13 ± 2
	C7	13 ± 2
	C8	12 ± 2
	TOTAL	13 ± 2
Distance >23.04 km/h (m)	C5/6	12 ± 4
	C7	12 ± 4
	C8	15 ± 4
	TOTAL	13 ± 4
$p < 0.05$ between sport classes for CP-Football		C8 > C7 and C5/6. - Total distance. - Distance covered > 23.04 km/h. No differences were observed between FT5/6 and FT7 classes.

Note: SC = sport class.

Table 4. Results for measures of total and distance covered at different speed ranges extracted from the literature research of studies on para-footballers with cerebral palsy.

Variables	SC	Gamonales et al. [28]	Henríquez et al. [29]	Reina et al. [30]	Reina et al. [31]	Yanci et al. [32]
Total distance (m/min)	FT5/6	-	-	-	-	93.12 ± 18.02
	FT7	-	-	-	-	92.88 ± 12.49
	FT8	-	-	-	-	91.57 ± 14.48
	TOTAL	-	76.81 ± 11.55 [a] 92.06 ± 12.47 [b] 84.43 ± 14.20 [c]	84.51 ± 16.50	-	92.63 ± 13.54
	FT1	60.55 ± 23.62	74.06 ± 11.36 [a] 84.36 ± 12.16 [b]	81.26 ± 15.35	-	-
	FT2	84.24 ± 17.27	79.30 ± 11.19 [a] 95.56 ± 11.05 [b]	85.23 ± 17.05	-	-
	FT3	106.42 ± 9.59	70.21 ± 11.21 [a] 88.01 ± 14.04 [b]	84.75 ± 5.13	-	-
Distance <0.4 km/h (m/min)	FT5/6	-	-	-	-	1.17 ± 0.64
	FT7	-	-	-	-	1.10 ± 0.76
	FT8	-	-	-	-	1.08 ± 0.19
	TOTAL	-	2.56 ± 1.05 [a] 1.23 ± 0.58 [b] 1.89 ± 1.08 [c]	2.68 ± 1.21	-	1.11 ± 0.68
	FT1	-	2.47 ± 1.04 [a] 1.43 ± 0.69 [b]	2.03 ± 0.85	-	-
	FT2	-	2.54 ± 1.11 [a] 1.09 ± 0.43 [b]	1.69 ± 0.99	-	-
	FT3	-	2.70 ± 0.96 [a] 1.51 ± 0.82 [b]	1.78 ± 1.11	-	-

Table 4. *Cont.*

Variables	SC	Gamonales et al. [28]	Henríquez et al. [29]	Reina et al. [30]	Reina et al. [31]	Yanci et al. [32]
Distance between 0.4–3 km/h (m/min)	FT5/6	-	-	-	-	9.47 ± 3.10
	FT7	-	-	-	-	8.32 ± 5.66
	FT8	-	-	-	-	6.73 ± 2.33
	TOTAL	-	11.74 ± 3.73 [a] 7.89 ± 2.72 [b] 9.81 ± 3.78 [c]	10.16 ± 5.03	-	8.30 ± 4.93
	FT1	-	11.75 ± 2.80 [a] 9.65 ± 2.97 [b]	12.21 ± 8.32	-	-
	FT2	-	11.96 ± 4.21 [a] 7.19 ± 1.90 [b]	9.92 ± 4.11	-	-
	FT3	-	10.87 ± 2.66 [a] 8.43 ± 4.09 [b]	9.10 ± 3.54	-	-
Distance between 0.6–6 km/h (m/min)	FT1	38.06 ± 8.72	-	-	-	-
	FT2	41.97 ± 3.21	-	-	-	-
	FT3	39.80 ± 5.08	-	-	-	-
Distance between 3–9 km/h (m/min)	FT5/6	-	-	-	-	40.26 ± 4.39
	FT7	-	-	-	-	40.15 ± 5.15
	FT8	-	-	-	-	39.23 ± 4.45
	TOTAL	-	38.30 ± 6.74 [a] 44.11 ± 5.67 [b] 41.20 ± 6.84 [c]	42.33 ± 8.52	-	40.02 ± 4.84
	FT1	-	36.91 ± 6.48 [a] 42.13 ± 6.20 [b]	39.45 ± 9.14	-	-
	FT2	-	38.66 ± 5.70 [a] 44.95 ± 5.09 [b]	42.54 ± 8.17	-	-
	FT3	-	38.35 ± 10.59 [a] 43.28 ± 7.07 [b]	44.40 ± 8.78	-	-
Distance between 6–12 km/h (m/min)	FT1	16.72 ± 12.90	-	-	-	-
	FT2	29.54 ± 10.28	-	-	-	-
	FT3	36.50 ± 4.43	-	-	-	-
Distance between 9–13 km/h (m/min)	FT5/6	-	-	-	-	27.28 ± 11.59
	FT7	-	-	-	-	28.40 ± 9.08
	FT8	-	-	-	-	26.30 ± 7.28
	TOTAL	-	14.68 ± 5.36 [a] 22.11 ± 6.90 [b] 18.39 ± 7.19 [c]	19.38 ± 25.45	-	27.87 ± 9.18
	FT1	-	15.03 ± 6.29 [a] 18.14 ± 5.43 [b]	17.21 ± 7.32	-	-
	FT2	-	15.28 ± 5.46 [a] 23.80 ± 6.65 [b]	20.33 ± 30.42	-	-
	FT3	-	12.07 ± 3.47 [a] 20.43 ± 7.74 [b]	17.47 ± 6.26	-	-
Distance between 12–18 km/h (m/min)	FT1	5.40 ± 5.95	-	-	-	-
	FT2	10.38 ± 6.58	-	-	-	-
	FT3	23.49 ± 6.26	-	-	-	-

Table 4. *Cont.*

Variables	SC	Gamonales et al. [28]	Henríquez et al. [29]	Reina et al. [30]	Reina et al. [31]	Yanci et al. [32]
Distance between 13–18 km/h (m/min)	FT5/6	-	-	-	11.34 ± 5.07	12.21 ± 5.76
	FT7	-	-	-	11.62 ± 4.53	11.64 ± 4.18
	FT8	-	-	-	13.70 ± 5.35	13.71 ± 4.95
	TOTAL	-	7.28 ± 4.11 [a] 12.89 ± 5.10 [b] 10.23 ± 5.32 [c]	9.47 ± 5.46	11.87 ± 4.71	12.00 ± 4.52
	FT1	-	6.42 ± 3.79 [a] 9.37 ± 4.74 [b]	8.08 ± 4.97	-	-
	FT2	-	8.52 ± 4.23 [a] 14.55 ± 4.74 [b]	9.81 ± 5.59	-	-
	FT3	-	5.24 ± 2.97 [a] 10.82 ± 4.38 [b]	9.45 ± 5.30	-	-
Distance >18 km/h (m/min)	FT5/6	-	-	-	2.65 ± 2.09	2.73 ± 2.09
	FT7	-	-	-	3.23 ± 1.60	3.20 ± 1.63
	FT8	-	-	-	4.97 ± 2.97	4.53 ± 3.01
	TOTAL	-	2.05 ± 1.62 [a] 3.96 ± 2.69 [b] 3.01 ± 2.41 [c]	3.05 ± 2.79	3.38 ± 2.01	3.27 ± 1.96
	FT1	-	1.42 ± 0.95 [a] 2.44 ± 1.94 [b]	2.04 ± 2.09	-	-
	FT2	-	2.40 ± 1.68 [a] 4.54 ± 2.87 [b]	3.18 ± 2.82	-	-
	FT3	-	1.39 ± 1.67 [a] 3.55 ± 2.17 [b]	3.56 ± 3.11	-	-
Distance between 18–21 km/h (m/min)	FT1	0.96 ± 1.76	-	-	-	-
	FT2	3.85 ± 3.60	-	-	-	-
	FT3	9.87 ± 3.65	-	-	-	-
Distance between 21–24 km/h (m/min)	FT1	0.06 ± 0.18	-	-	-	-
	FT2	0.54 ± 0.76	-	-	-	-
	FT3	1.79 ± 1.14	-	-	-	-
Distance >24 km/h (m/min)	FT1	0.00 ± 0.00	-	-	-	-
	FT2	0.11 ± 0.25	-	-	-	-
	FT3	0.32 ± 0.23	-	-	-	-
$p < 0.05$ between sport classes for CP-Football		FT3 > FT2 > FT1. - Total distance. - Distance covered between 12–18, 18–21, and 21–24 km/h. FT3 = FT2 > FT1 in distance covered >24 km/h. FT3 > FT2 in distance covered bet-ween 6–12 km/h. FT2 > FT1 in distance covered bet-ween 6–12 km/h.	Does not analyze the significant differences between CP-Football classes without taking into account the place of the competition.	FT1 > FT3 = FT2 in distance covered between 0.4–3 km/h. FT3 = FT2 > FT1 in distance covered >18 km/h. FT3 > FT1 in distance covered between 3–9 km/h. No differences were observed between FT2 and FT3 classes.	FT8 > FT5/6 in distance covered >18 km/h. No differences were observed between FT8 and FT7 classes.	No differences were observed between sport classes.

Note: SC = sport class; [a] = moderate altitude group; [b] = sea level group; [c] = overall sample.

Maximum speed variables are shown in Tables 5 and 6, respectively. Table 6 also shows accelerations, decelerations, impacts, and change directions (COD) values (total and in different ranges of intensity), as well as player load and metabolic power, all expressed in relative terms.

Table 5. Results for measures of maximal speed extracted from literature research of studies on para-footballers with cerebral palsy.

Variables	SC	Boyd et al. [27]	Henríquez et al. [29]	Reina et al. [30]	Reina et al. [31]	Yanci et al. [32]
Maximal speed (km·h^{-1})	FT5/6	24.23 ± 1.58	-	-	21.86 ± 2.04	21.79 ± 1.92
	FT7	25.09 ± 2.02	-	-	22.94 ± 1.90	22.81 ± 2.41
	FT8	27.86 ± 1.22	-	-	24.41 ± 1.83	23.96 ± 2.12
	TOTAL	25.74 ± 1.62	21.96 ± 2.62 [a] 23.22 ± 2.41 [b] 22.59 ± 2.58 [c]	22.58 ± 3.18	22.95 ± 2.01	22.81 ± 2.34
	FT1	-	20.89 ± 2.37 [a] 22.36 ± 2.66 [b]	21.28 ± 2.86	-	-
	FT2	-	22.52 ± 2.06 [a] 23.46 ± 2.33 [b]	22.74 ± 3.05	-	-
	FT3	-	20.94 ± 4.16 [a] 23.36 ± 2.51 [b]	23.22 ± 3.75	-	-
$p < 0.05$ between sport classes for CP-Football		FT8 > FT5/6 and FT7 in maximal speed. No differences were observed between FT5/6 and FT7 classes.	Does not analyze the significant differences between CP-Football classes without taking into account the place of the competition.	FT3 = FT2 > FT1 in maximal speed. No differences were observed between FT2 and FT3 classes.	FT8 > FT7 and FT5/6 in maximal speed. No differences were observed between FT7 and FT5/6 classes.	No differences were observed between sport classes.

Note: SC = sport class; [a] = moderate altitude group; [b] = sea level group; [c] = overall sample.

Table 6. Results for measures of accelerations, decelerations, player load, metabolic power, change of directions (COD), and impacts per minute, extracted from literature research of studies on para-footballers with cerebral palsy.

Variables	SC	Gamonales et al. [28]	Henríquez et al. [29]	Reina et al. [30]	Reina et al. [31]	Yanci et al. [32]
Mean speed (km·h^{-1})	TOTAL	-	-	5.07 ± 0.99	-	-
	FT1	-	-	4.87 ± 0.93	-	-
	FT2	-	-	5.12 ± 1.02	-	-
	FT3	-	-	5.09 ± 0.91	-	-
Total accelerations (n/min)	FT1	11.75 ± 5.26	-	-	-	-
	FT2	13.91 ± 2.93	-	-	-	-
	FT3	14.93 ± 2.29	-	-	-	-
Accelerations 1 to 2 m·seg^{-2} (n/min)	FT1	9.63 ± 4.20	-	-	-	-
	FT2	10.47 ± 2.08	-	-	-	-
	FT3	10.77 ± 1.74	-	-	-	-
Accelerations 1 to 2.78 m·seg^{-2} (n/min)	FT5/6	-	-	-	1.08 ± 0.60	1.15 ± 0.64
	FT7	-	-	-	0.88 ± 0.33	0.98 ± 0.52
	FT8	-	-	-	1.29 ± 0.83	1.34 ± 0.79
	TOTAL	-	5.43 ± 1.57 [a] 7.21 ± 1.42 [b] 6.32 ± 1.74 [c]	5.55 ± 3.81	0.98 ± 0.50	1.06 ± 0.58
	FT1	-	5.46 ± 1.24 [a] 6.38 ± 1.37 [b]	4.82 ± 2.78	-	-
	FT2	-	5.63 ± 1.72 [a] 7.54 ± 1.42 [b]	5.78 ± 4.14	-	-
	FT3	-	4.64 ± 1.13 [a] 6.93 ± 1.16 [b]	5.29 ± 3.11	-	-

Table 6. *Cont.*

Variables	SC	Gamonales et al. [28]	Henríquez et al. [29]	Reina et al. [30]	Reina et al. [31]	Yanci et al. [32]
Accelerations 2 to 3 m·seg^{-2} (*n*/min)	FT1	1.67 ± 0.97	-	-	-	-
	FT2	2.46 ± 0.85	-	-	-	-
	FT3	2.67 ± 0.80	-	-	-	-
Accelerations >2.78 m·seg^{-2} (*n*/min)	FT5/6	-	-	-	0.03 ± 0.03	0.03 ± 0.04
	FT7	-	-	-	0.06 ± 0.05	0.07 ± 0.06
	FT8	-	-	-	0.15 ± 0.11	0.14 ± 0.10
	TOTAL	-	1.09 ± 0.38 [a] 1.32 ± 0.39 [b] 1.20 ± 0.40 [c]	1.08 ± 0.66	0.07 ± 0.07	0.07 ± 0.07
	FT1	-	0.96 ± 0.40 [a] 1.22 ± 0.50 [b]	0.87 ± 0.64	-	-
	FT2	-	1.12 ± 0.40 [a] 1.37 ± 0.33 [b]	1.09 ± 0.59	-	-
	FT3	-	1.08 ± 0.30 [a] 1.25 ± 0.45 [b]	1.26 ± 0.90	-	-
Accelerations 3 to 4 m·seg^{-2} (*n*/min)	FT1	0.36 ± 0.29	-	-	-	-
	FT2	0.77 ± 0.43	-	-	-	-
	FT3	1.12 ± 0.36	-	-	-	-
Accelerations 4 to 100 m·seg^{-2} (*n*/min)	FT1	0.08 ± 0.11	-	-	-	-
	FT2	0.21 ± 0.15	-	-	-	-
	FT3	0.38 ± 0.10	-	-	-	-
Total decelerations (*n*/min)	TOTAL	-	-	-	-	-
	FT1	10.28 ± 5.29	-	-	-	-
	FT2	12.14 ± 2.83	-	-	-	-
	FT3	11.97 ± 2.13	-	-	-	-
Decelerations −1 to −2 m·seg^{-2} (*n*/min)	FT1	8.58 ± 4.35	-	-	-	-
	FT2	9.39 ± 2.01	-	-	-	-
	FT3	8.44 ± 1.50	-	-	-	-
Decelerations −1 to −2.78 m·seg^{-2} (*n*/min)	FT5/6	-	-	-	0.86 ± 0.28	0.95 ± 0.36
	FT7	-	-	-	0.89 ± 0.32	0.99 ± 0.44
	FT8	-	-	-	1.37 ± 0.71	1.36 ± 0.65
	TOTAL	-	4.20 ± 1.26 [a] 5.77 ± 1.22 [b] 4.99 ± 1.46 [c]	4.49 ± 3.15	0.95 ± 0.42	1.03 ± 0.47
	FT1	-	4.03 ± 0.98 [a] 5.44 ± 1.65 [b]	3.89 ± 2.38	-	-
	FT2	-	4.43 ± 1.37 [a] 6.00 ± 1.05 [b]	4.69 ± 3.44	-	-
	FT3	-	3.49 ± 0.78 [a] 5.34 ± 1.21 [b]	4.24 ± 2.33	-	-
Decelerations −2 to −3 m·seg^{-2} (*n*/min)	FT1	1.30 ± 0.80	-	-	-	-
	FT2	1.91 ± 0.75	-	-	-	-
	FT3	2.36 ± 0.62	-	-	-	-
Decelerations >−2.78 m·seg^{-2} (*n*/min)	FT5/6	-	-	-	0.05 ± 0.03	0.08 ± 0.11
	FT7	-	-	-	0.12 ± 0.08	0.13 ± 0.09
	FT8	-	-	-	0.14 ± 0.09	0.15 ± 0.09
	TOTAL	-	0.74 ± 0.30 [a] 0.96 ± 0.35 [b] 0.85 ± 0.35 [c]	0.76 ± 0.72	0.11 ± 0.08	0.12 ± 0.09
	FT1	-	0.68 ± 0.26 [a] 0.77 ± 0.41 [b]	0.55 ± 0.42	-	-
	FT2	-	0.76 ± 0.31 [a] 1.03 ± 0.33 [b]	0.80 ± 0.81	-	-
	FT3	-	0.74 ± 0.35 [a] 0.93 ± 0.34 [b]	0.79 ± 0.54	-	-

Table 6. *Cont.*

Variables	SC	Gamonales et al. [28]	Henríquez et al. [29]	Reina et al. [30]	Reina et al. [31]	Yanci et al. [32]
Decelerations -3 to -4 m·seg^{-2} (n/min)	FT1	0.30 ± 0.22	-	-	-	-
	FT2	0.60 ± 0.33	-	-	-	-
	FT3	0.85 ± 0.18	-	-	-	-
Decelerations -4 to -100 m·seg^{-2} (n/min)	FT1	0.11 ± 0.10	-	-	-	-
	FT2	0.25 ± 0.14	-	-	-	-
	FT3	0.32 ± 0.15	-	-	-	-
Player load (A.U./min)	FT5/6	-	-	-	10.86 ± 1.83	10.76 ± 2.02
	FT7	-	-	-	10.39 ± 2.57	10.55 ± 2.39
	FT8	-	-	-	10.46 ± 1.43	10.55 ± 1.35
	TOTAL	-	-	9.85 ± 2.26	10.49 ± 2.28	10.56 ± 2.19
	FT1	-	-	10.05 ± 1.77	-	-
	FT2	-	-	9.87 ± 2.40	-	-
	FT3	-	-	9.53 ± 2.10	-	-
Metabolic Power (W/min)	FT5/6	-	-	-	106.91 ± 47.25	106.74 ± 42.43
	FT7	-	-	-	117.84 ± 36.31	114.64 ± 35.75
	FT8	-	-	-	113.51 ± 37.48	108.57 ± 37.41
	TOTAL	-	-	-	115.16 ± 38.04	113.21 ± 36.94
Low-intensity COD forward (n/min)	FT5/6	-	-	-	-	0.50 ± 0.14
	FT7	-	-	-	-	0.69 ± 0.43
	FT8	-	-	-	-	0.46 ± 0.13
	TOTAL	-	-	-	-	0.62 ± 0.38
Low-intensity COD backward (n/min)	FT5/6	-	-	-	-	0.77 ± 0.39
	FT7	-	-	-	-	1.03 ± 0.41
	FT8	-	-	-	-	0.67 ± 0.29
	TOTAL	-	-	-	-	0.94 ± 0.41
Low-intensity COD left (n/min)	FT5/6	-	-	-	-	3.87 ± 3.84
	FT7	-	-	-	-	2.38 ± 0.83
	FT8	-	-	-	-	2.08 ± 0.55
	TOTAL	-	-	-	-	2.64 ± 1.82
Low-intensity COD right (n/min)	FT5/6	-	-	-	-	3.35 ± 3.14
	FT7	-	-	-	-	3.35 ± 1.37
	FT8	-	-	-	-	2.81 ± 0.77
	TOTAL	-	-	-	-	3.27 ± 1.73
Medium-intensity COD forward (n/min)	FT5/6	-	-	-	-	0.11 ± 0.09
	FT7	-	-	-	-	0.18 ± 0.11
	FT8	-	-	-	-	0.18 ± 0.07
	TOTAL	-	-	-	-	0.17 ± 0.10
Medium-intensity COD backward (n/min)	FT5/6	-	-	-	-	0.26 ± 0.16
	FT7	-	-	-	-	0.35 ± 0.17
	FT8	-	-	-	-	0.37 ± 0.13
	TOTAL	-	-	-	-	0.34 ± 0.17
Medium-intensity COD left (n/min)	FT5/6	-	-	-	-	0.48 ± 0.30
	FT7	-	-	-	-	0.40 ± 0.23
	FT8	-	-	-	-	0.39 ± 0.15
	TOTAL	-	-	-	-	0.42 ± 0.24
Medium-intensity COD right (n/min)	FT5/6	-	-	-	-	0.48 ± 0.35
	FT7	-	-	-	-	0.53 ± 0.24
	FT8	-	-	-	-	0.52 ± 0.21
	TOTAL	-	-	-	-	0.52 ± 0.26
High-intensity COD forward (n/min)	FT5/6	-	-	-	-	0.08 ± 0.09
	FT7	-	-	-	-	0.08 ± 0.06
	FT8	-	-	-	-	0.11 ± 0.06
	TOTAL	-	-	-	-	0.09 ± 0.07

Table 6. *Cont.*

Variables	SC	Gamonales et al. [28]	Henríquez et al. [29]	Reina et al. [30]	Reina et al. [31]	Yanci et al. [32]
High-intensity COD backward (*n*/min)	FT5/6	-	-	-	-	0.17 ± 0.17
	FT7	-	-	-	-	0.13 ± 0.09
	FT8	-	-	-	-	0.17 ± 0.14
	TOTAL	-	-	-	-	0.14 ± 0.11
High-intensity COD left (*n*/min)	FT5/6	-	-	-	-	0.11 ± 0.09
	FT7	-	-	-	-	0.12 ± 0.12
	FT8	-	-	-	-	0.08 ± 0.07
	TOTAL	-	-	-	-	0.11 ± 0.11
High-intensity COD right (*n*/min)	FT5/6	-	-	-	-	0.11 ± 0.10
	FT7	-	-	-	-	0.13 ± 0.09
	FT8	-	-	-	-	0.17 ± 0.08
	TOTAL	-	-	-	-	0.13 ± 0.09
Total impacts (*n*/min)	FT1	45.45 ± 40.24	-	-	-	-
	FT2	76.75 ± 39.22	-	-	-	-
	FT3	94.95 ± 45.77	-	-	-	-
Impacts 2 to 5 G (*n*/min)	FT1	38.97 ± 34.81	-	-	-	-
	FT2	69.35 ± 34.21	-	-	-	-
	FT3	83.10 ± 42.36	-	-	-	-
Impacts 5 to 7 G (*n*/min)	FT1	5.34 ± 5.37	-	-	-	-
	FT2	6.29 ± 5.91	-	-	-	-
	FT3	10.15 ± 3.68	-	-	-	-
Impacts 7 to 8 G (*n*/min)	FT1	0.67 ± 0.58	-	-	-	-
	FT2	0.65 ± 0.58	-	-	-	-
	FT3	1.06 ± 0.12	-	-	-	-
Impacts 8 to 9 G (*n*/min)	FT1	0.22 ± 0.19	-	-	-	-
	FT2	0.25 ± 0.27	-	-	-	-
	FT3	0.35 ± 0.11	-	-	-	-
Impacts 9 to 10 G (*n*/min)	FT1	0.11 ± 0.12	-	-	-	-
	FT2	0.11 ± 0.12	-	-	-	-
	FT3	0.12 ± 0.04	-	-	-	-
Impacts 10 to 100 G (*n*/min)	FT1	0.13 ± 0.12	-	-	-	-
	FT2	0.11 ± 0.09	-	-	-	-
	FT3	0.17 ± 0.09	-	-	-	-
$p < 0.05$ between sport classes for CP-Football		FT3 > FT2 > FT1. -Accelerations 2 to 3 and 3 to 4 m·seg^{-2}. -Decelerations between −2 to −3 and −3 to −4 m·seg^{-2}. FT3 = FT2 > FT1. -Accelerations 1 to 100 m·seg^{-2}. -Decelerations −1 to −100 m·seg^{-2}. -Total impacts. -Impacts 2 to 5 G.	Does not analyze the significant differences between CP-Football classes without taking into account the place of the competition.	FT3 > FT1 in accelerations >2.78 m·seg^{-2}. No differences were observed between FT2 and FT3 classes.	FT8 > FT7 and FT5/6. - Accelerations >2.78 m·seg^{-2}. - Decelerations −1 to −2.78 m·seg^{-2}. No differences were observed between FT7 and FT5/6 classes.	FT8 > FT7 and FT5/6 in accelerations >2.78 m·seg^{-2}. FT5/6 > FT8 and FT7 in low-intensity COD to the left. FT7 > FT8 in low-intensity COD backward.

Note: SC = sport class; *n* = number; COD = change of direction; A.U. = Arbitrary units; [a] = moderate altitude group; [b] = sea level group; [c] = overall sample.

Finally, Table 7 shows the physiological responses recorded by the players with CP during the competition.

Table 7. Results for measures of physiological responses extracted from literature research of studies on para-footballers with cerebral palsy.

Variables	SC	Boyd et al. [27]
Maximum heart rate (bpm)	C5/6	196 ± 18
	C7	194 ± 11
	C8	200 ± 6
	TOTAL	197 ± 12
Average heart rate (bpm)	C5/6	161 ± 20 [a] ǀ 157 ± 19 [b] ǀ 153 ± 19 [c] ǀ 158 ± 18 [d]
	C7	164 ± 14 [a] ǀ 166 ± 13 [b] ǀ 159 ± 14 [c] ǀ 160 ± 13 [d]
	C8	170 ± 5 [a] ǀ 171 ± 7 [b] ǀ 168 ± 7 [c] ǀ 169 ± 10 [d]
	TOTAL	165 ± 13 [a] ǀ 165 ± 13 [b] ǀ 160 ± 13 [c] ǀ 162 ± 14 [d]
Time < 75% Maximum HR (min)	C5/6	3.5 [a] ǀ 4.5 [b] ǀ 5.6 [c] ǀ 8.0 [d]
	C7	2.3 [a] ǀ 1.8 [b] ǀ 3.6 [c] ǀ 2.7 [d]
	C8	1.0 [a] ǀ 1.6 [b] ǀ 1.9 [c] ǀ 2.9 [d]
Time between 75–85% Maximum HR (min)	C5/6	4.4 [a] ǀ 4.7 [b] ǀ 5.0 [c] ǀ 3.9 [d]
	C7	6.0 [a] ǀ 6.0 [b] ǀ 6.8 [c] ǀ 7.4 [d]
	C8	3.9 [a] ǀ 4.0 [b] ǀ 5.0 [c] ǀ 3.7 [d]
Time > 85% Maximum HR (min)	C5/6	7.1 [a] ǀ 5.8 [b] ǀ 4.4 [c] ǀ 3.3 [d]
	C7	6.6 [a] ǀ 7.1 [b] ǀ 4.4 [c] ǀ 4.8 [d]
	C8	10.4 [a] ǀ 9.4 [b] ǀ 8.0 [c] ǀ 9.0 [d]
$p < 0.05$ between sport classes for CP-Football		No differences were observed between sport classes for maximum or mean HR. C8 > C7 and C5/6 in time spent > 85% Max HR. No differences were observed between C5/6 and C7 classes.

Note: SC = sport class; [a] = between 0–15 min of the match; [b] = between 16–30 min of the match; [c] = between 31–45 min of the match; [d] = between 46–60 min of the match.

4. Discussion

Analyzing match responses in footballers with CP has a two-fold purpose. On the one hand, coaches and strength and conditional coaches can design training drills that allow replicable competitive situations, under-stimulated or over-stimulated; and on the other hand, help classifiers to make decisions when assigning a player to a certain sport class. Therefore, the aim of this systematic review was to summarize the physical and physiological responses encountered by para-footballers with CP during the competition according to sport classes. To our knowledge, this is the first review that analyzes these locomotor and physiological responses in CP players during official matches. The main results showed that players with less physical impairment cover greater total and distance at high speeds, perform greater high-intensity acceleration and deceleration per minute, and achieve greater maximal speed. However, the physiological responses do not seem to be influenced by the sport class assigned.

To gain a comprehensive understanding of the responses of football PC and to optimize performance, it is necessary to consider not only locomotor responses but also the physiological responses of players during match-play [33]. Only one study included in this review analyzes the HR, dividing the sample by sport classes [27]. In the selected study, maximum HR values range from 200 ± 6 to 196 ± 18 bpm, and average heart rate values range from 153 ± 19 to 171 ± 7 bpm. These values were obtained by the sport classes with the least impairment (C8) and the maximum values obtained by other studies which the sample is not divided are similar [34,35]: the values of maximum and average heart rate have been shown 194 ± 13 and 154.4 ± 22 bpm, respectively. This similar physiological response during matches can be attributed to several factors. On one hand, it may be due to the great variability existing among players in terms of muscle glycogen, free fatty acid levels, insulin levels, and so forth, during a game [36]. On the other hand, it could be because CP players with less physical impairment have higher levels of physical fitness [37]. Therefore, despite demonstrating higher physical performance (i.e., covering greater total distance and distance at high speeds), their physiological response during matches is similar, as occurs in non-disabled soccer players [38]. However, the relationship between physical fitness and match running performance was shown to be playing position-dependent [39] and, therefore, more studies with CP players are necessary to analyze this aspect.

Only one study included in the review analyzes the total distance covered in absolute terms dividing the sample by sport classes [27]. This study indicates that total distance covered was 6343 $\pm$ 551 m, 5642 $\pm$ 674 m, and 5532 $\pm$ 814 m for classes C8, C7, and C5/6, respectively [27]. The highest values of total distance covered in relative terms in para-footballers were 106.42 $\pm$ 9.59 $m \cdot min^{-1}$, 95.56 $\pm$ 11.05 $m \cdot min^{-1}$, and 60.55 $\pm$ 23.62 $m \cdot min^{-1}$ for FT3, FT2, and FT1, respectively [28,29]. Therefore, the total distance covered seems to be related to the degree of physical impairment of footballers with CP [27–29], as the para-footballers with minimal impairment are the ones who complete the greatest total distance in absolute terms and per minute of play. Among the players classified according to the previous classification system (C5/6-C8) there are significant differences between sport classes regarding the total distance covered in absolute terms, the same as occurs with the players classified according to the current system (FT1-FT3) with respect to the total distance covered in relative terms. These differences between sport classes could occur because C5/6, FT5/6, and FT1, regardless of the classification system used, are the sport classes with the greatest physical impairments to move due to diplegic, hemiplegia, ataxia, athetosis, dyskinesia or dystonia, unlike C8, FT8, and FT3, which are the sport classes with the least physical impairment and the greatest locomotion capacity.

In relation to the distance covered in different speed ranges in absolute terms, only one study included in this review analyzes these variables dividing the sample by sport class [28]. The results showed that C8 players covered more distance above 23.04 $km \cdot h^{-1}$. Considering the correlation between the distance covered at high speeds and the effectiveness of attacking moves during the match [40], it appears that being able to go a greater distance at these speeds helps players become more competent in-game. On the other hand, an analysis of the distances covered at different speeds shows a disparity in the results obtained in relative terms [41]. While some studies show a relationship between the distance covered at high speeds and the degree of physical impairment of para-footballers [28], others show no such results [29,31,32]. The establishment of arbitrary values for the speed ranges may have influenced the results obtained by the different studies [42]. More studies are needed using individualized ranges in CP footballers, which allow us to obtain a clearer vision of the activity levels of the players in all-time motion analysis studies using GPS devices as occurs in conventional football [43]. To our knowledge, only the study of Goh et al. [35] analyzed match responses in para-footballers using individualized thresholds, i.e., below 25%, between 25 and 50%, between 50 and 70%, between 70 and 90%, and above 90% of maximum speed.

In addition to the relevance of recording the distance covered at high speeds, it is also necessary to pay attention to the maximum speed achieved by the players, since one of the most frequent actions preceded by goal situations in soccer is the sprint [44]. In the studies included in this review, the maximum speed values were 27.86 $\pm$ 1.22 $km \cdot h^{-1}$. Previous studies have indicated that as the level of physical impairment decrease (i.e., C8, FT8, or FT3, depending on the classification system in force at the time of each investigation), maximum speed values tend to be higher [27,30,31]. This variable in football is closely associated with physical and locomotor performance [43,45]. Therefore, players with less motor impairment are likely to generate force more efficiently and move at faster speeds.

The intermittent nature of PC football underscores the importance of short-term high-intensity actions, such as accelerations, decelerations and change of direction [46,47].

The intensity zones for the accelerations and decelerations are arbitrary and vary depending on the authors. Different ranges have been proposed, including 1–2 $m \cdot s^{-2}$ [28], 1–2.78 $m \cdot s^{-2}$ [29–32], 2–3 $m \cdot s^{-2}$ [28], >2.78 $m \cdot s^{-2}$ [29–32], 3–4 and >4 $m \cdot s^{-2}$ [28]. Like the distance covered in different speed zones, there should be unanimity in the scientific community for the presentation of the results in the research studies that analyze the intensity zones of the external load variables collected by GPS devices and facilitate the understanding and comparison of the activity levels of athletes, as pointed out by Malone et al. [48].

In the reviewed studies, it is observed that sports classes with lesser impairment (FT3-FT2 and FT8-FT7) exhibit higher values of accelerations and decelerations compared to FT1 and FT5/6 classes [28,30–32]. This trend can be attributed to greater neuromuscular impairment, poorer coordination, and reduced functional capacity resulting from spasticity, ataxia, athetosis, dyskinesia, or dystonia [6]. In addition, this difference is conditioned by playing time, which significantly affects the external load of PC players since those who play more minute's (i.e., <20, 20–40, and <40 min) experience a higher match load [18]. Additionally, regarding Metabolic Power, Player Load, and change of direction, no significant differences were observed between sport classes [30–32].

While the present review provides novel outcomes in physical and physiological match-play load in CP footballers, the limitations of our findings should be acknowledged, therefore, the results should be interpreted with caution. Firstly, studies included in this systematic review are subject to different classification systems for para-footballers, which has made it impossible to relate the variation in physical and physiological responses during official matches from all the studies, according to the same sport classes. This limitation can likely persist over time, considering that the classification process is dynamic and subject to continuous and necessary changes to ensure competitive equality. Secondly, it is difficult to establish a consensus regarding physical and physiological responses during match-play, as the competitive levels included in this review are different. In this sense, while some studies have reported data from national championships, others have focused on international championships. Thirdly, only one study has analyzed the physiological responses according to the sport classes of different classification systems. As such, it is impossible to compare the results obtained. Fourth, the speed ranges and thresholds for accelerations and decelerations vary among studies, making it challenging to compare them. Lastly, given that all the studies are carried out in male competitions, and considering that gender determines the physical responses of competition in conventional soccer [49], and the participation of women football players with CP and the organization of different events is becoming relevant, it would be necessary to analyze this aspect in future studies. We acknowledge that subsequent to the completion of our review process, additional relevant studies have been published. While our review was conducted up to 31 January 2023, we are aware of the inclusion of one additional study that was not part of our original review [50] (online, ahead of print). Despite our efforts to capture all relevant literature available at the time of our review, the dynamic nature of research in this field may result in the emergence of new studies post-review.

Strength and conditions coaches, along with performance staff, working across para-footballers with CP must know what the physical and physiological demands of match-play are. Previous studies have analyzed competition demands based on different contextual variables, such as moderate altitude [29], sport classes [32], simulated games [29], or even in a 3-day national tournament [35]. However, to our knowledge, this is the first systematic review to analyze the physical and physiological responses encountered by para-footballers with CP during the competition, according to sport classes. This knowledge is essential for adequately preparing athletes for competition and simulating competition situations during training tasks.

5. Conclusions

The main conclusions of this systematic review suggest that para-footballers with CP and less physical impairment (i.e., current FT3 or FT8 in the previous classification system) tend to cover a greater total distance, achieve higher maximum speeds, and cover more distance above 23.04 km·h^{-1} during match-play, indicating potentially greater competence during a game. However, it is essential to interpret these findings with caution due to the limited number of studies examining the physiological response of para-footballers. Furthermore, players with an intermediate degree of impairment (i.e., current FT2 or FT7 in the previous classification system) demonstrate the highest relative values in specific performance metrics such as accelerations from 1 to 2.78 m·s^{-2} and above 2.78 m·s^{-2}, decelerations from −1 to −2.78 m·s^{-2} and above 2.78 m·s^{-2}, as well as greater peak metabolic power suggesting unique strengths in certain aspects of play. Conversely, players with severe physical impairment (FT1 or FT5/6 in the previous classification system) exhibit higher player load, which may reflect different physical demands. Despite these insights, the conclusions are constrained by the scarcity of studies directly comparing physical and physiological demands across classification groups. Therefore, while the findings provide valuable insights into the performance characteristics of para-footballers with CP, further research is needed to draw definitive conclusions and inform training and classification strategies.

Funding: This research received no external funding.

Conflicts of Interest: The authors declare no conflicts of interest.

References

1. IFCPF. Classification Rules and Regulations. Available online: https://www.ifcpf.com/static/upload/raw/8ce6fab2-257c-43a7-a22d-db0e74f7b089/IFCPF+Classification+Rules+2018.pdf (accessed on 26 August 2021).
2. Tweedy, S.M.; Connick, M.J.; Beckman, E.M. Applying Scientific Principles to Enhance Paralympic Classification Now and in the Future: A Research Primer for Rehabilitation Specialists. *Phys. Med. Rehabil. Clin.* **2018**, *29*, 313–332. [CrossRef] [PubMed]
3. Jaeken, D. Classification in the Paralympics: The Relationship between Impairment and Participation. *Dev. Med. Child. Neurol.* **2020**, *62*, 769. [CrossRef] [PubMed]
4. Tweedy, S.M.; Vanlandewijck, Y.C. International Paralympic Committee Position Stand--Background and Scientific Principles of Classification in Paralympic Sport. *Br. J. Sports Med.* **2011**, *45*, 259–269. [CrossRef] [PubMed]
5. Reina, R. Evidence-Based Classification in Paralympic Sport: Application to Football-7-a-Side. *Eur. J. Hum. Mov.* **2014**, *32*, 161–185.
6. Reina, R.; Sarabia, J.M.; Yanci, J.; García-Vaquero, M.P.; Campayo-Piernas, M. Change of Direction Ability Performance in Cerebral Palsy Football Players According to Functional Profiles. *Front. Physiol.* **2015**, *6*, 409. [CrossRef] [PubMed]
7. Reina, R.; Sarabia, J.M.; Caballero, C.; Yanci, J. How Does the Ball Influence the Performance of Change of Direction and Sprint Tests in Para-Footballers with Brain Impairments? Implications for Evidence-Based Classification in CP-Football. *PLoS ONE* **2017**, *12*, e0187237. [CrossRef] [PubMed]
8. Sarabia, J.M.; Roldan, A.; Henríquez, M.; Reina, R. Using Decision Trees to Support Classifiers' Decision-Making about Activity Limitation of Cerebral Palsy Footballers. *Int. J. Environ. Res. Public Health* **2021**, *18*, 4320. [CrossRef] [PubMed]
9. Roldan, A.; Sarabia, J.M.; Gómez-Marcos, G.; Reina, R. An Observational Tool to Assess Activity Limitation in Ambulatory People with Cerebral Palsy When Performing Motor Skills. *Int. J. Environ. Res. Public Health* **2020**, *17*, 1896. [CrossRef]
10. Pastor, D.; Campayo-Piernas, M.; Pastor, J.T.; Reina, R. A Mathematical Model for Decision-Making in the Classification of Para-Footballers with Different Severity of Coordination Impairments. *J. Sports Sci.* **2019**, *37*, 1403–1410. [CrossRef]
11. Sarabia, J.M.; Doménech, C.; Roche, E.; Vicente-Salar, N.; Reina, R. Anthropometrical Features of Para-Footballers According to Their Cerebral Palsy Profiles and Compared to Controls. *Int. J. Environ. Res. Public Health* **2020**, *17*, 9071. [CrossRef]
12. Roldan, A.; Henríquez, M.; Iturricastillo, A.; Castillo, D.; Yanci, J.; Reina, R. To What Degree Does Limb Spasticity Affect Motor Performance in Para-Footballers With Cerebral Palsy? *Front. Physiol.* **2022**, *12*, 807853. [CrossRef]
13. Peña-González, I.; Sarabia, J.M.; Roldan, A.; Manresa-Rocamora, A.; Moya-Ramón, M. Physical Performance Differences between Spanish Selected and Nonselected Para-Footballers With Cerebral Palsy for the National Team. *Int. J. Sports Physiol. Perform.* **2021**, *16*, 1676–1683. [CrossRef]
14. Yanci, J.; Castagna, C.; Los Arcos, A.; Santalla, A.; Grande, I.; Figueroa, J.; Camara, J. Muscle Strength and Anaerobic Performance in Football Players with Cerebral Palsy. *Disabil. Health J.* **2016**, *9*, 313–319. [CrossRef] [PubMed]
15. Cámara, J.; Grande, I.; Mejuto, G.; Los Arcos, A.; Yanci, J. Jump Landing Characteristics in Elite Soccer Players with Cerebral Palsy. *Biol. Sport* **2013**, *30*, 91–95. [CrossRef] [PubMed]

16. Reina, R.; Barbado, D.; Hernández-Davó, H.; Roldan, A. Dynamic and Static Stability in Para-Athletes with Cerebral Palsy Considering Their Impairment Profile. *PM&R* **2022**, *14*, 366–376. [CrossRef]
17. Peña-González, I.; Javaloyes, A.; Manuel Sarabia, J.; Moya-Ramón, M. Assessing the Sprint Force-Velocity Profile in International Football Players with Cerebral Palsy: Validity, Reliability and Sport Class' Profiles. *J. Hum. Kinet.* **2022**, *82*, 253–262. [CrossRef] [PubMed]
18. Yanci, J.; Castillo, D.; Iturricastillo, A.; Reina, R. Evaluation of the Official Match External Load in Soccer Players with Cerebral Palsy. *J. Strength Cond. Res.* **2019**, *33*, 866–873. [CrossRef]
19. Barbero-Alvarez, J.C.; Lopez, M.G.; Castagna, C.; Barbero-Alvarez, V.; Romero, D.V.; Blanchfield, A.W.; Nakamura, F.Y. Game Demands of 7-a-Side Soccer in Young Players. *J. Strength Cond. Res.* **2015**, *31*, 1771–1779. [CrossRef]
20. Yanci, J.; Castillo, D.; Iturricastillo, A.; Henríquez, M.; Roldan, A.; Reina, R. Comparison of the Physical Response During Official Matches and Small-Sided Games in International Cerebral Palsy Footballers: Implications for Evidence-Based Classification. *Adapt. Phys. Act. Q.* **2023**, *40*, 4–18. [CrossRef]
21. Rico-González, M.; Pino-Ortega, J.; Clemente, F.M.; Arcos, A.L. Guidelines for Performing Systematic Reviews in Sports Science. *Biol. Sport* **2022**, *39*, 463–471. [CrossRef]
22. Page, M.J.; McKenzie, J.E.; Bossuyt, P.M.; Boutron, I.; Hoffmann, T.C.; Mulrow, C.D.; Shamseer, L.; Tetzlaff, J.M.; Moher, D. Updating Guidance for Reporting Systematic Reviews: Development of the PRISMA 2020 Statement. *J. Clin. Epidemiol.* **2021**, *134*, 103–112. [CrossRef] [PubMed]
23. Moher, D.; Liberati, A.; Tetzlaff, J.; Altman, D.G.; The PRISMA Group. Preferred Reporting Items for Systematic Reviews and Meta-Analyses: The PRISMA Statement. *PLoS Med.* **2009**, *6*, e1000097. [CrossRef] [PubMed]
24. Palucci Vieira, L.H.; Carling, C.; Barbieri, F.A.; Aquino, R.; Santiago, P.R.P. Match Running Performance in Young Soccer Players: A Systematic Review. *Sports Med.* **2019**, *49*, 289–318. [CrossRef] [PubMed]
25. Castellano, J.; Alvarez-Pastor, D.; Bradley, P.S. Evaluation of Research Using Computerised Tracking Systems (Amisco® and Prozone®) to Analyse Physical Performance in Elite Soccer: A Systematic Review. *Sports Med.* **2014**, *44*, 701–712. [CrossRef] [PubMed]
26. Bishop, C.; Turner, A.; Read, P. Effects of Inter-Limb Asymmetries on Physical and Sports Performance: A Systematic Review. *J. Sports Sci.* **2018**, *36*, 1135–1144. [CrossRef] [PubMed]
27. Boyd, C.; Barnes, C.; Eaves, S.J.; Morse, C.I.; Roach, N.; Williams, A.G. A Time-Motion Analysis of Paralympic Football for Athletes with Cerebral Palsy. *Int. J. Sports Sci. Coach.* **2016**, *11*, 552–558. [CrossRef]
28. Gamonales, J.M.; Muñoz-Jiménez, J.; Gómez-Carmona, C.D.; Ibáñez, S.J. Comparative External Workload Analysis Based on the New Functional Classification in Cerebral Palsy Football 7-a-Side. A Full-Season Study. *Res. Sports Med.* **2022**, *30*, 295–307. [CrossRef] [PubMed]
29. Henríquez, M.; Castillo, D.; Yanci, J.; Iturricastillo, A.; Reina, R. Physical Responses by Cerebral Palsy Footballers in Matches Played at Sea Level and Moderate Altitude. *Res. Sports Med.* **2021**, *31*, 296–308. [CrossRef] [PubMed]
30. Reina, R.; Iturricastillo, A.; Castillo, D.; Roldan, A.; Toledo, C.; Yanci, J. Is Impaired Coordination Related to Match Physical Load in Footballers with Cerebral Palsy of Different Sport Classes? *J. Sports Sci.* **2021**, *39*, 140–149. [CrossRef]
31. Reina, R.; Iturricastillo, A.; Castillo, D.; Urbán, T.; Yanci, J. Activity Limitation and Match Load in Para-Footballers with Cerebral Palsy: An Approach for Evidence-Based Classification. *Scand. J. Med. Sci. Sports* **2020**, *30*, 496–504. [CrossRef]
32. Yanci, J.; Castillo, D.; Iturricastillo, A.; Urbán, T.; Reina, R. External Match Loads of Footballers with Cerebral Palsy: A Comparison among Sport Classes. *Int. J. Sports Physiol. Perform.* **2018**, *13*, 590–596. [CrossRef] [PubMed]
33. Impellizzeri, F.M.; Marcora, S.M.; Coutts, A.J. Internal and External Training Load: 15 Years On. *Int. J. Sports Physiol. Perform.* **2019**, *14*, 270–273. [CrossRef] [PubMed]
34. Peña-Gónzalez, I.; Sarabia, J.M.; Mancha-Triguero, D.; Moya-Ramón, M.; Gamonales, J.M. Relationship between Physical Performance and Match Load and Effects of Two Consecutive Matches in Cerebral Palsy Footballers. *Retos* **2021**, *41*, 728–734. [CrossRef]
35. Goh, A.M.; Ma, F.; Harms, C.A.; Newton, R.U.; Drinkwater, E.J.; Goh, A. Global Positioning System Activity Profile in Male Para Footballers with Cerebral Palsy: Does Training Meet the Match-Play Intensity in a Three-Day National Tournament? *Am. J. Phys. Med. Rehabil.* **2022**, *101*, 1163–1167. [CrossRef] [PubMed]
36. Krustrup, P.; Mohr, M.; Steensberg, A.; Bencke, J.; Klær, M.; Bangsbo, J. Muscle and Blood Metabolites during a Soccer Game: Implications for Sprint Performance. *Med. Sci. Sports Exerc.* **2006**, *38*, 1165–1174. [CrossRef] [PubMed]
37. Yanci, J.; Castillo, D.; Iturricastillo, A.; Aracama, A.; Roldan, A.; Reina, R. Performance Analysis in Football-Specific Tests by Para-Footballers with Cerebral Palsy: Implications for Evidence-Based Classification. *Int. J. Sports Physiol. Perform.* **2021**, *16*, 1328–1334. [CrossRef] [PubMed]
38. Rice, J.; Brownlee, T.E.; McRobert, A.P.; Ade, J.; Drust, B.; Malone, J.J. The Association between Training Load and Physical Development in Professional Male Youth Soccer Players: A Systematic Review. *Int. J. Sports Sci. Coach.* **2022**, *17*, 1488–1505. [CrossRef]
39. Buchheit, M.; Mendez-Villanueva, A.; Simpson, B.M.; Bourdon, P.C. Match Running Performance and Fitness in Youth Soccer. *Int. J. Sports Med.* **2010**, *31*, 818–825. [CrossRef] [PubMed]
40. Castellano, J.; Echeazarra, I. Network-Based Centrality Measures and Physical Demands in Football Regarding Player Position: Is There a Connection? A Preliminary Study. *J. Sports Sci.* **2019**, *37*, 2631–2638. [CrossRef]

41. Gabbett, T.J. Use of Relative Speed Zones Increases the High-Speed Running Performed in Team Sport Match Play. *J. Strength Cond. Res.* **2015**, *29*, 3353–3359. [CrossRef]
42. Clemente, F.M.; Ramirez-Campillo, R.; Beato, M.; Moran, J.; Kawczynski, A.; Makar, P.; Sarmento, H.; Alfonso, J. Arbitrary Absolute vs. Individualized Running Speed Thresholds in Team Sports: A Scoping Review with Evidence Gap Map. *Biol. Sport* **2023**, *40*, 919–943. [CrossRef]
43. Snyder, B.J.; Maung-Maung, C.; Whitacre, C. Indicators of Fatigue during a Soccer Match Simulation Using GPS-Derived Workload Values: Which Metrics Are Most Useful? *Sports* **2024**, *12*, 9. [CrossRef] [PubMed]
44. Faude, O.; Koch, T.; Meyer, T. Straight Sprinting Is the Most Frequent Action in Goal Situations in Professional Football. *J. Sports Sci.* **2012**, *30*, 625–631. [CrossRef] [PubMed]
45. Gualtieri, A.; Rampinini, E.; Dello Iacono, A.; Beato, M. High-Speed Running and Sprinting in Professional Adult Soccer: Current Thresholds Definition, Match Demands and Training Strategies. A Systematic Review. *Front. Sports Act. Living* **2023**, *5*, 1116293. [CrossRef] [PubMed]
46. Akenhead, R.; Nassis, G.P. Training Load and Player Monitoring in High-Level Football: Current Practice and Perceptions. *Int. J. Sports Physiol. Perform.* **2016**, *11*, 587–593. [CrossRef] [PubMed]
47. Mara, J.K.; Thompson, K.G.; Kate, L.; Morgan, S. The Acceleration and Deceleration Profiles of Elite Female Soccer Players during Competitive Matches. *J. Sci. Med. Sport* **2017**, *20*, 867–872. [CrossRef] [PubMed]
48. Malone, J.J.; Lovell, R.; Varley, M.C.; Coutts, A.J. Unpacking the Black Box: Applications and Considerations for Using GPS Devices in Sport. *Int. J. Sports Physiol. Perform.* **2017**, *12*, S218–S226. [CrossRef] [PubMed]
49. McFadden, B.A.; Walker, A.J.; Bozzini, B.N.; Sanders, D.J.; Arent, S.M. Comparison of Internal and External Training Loads in Male and Female Collegiate Soccer Players During Practices vs. Games. *J. Strength Cond. Res.* **2020**, *34*, 969–974. [CrossRef]
50. Henríquez, M.; Reina, R.; Castillo, D.; Iturricastillo, A.; Yanci, J. Contextual Factors and Match-Physical Performance of International-Level Footballers with Cerebral Palsy. *Sci. Med. Foot* **2023**, *27*, 1–10. [CrossRef]

MDPI AG
Grosspeteranlage 5
4052 Basel
Switzerland
Tel.: +41 61 683 77 34

Applied Sciences Editorial Office
E-mail: applsci@mdpi.com
www.mdpi.com/journal/applsci

www.ingramcontent.com/pod-product-compliance
Lightning Source LLC
Chambersburg PA
CBHW040316270926
51850CB00007BC/1495